Polyether Antibiotics

Polyether Antibiotics

Naturally Occurring Acid Ionophores

VOLUME 2

Chemistry

edited by JOHN W. WESTLEY
Hoffmann-La Roche Inc.
Nutley, New Jersey

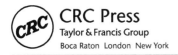

CRC Press
Taylor & Francis Group
Boca Raton London New York

CRC Press is an imprint of the
Taylor & Francis Group, an **informa** business

First published 1983 by Marcel Dekkar, Inc.

Published 2019 by CRC Press
Taylor & Francis Group
6000 Broken Sound Parkway NW, Suite 300
Boca Raton, FL 33487-2742

© 1983 by Taylor & Francis Group, LLC
CRC Press is an imprint of Taylor & Francis Group, an Informa business

First issued in paperback 2019

No claim to original U.S. Government works

ISBN 13: 978-0-367-45192-9 (pbk)
ISBN 13: 978-0-8247-1888-6 (hbk)

Visit the Taylor & Francis Web site at
http://www.taylorandfrancis.com

and the CRC Press Web site at
http://www.crcpress.com

Library of Congress Cataloging in Publication Data
(Rev. for volume 2)
Main entry under title:

Polyether antibiotics.

    Contents: --v. 2. Chemistry.
    1. Antibiotics. 2. Ionophores. 3. Carboxylic
acids. 4. Ethers. [DNLM: 1. Antibiotics. 2. Carbo-
xylic Acids. 3. Ionophores. QV 350 P782 (P)]
QP801.A63P64 1983   615'.329   82-10004
ISBN 0-8247-1655-8 (v. 1)
ISBN 0-8247-1888-7 (v. 2)

FOREWORD

Sourcebooks of specific scientific information are of tremendous value. They provide orientation for investigators who wish to use a technique, an organism, or a new series of chemical compounds with which they are not familiar. For the expert, they provide assurance that no important discoveries, reported in obscure journals, have been overlooked. And for the intellectually curious, they provide an introduction to concepts that may be far afield from the reader's area of research; it is just such reading that enriches one's understanding and may contribute new experimental approaches.

To find, a quarter-century after we first reported their biological activity, that the carboxylic ionophores deserve a two-volume appraisal is gratifying. These agents have become essential tools for cell biologists, physiologists, and biochemists. (The assumption that one can categorize these investigators is arbitrary.) The careful chemical work that led to the elucidation of the structures of these compounds and the elegant studies that show us the conformation of their metal ion-complexed forms in solution provide a firm background for understanding their effects on various biological systems. Nature has provided an abundance of types of ionophores; the experimenter can choose individuals with remarkable specificity for a given alkali metal ion. A 23187 is no longer the only agent with relatively high selectivity for divalent cations. Where nature's products are not sufficiently specific for individual cations in this group, chemical modification can improve specificity. This has already been demonstrated with a few halogenated ionophores and undoubtedly even greater selectivity will be achieved as more derivatives are made.

   This remarkable collection of essays should stimulate the use of ionophores in many different research areas. Dr. Westley and his co-authors will earn the gratitude of all investigators whose work will benefit from ideas sparked by these chapters.

Henry Lardy
Vilas Professor of Biological Science
Institute for Enzyme Research
University of Wisconsin
Madison, Wisconsin

PREFACE

The chemistry of the polyether antibiotics is not simple. For instance, the synthesis of a typical member of this class confronts one with the problem of twenty asymmetric centers representing more than a million possible stereoisomers. The characteristic structural features of this unique class of natural products include β-hydroxy ketones, spiro-ketals, tetrahydrofurans, and tetrahydropyrans. The construction of these different moieties has led to a reevaluation of the stereo-, regio-, and chemiselectivity of such familiar synthetic methods as the crossed aldol and Grignard reactions, intramolecular ketalization, epoxidation and cyclization of bishomoallylic alcohols, and the Claisen rearrangement of glycans.

The chemical transformation of polyether antibiotics into derivatives with enhanced therapeutic indexes has proved an elusive goal, but potential breakthroughs have been obtained with the halogenated derivatives of lasalocid and the ethers of antibiotic A204A.

The final four chapters of this second volume devoted to the polyethers deal primarily with the different analytical techniques used to unravel their complex structures. The single most powerful technique to date has been x-ray crystallography, which has revealed the structure, absolute configuration, and conformation of both the solvated antibiotics and their metal ion complexes. Interestingly, in many cases, there is very little change in conformation between the free acid and salt forms of the antibiotics. Antibiotic A23187 is an outstanding exception to this generalization.

Mass spectrometry was first utilized in this field to determine the structure of the minor factors in the monesin complex and represents a rapid means of structure elucidation, provided that the new compound can be related to a known one of similar type. This is particularly useful in metabolism studies, where many noncrystalline, somewhat impure samples are generated, often in minute quantities. An unusual feature of the mass spectrometry of polyether antibiotics is that their salts usually yield more information than the free acids and are often the only derivative required to obtain a reliable molecular weight, particularly if the technique of field desorption is employed.

Nuclear magnetic resonance (NMR) spectroscopy offers the opportunity to study the conformation of the polyethers and their salts *in solution*. This ultimately could lead to the elucidation of the details of their mode of action. For instance, proton NMR has suggested that the water molecules on a hydrated cation are removed sequentially by a polyether antibiotic like lonomycin in a consecutive, competitive manner. ^{13}C NMR has advantages over proton NMR in providing information on the number of carbon atoms in the molecule and their directly bonded protons. The assignment of the rather complex ^{13}C spectra of polyethers has been helped by the earlier biosynthetic labeling results and the extensive proton NMR studies. This has made it possible to establish correlations between specific moieties and the chemical shifts of the relevant carbons in their ^{13}C NMR spectra. The first antibiotic in the class to be structurally assigned by ^{13}C NMR was antibiotic 6016. The empirical rules by which this structure was elucidated are outlined in the last chapter of the book.

Finally, the editor would like to acknowledge the close cooperation of all the contributing authors and the editorial staff of Marcel Dekker in the production of these two volumes.

John W. Westley

CONTENTS

CONTRIBUTORS

Marc J. O. Anteunis, Ph.D., NMR Spectroscopic Unit, Laboratory of
Organic Chemistry, State University of Ghent, Ghent, Belgium

Eileen N. Duesler, Ph.D.,* Department of Chemistry, School of Chemical Sciences, University of Illinois, Urbana, Illinois

R. L. Hamill, Ph.D., Microbiological and Fermentation Products
Research, Lilly Research Laboratories, Indianapolis, Indiana

Yoshito Kishi, Ph.D., Department of Chemistry, Harvard University,
Cambridge, Massachusetts

J. L. Occolowitz, M.Sc., Molecular Structure Research, Lilly Research
Laboratories, Indianapolis, Indiana

Noboru Ōtake, Ph.D., Division of Antibiotics, Institute of Applied
Microbiology, University of Tokyo, Tokyo, Japan

Iain C. Paul., Ph.D., Department of Chemistry, School of Chemical
Sciences, University of Illinois, Urbana, Illinois

Haruo Seto, Ph.D., Department of Antibiotics, Institute of Applied
Microbiology, University of Tokyo, Tokyo, Japan

John W. Westley, Ph.D., Department of Chemical Research, Hoffmann-
La Roche Inc., Nutley, New Jersey

Present affiliation: The University of New Mexico, Albuquerque,
New Mexico

CONTENTS OF VOLUME 1
BIOLOGY

Polyether Antibiotics

chapter 1

CHEMICAL SYNTHESIS

Yoshito Kishi
Harvard University, Cambridge, Massachusetts

I. INTRODUCTION

For the past three years or so an increasing number of papers have addressed the total synthesis of polyether antibiotics or synthetic methods to construct their structural units. Besides the important biological activity of polyether antibiotics there seem to be two major reasons for these reaearch efforts. First, polyether antibiotics present a formidable challenge to synthetic chemists. For representative polyether antibiotics are listed in Table 1. There are 17 asymmetric centers present in monensin, for example, which means that in principle 131,072 stereoisomers exist for the antibiotic. In the case of lonomycin, the number of stereoisomers exceeds 8 million! The total number of isomers for these antibiotics will be infinite if constitutional isomers are counted. Thus to achieve the total synthesis of one of these antibiotics it is essential to have a high degree of stereo-, regio-, and chemoselectivity for each step of the synthesis. Second, polyether antibiotics present almost perfect cases for testing principles or reactions for controlling stereo-, regio-, and chemoselectivity in acyclic systems.

In reviewing total syntheses of polyether antibiotics, first a brief survey of synthetic methods proven effective in constructing some functionalities commonly found in naturally occurring polyether antibiotics will be presented.

II. SYNTHETIC METHODS

A. β-Hydroxy Ketone

A β-hydroxy ketone group (or groups) exists as the structural unit (or units) in all but one of the naturally occurring polyether antibiotics, although in some cases it is hidden. Crossed aldol reaction seems to be one of the most attractive choices to disconnect this functionality. The magnitude of difficulty encountered in the synthesis of polyether antibiotics should be decreased dramatically by this single, convergent disconnection.

In order to test the feasibility of this disconnection, the crossed aldol reaction between the aldehyde [1] and the ketone [2] (scheme 1) was investigated by Kishi (Nakata et al, 1978). Based on Cram's rule (for example, see Morrison and Mosher (1976), *Asymmetric Organic Reactions*, American Chemical Society, p. 87 ff) and also on House's observations (House et al., 1973), the relative sterochemistry at C-10, C-11, and C-12 of the major product was anticipated to be the desired one. The stereochemistry of the remote positions, for example, at C-10 and C-14, could be controlled by using both components in an optically active form with the correct absolute configuration. The crossed aldol reaction between [1] and [2] was realized under the conditions indicated. The major product was proven to be [3].

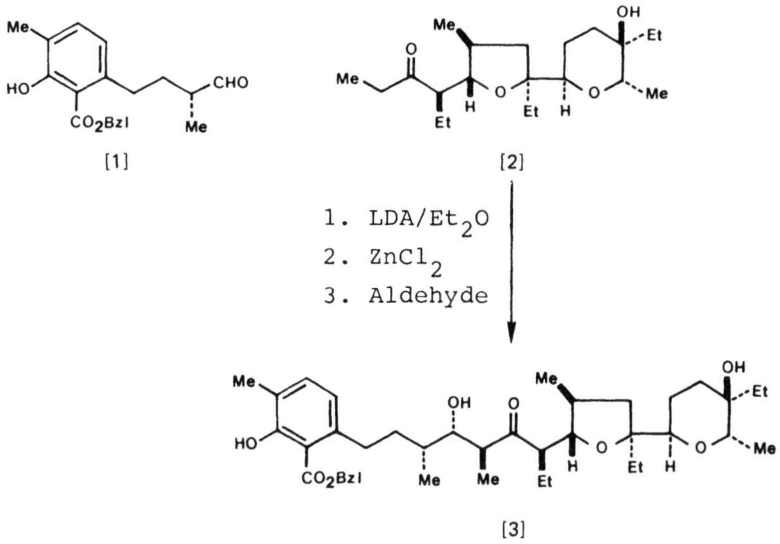

Scheme 1

Stereoselectivity increased in DMF, while the chemical yield decreased. The best conditions proved later to be magnesium dicyclohexylamide as a base in THF, yielding an 8:1:1 ratio with a chemical yield of over 65% (Hatekeyama et al., 1982).

A crossed aldol reaction has successfully been used as the key step in the total synthesis of lasalocid A (Nakata et al, 1978a; Ireland et al., 1980), monensin (Fukuyama et al., 1979b; Collum et al., 1980c), A23187 (Evans et al., 1979a), and also narasin and salinomycin (Hatekeyama et al., 1982). Related to the observed stereochemical outcome, it is important to note the recent publications of a crossed aldol reaction by Heathcock et al. (1979), Masamune (1979), Evans et al. (1979b), and others.

B. Spiroketal

Spiroketal groups are quite often found as functional groups of poly-ether antibiotics. Monensin and antibiotic A23187 present a representative example. Based on an analysis using the anomeric effect well known in carbohydrate chemistry, it was anticipated that the intramolecular ketalization of the corresponding dihydroxy ketone under thermodynamically controlled conditions should result in the spiroketal with the desired stereochemistry. Indeed, using a simple model synthesis, this was shown to be true for the monensin type (Scheme 2) by

Table 1 Four Representative Polyether Antibiotics

| Polyether antibiotics | | Number of | |
Name	Structure	Asymmetric centers	Stereoisomers
Lasalocid A	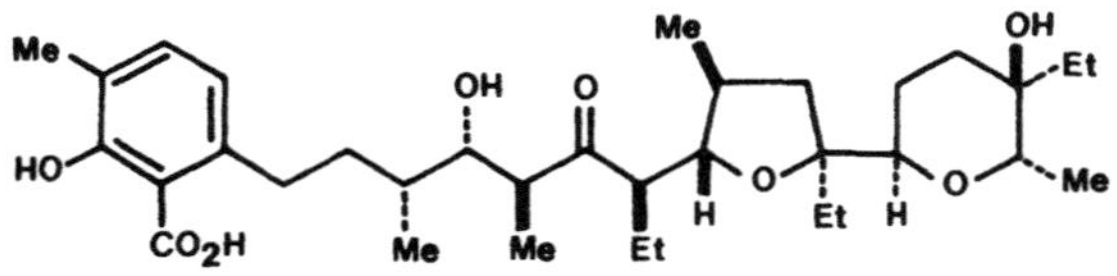	10	1,024
Monensin	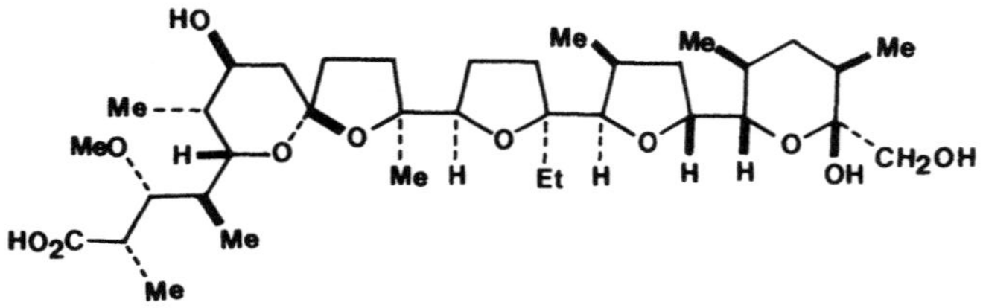	17	131,072

Narasin   19   524,288

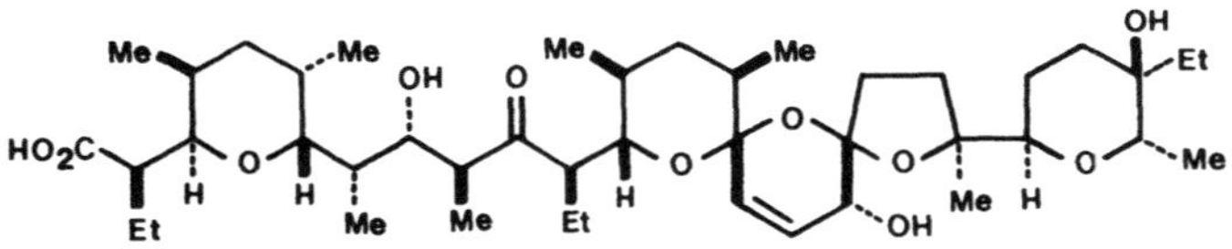

Lonomycin   23   8,388,608

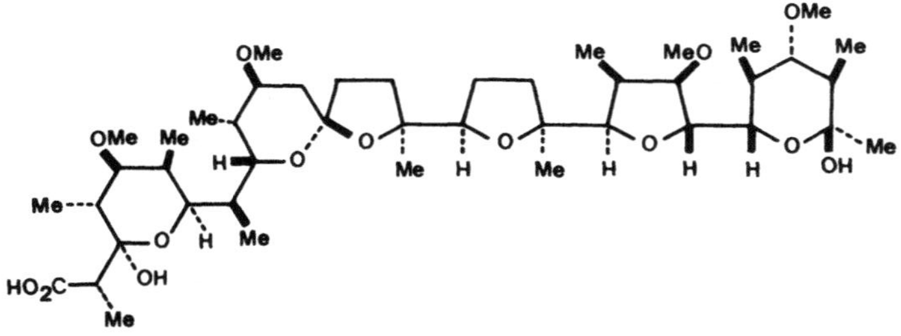

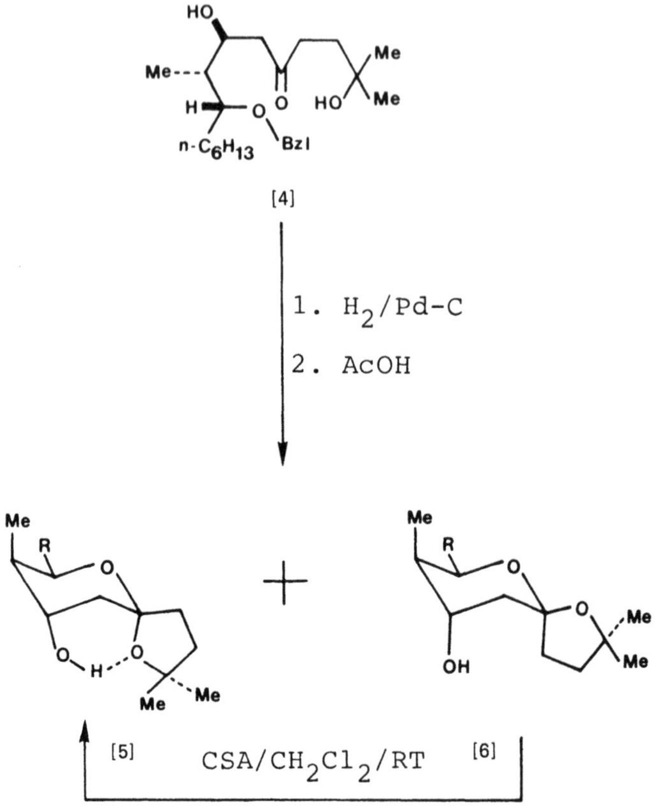

[4]

1. H_2/Pd–C

2. AcOH

[5]   +   [6]

CSA/CH_2Cl_2/RT

20 > 1

Scheme 2

Fukuyama et al. (1979b), and for the A23187 type (Scheme 3) by
Evans et al. (1978) and also Crespe et al. (1978). Successful total
syntheses of monensin and of A23187 used this reaction.

Different approaches to the spiroketal system have also been stud-
ied. Ireland and Häbach (1980) have shown that the hetero Diels-
Alder reaction of, for example [10] (Scheme 4) and acrolein, followed
by oxidation with m-chloroperbenzoic acid yields the spiroketal [12].
Decotes and Cottier (1979) have investigated a photochemical approach
(Scheme 5).

This bis-spiroketal ring system existing in salinomycin and narasin
requires special comment. There are two different kinds of relative
stereochemistry known: one of them is found in narasin and salinomycin, the other in 17-deoxysalinomycin. It was suggested
by Hatakeyama et al. (1982) that the indicated hydrogen bond
would be an important factor in (Scheme 6) compensating for

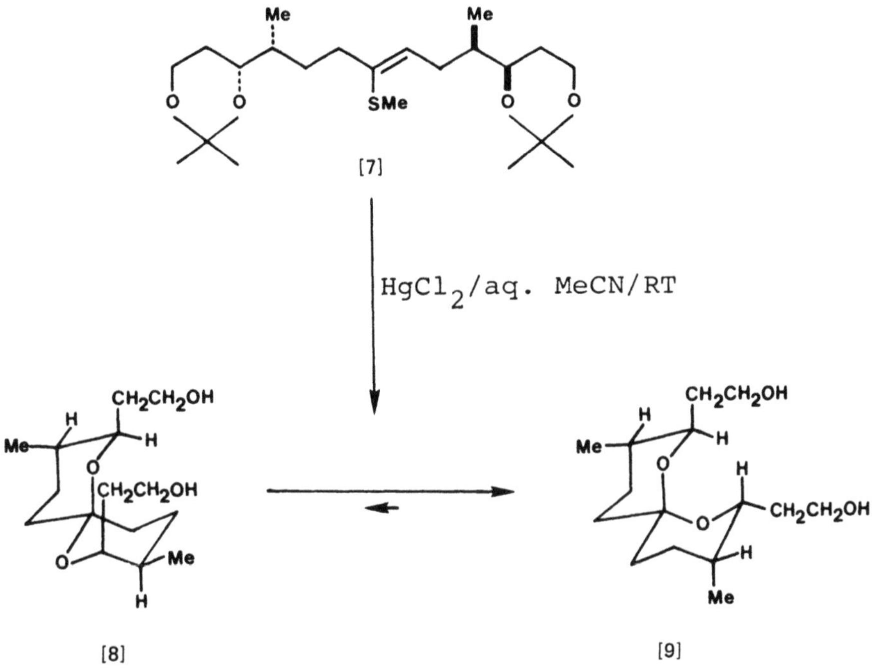

Scheme 3

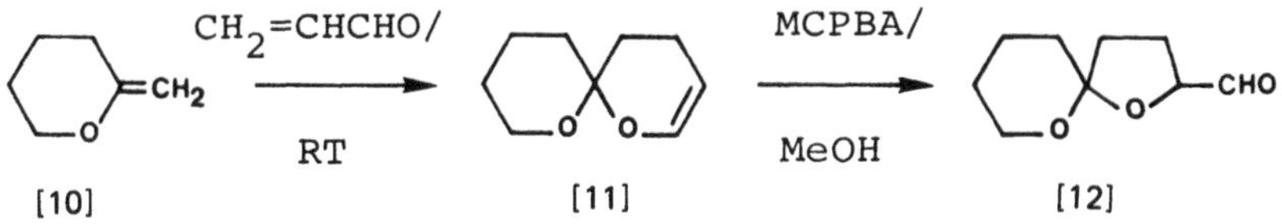

Scheme 4

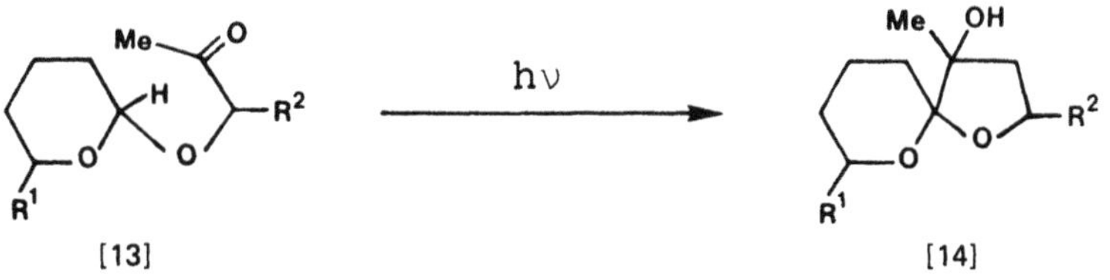

Scheme 5

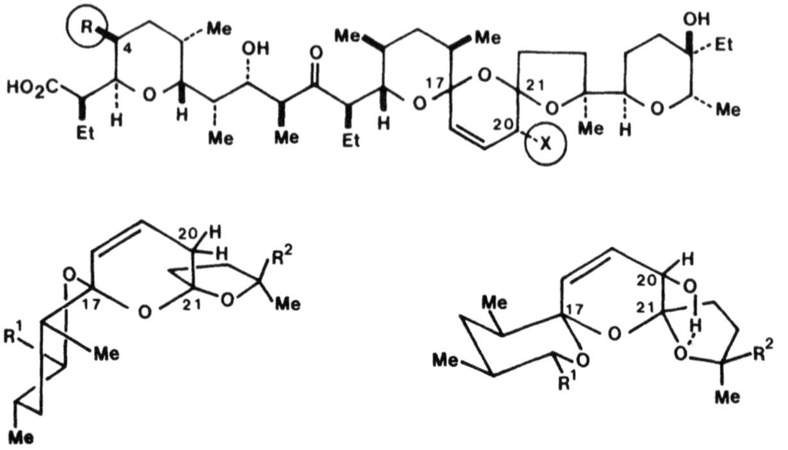

Scheme 6

a seemingly unfavorable dipole-dipole interaction at the bis-spiro centers of the salinomycin and narasin series. Indeed, it was shown that while the O-17 acetate of [15a] (Scheme 7) isomerized completely to the deoxy type under acidic conditions, the compound [15b] exists as an equilibrium mixture of normal and deoxy series.

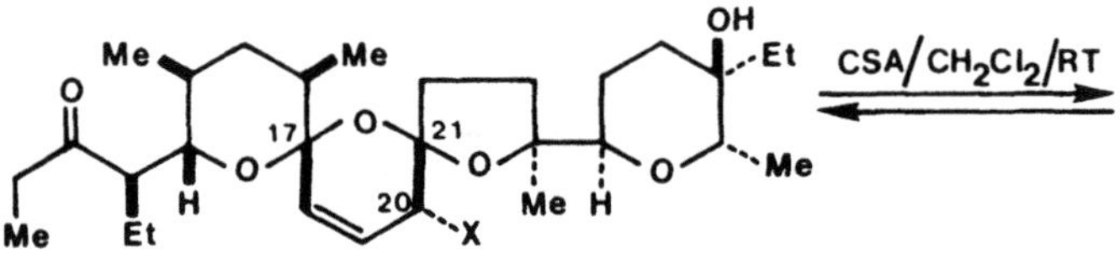

[15a,b]

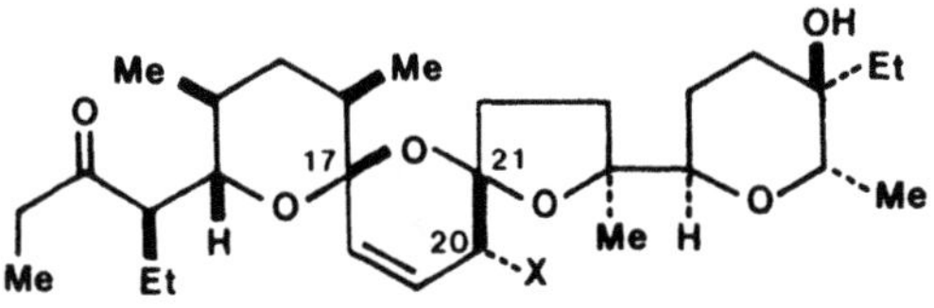

[16a,b]

Scheme 7

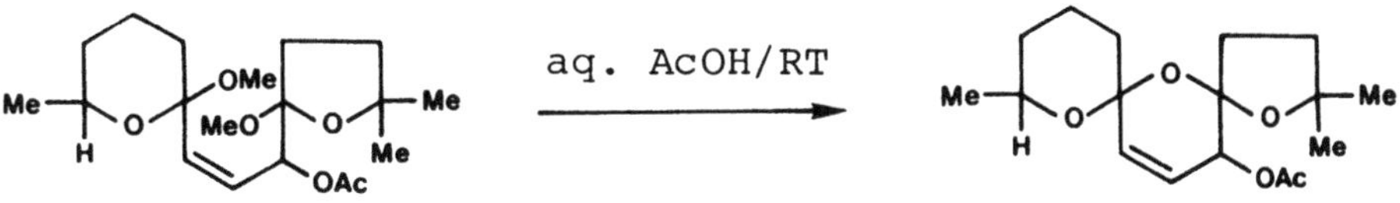

[17]   [18]

Scheme 8

Intramolecular bis-spiroketalization of the acetate [17] (Scheme 8) was shown by R. W. Freerksen and Y. Kishi (unpublished data, 1980) to yield the bis-spiroketal [18] belonging to the deoxy series.

C. Tetrahydrofurans

Almost all polyether antibiotics contain a tetrahydrofuran ring(s) with two chains extended at the 2 and 5 positions. Usually, at least one of the α'-carbon atoms of these chains carries an ether or an alcohol oxygen atom. Thus, with respect to their relative stereochemistry, there are four different types (Scheme 9; [19], [20], [21], and [22]) of tetrahydrofurans considered, among which the first two are most commonly found in the naturally occurring polyether antibiotics. Various methods have been investigated to control the relative stereochemistry of these tetrahydrofurans.

Certain oxidative cyclization reactions of bishomoallylic alcohols to tetrahdrofurans are known to take place stereoselectively. For example, cyclosporin A, a part of which is shown below, is known to yield the iodide [24] (Scheme 10) (Petcher et al., 1976). A similar method has been used in the monesin synthesis by Fukuyama et al. (1979a), for example, [25] to [26] (Scheme 11).

Overall stereoselectivity of epoxidation of bishomallylic alcohols, followed by acid-catalyzed cyclization to tetrahydrofurans, was investigated by Fukuyama et al. (1978). The results are summarized in Table 2. This method was used in Kishi's first lasalocid A synthesis (Nakata et al., 1978).

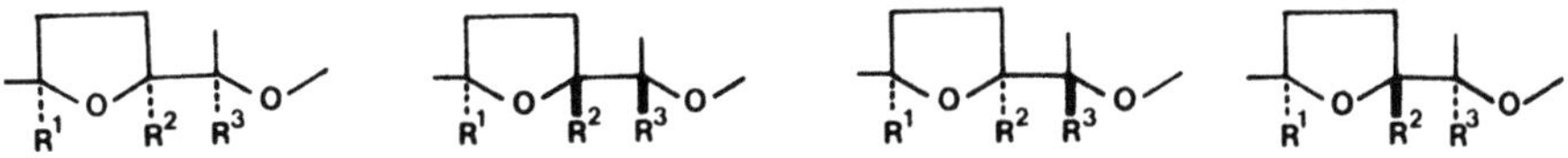

[19]   [20]   [21]   [22]

Scheme 9

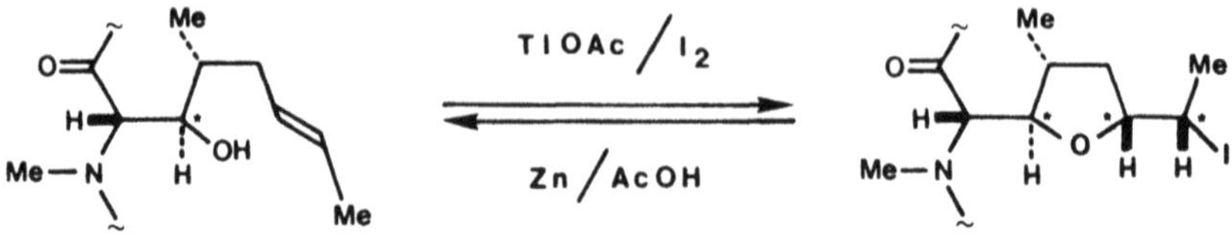

[23]   [24]

Scheme 10

An effective method for constructing the type B tetrahydrofurans has also been developed by Fukuyama et al. (1978). The overall stereoselectivity is excellent by using a combination of lithium aluminum hydride and racemic diamine [31] (Table 3), but its detailed mechanistic aspect has not yet been unveiled. This method was used in Kishi's second lasalocid A synthesis (Nakata and Kishi, 1978) and also in Kishi's monensin synthesis (Fukuyama et al, 1979a).

Cyclization of the properly functionalized halo alcohols or their equivalents to tetrahydrofurans has been known for many years. This method was effectively used in Still's monensin synthesis (Collum et al., 1908b,c), for example, [32] to [33] (Scheme 12).

Walba et al. (1979) have recently demonstrated that oxidation of 1,5-diene to tetrahydrofurans by permangante is highly stereoselective. This method or its variants seem to have good potential. Similar results have been published also by Baldwin et al. (1979).

D. Tetrahydropyrans

The synthesis of tetrahydropyrans is somewhat more difficult than that of tetrahydrofurans; for example, cyclization of halo alcohols is less effective. One of the successful methods used to solve this problem was the solvolysis reaction of the methanesulfonate of [36] (Scheme 14) in an about 4 ∿ 5:1 mixture of [37] and [36]. This reaction was used for the Kishi lasalocid synthesis (Nakata et al., 1978).

Ireland et al. (1980) used glycals to solve this problem. For example, the glycal [39] (Scheme 15) prepared from 6-deoxy-L-glucose

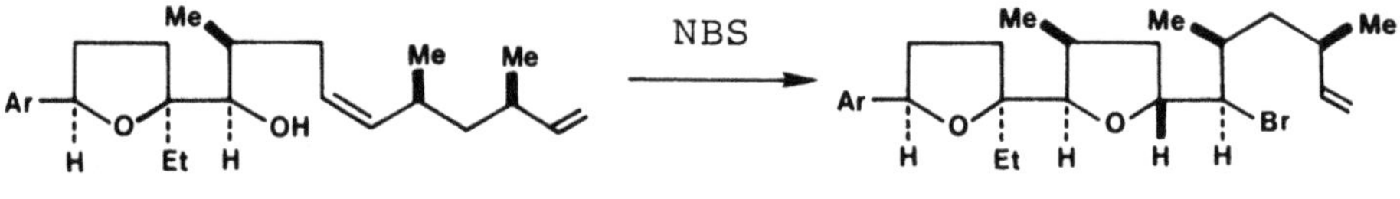

[25]   [26]

Scheme 11

Table 2

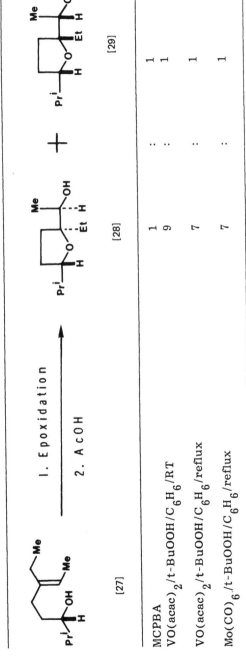

	[28]		[29]	
MCPBA	1	:	1	
VO(acac)₂/t-BuOOH/C₆H₆/RT	9	:	1	
VO(acac)₂/t-BuOOH/C₆H₆/reflux	7	:	1	
Mo(CO)₆/t-BuOOH/C₆H₆/reflux	7	:	1	

Table 3

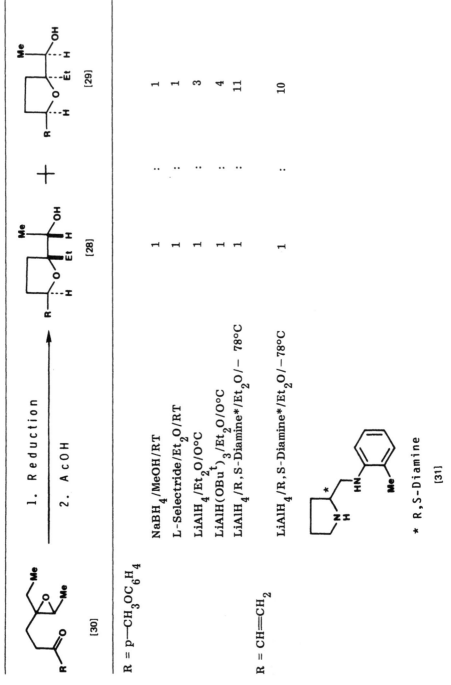

	[28]		[29]
NaBH₄/MeOH/RT	1	:	1
L-Selectride/Et₂O/RT	1	:	1
LiAlH₄/Et₂O/O°C	1	:	3
LiAlH(OBuᵗ)₃/Et₂O/O°C	1	:	4
LiAlH₄/R,S-Diamine*/Et₂O/−78°C	1	:	11
LiAlH₄/R,S-Diamine*/Et₂O/−78°C	1	:	10

$R = p-CH_3OC_6H_4$

$R = CH=CH_2$

* R,S-Diamine
[31]

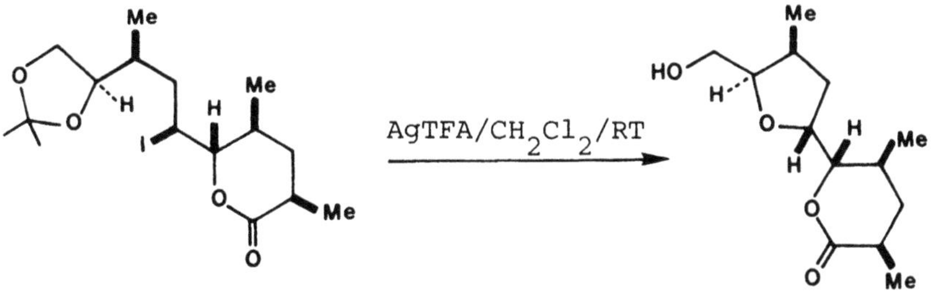

[32]   [33]

Scheme 12

was subjected to an enolate Claisen rearrangement to yield [40] and [41] in a ratio of 76:24. [The reagents were the following: (a), $(COCl)_2/C_6H_6$; (b), BuLi, THF, LDA, THF, TMSCl, RT, H_2O, OH⁻, CH_2N_2.]

E. 1,2-Stereochemistry

In addition to the crossed aldol reactions described, Grignard reactions of α-alkoxy aldehydes or ketones are extremely useful in controlling the stereochemistry of 1,2-positions. The stereochemical outcome can be predicted by using Cram's cyclic model. The usefulness of this type of reaction for the synthesis of polyether antibiotics was first demonstrated in the Kishi lasalocid A synthesis (Nakata and Kishi, 1978), i.e., [42] to [43]. (Scheme 16).

Still and McDonald (1980) studied the stereoselectivity of Grignard reactions or various protected α-hydroxy ketones and confirmed that numerous protecting groups yielded excellent stereoselectivity. This method was extensively used in Still's monensin synthesis (Collum et al., 1980b,c). Still and Schneider (1980) have also found that organocuprates add highly stereoselectively to α-asymmetric aldehydes bearing β-oxygen substituents. (Scheme 17).

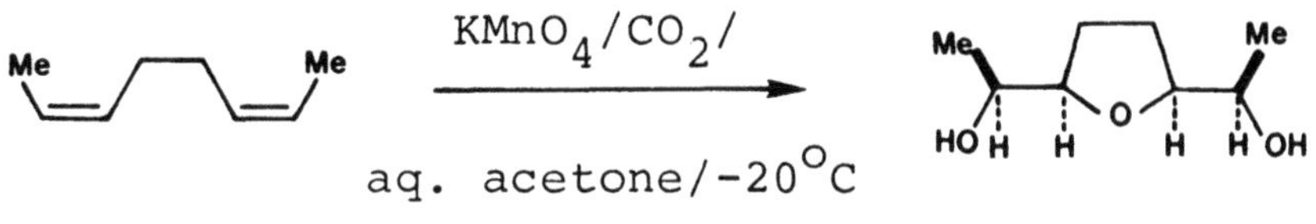

[34]   [35]

Scheme 13

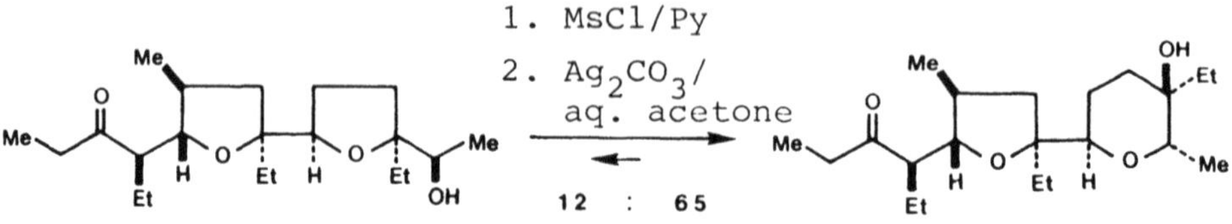

1. MsCl/Py

2. Ag$_2$CO$_3$/
    aq. acetone

12 : 65

[36]   [37]

Scheme 14

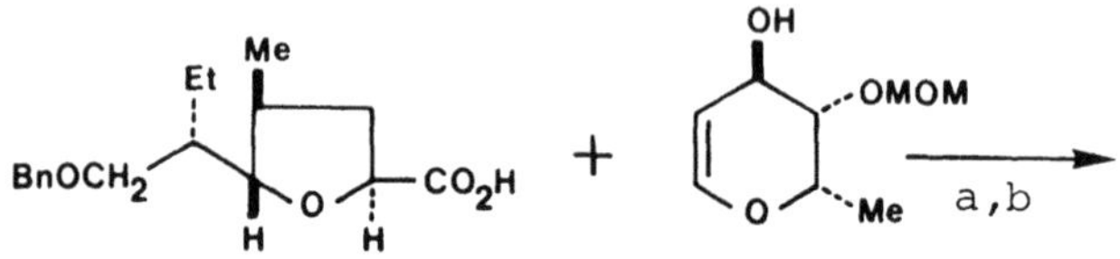

[38]   [39]   a,b

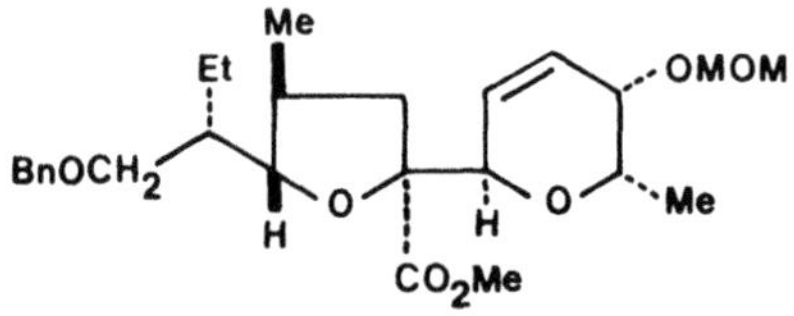

+   [41]

antiepimer

[40]

Scheme 15

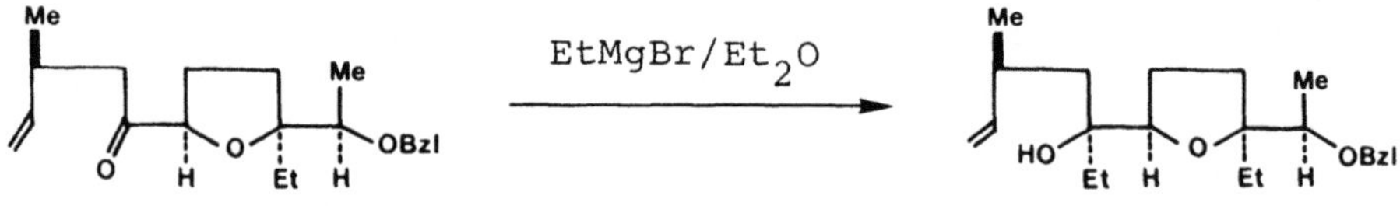

EtMgBr/Et$_2$O

[42]   [43]

Scheme 16

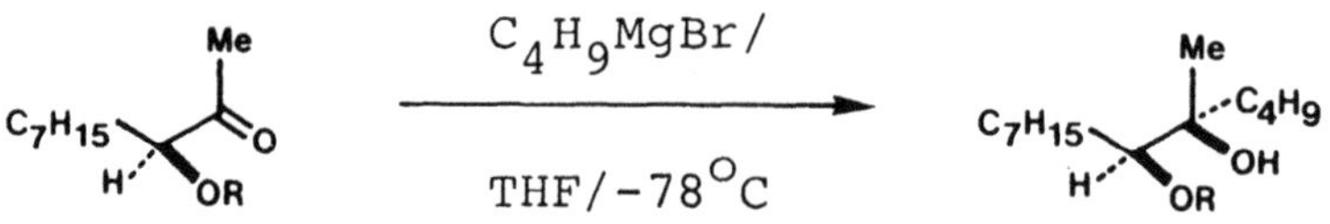

C$_4$H$_9$MgBr/

THF/$-78°$C

[44]   [45] (threo)

Scheme 17

F. Chiral Starting Materials

Because convergent disconnections are often used, the choice of the chiral starting materials becomes rather important, especially in practical terms. The following chiral starting materials (Scheme 18) have been used in the total synthesis of polyether antibiotics.

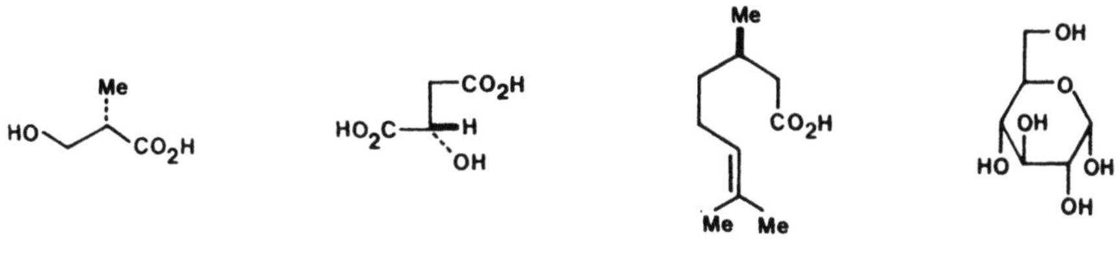

[46]	[47]	[48]	[49]

Scheme 18

III. TOTAL SYNTHESES

A. A23187 (Calcimycin)

The first total synthesis of antibiotic A23187 (calcimycin) was achieved by Evans et al. (1979a). Grieco et al. (1980) synthesized the key intermediate of the Evans synthesis from a bicyclo precursor. Nakahara et al. (1979) have made considerable progress in the total synthesis of the antibiotic from D-glucose.

B. Evans Synthesis

Based on the analysis counting anomeric effect and supported by the aforementioned model studies, the antibiotic A23187 was considered equivalent to the corresponding open form [51] (Scheme 19). Furthermore, it was anticipated, and confirmed, that the stereochemistry of the C-15 methyl group of the antibiotic is thermodynamically more preferred, and hence the stereochemistry control of this center is not necessarily required. The intermediate [51] was then disconnected into three segments, [52], [53], and [54], by using crossed aldol reactions.

Segment [54] was synthesized by the method summarized in Scheme 20. Nitration of [56] yielded a 2:1 mixture of [58] and its position isomer. [The reagents were the following: (a), TFAA/Py, (b), HNO_3/Et_2O; (c), $H_2/Pd-C$; (d), MeCOCl/xylene/140°C; (e), MeI/ K_2CO_3/acetone.]

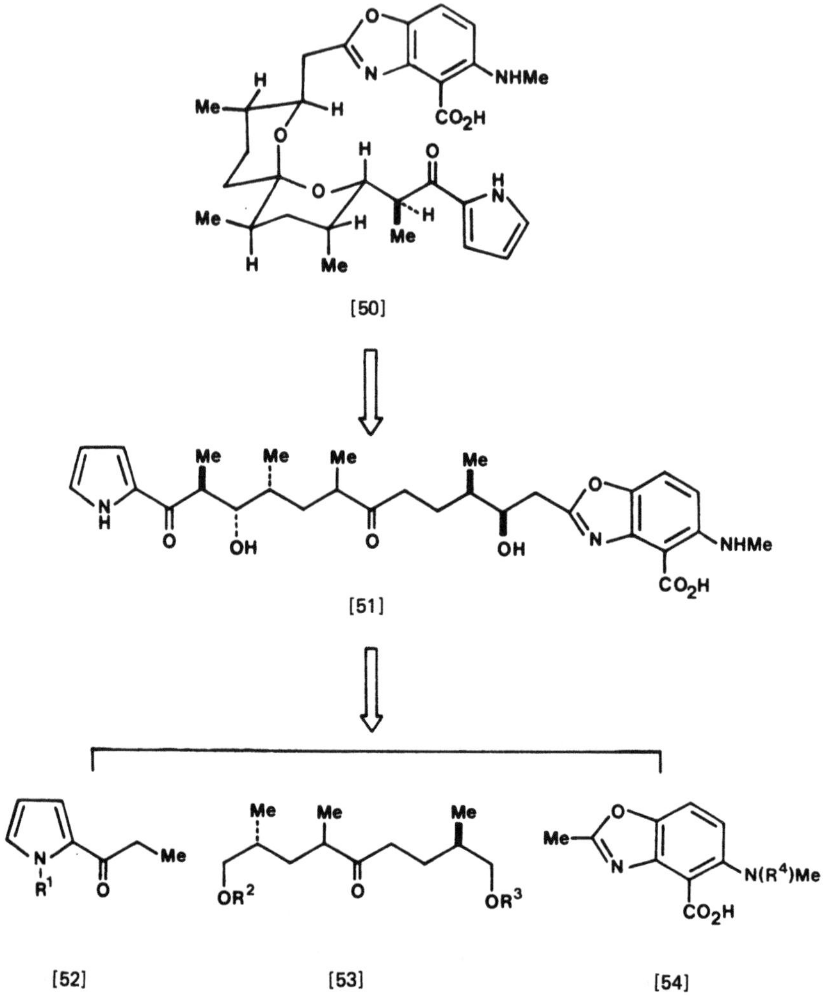

[50]

[51]

[52]   [53]   [54]

Scheme 19

(S)-(+)-β-Hydroxyisobutyric acid [46] was used as the chiral starting material for segment [53]; [46] was converted to the iodides [60] and [61], respectively (Scheme 21).

The two iodides [60] and [61] were then joined by using hydrazone [62]. This synthesis is summarized in Scheme 22. [The reagents were the following: (a), KH/KOBu^t/THF/reflux, [60]/0°C to RT; (b), Li/NH$_3$; (c), LDA/THF/0°C, [61]; (d), CuCl$_2$/aq. THF; (e), C(Me)$_2$(CH$_2$OH)$_2$/p-TSA; (f), sec-BuLi/THF/−78°C, B(OMe)$_3$/−78°C to RT, H$_2$O$_2$/NaOH; (g), CrO$_3$/Py; (h), [54]/LDA/THF/−100°C, [65]; (i), (CO$_2$H)$_2$/MeOH/RT; (j), Bu$_4$N$^+$F$^-$/THF; (k), Collins reagent; (l),

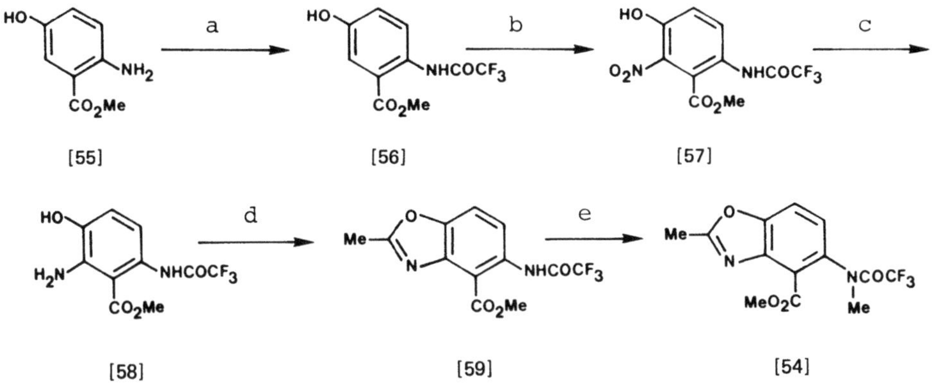

Scheme 20

zinc enolate of [52]/Et_2O-DME/0°C, [68]; (m), Bio Rad Ag 50W-X8/ toluene/100°C, Li propylmercaptide/HMPA.] Deprotection of the benzyl group of [64] was effected by benzylic metalation, followed by oxidation. The crossed aldollike reaction of [54] and [65] resulted in an 88:12 mixture of [66] and its diastereomer. The alcohol [66] was then transformed to the aldehyde [68] in three steps.

Crossed aldol reaction of [68] and zinc enolate prepared from [52] gave a 70.30 mixture of [69] and its diastereomer. The aldol [69] was then transformed to the methyl ester of A23187 under acidic conditions. The methyl ester was hydrolyzed with lithium n-propylmercaptide to complete the total synthesis. Since the sign of the rotation of the synthetic substance was the same as that of natural A23187, the absolute configuration previously assigned to the antibiotic was confirmed by this total synthesis.

C. Grieco Synthesis

The Grieco synthesis started with the bicyclo[2,2,1]heptenone [70] (Scheme 23), which was converted to the segment [76] by the methods summarized. [The reagents were the following: (a), H_2O_2/OH^-; (b), $BF_3 \cdot Et_2O/CH_2Cl_2$; (c), LAH/Et_2O; (d), $H_2/PtO_2/EtOAc$; (e),

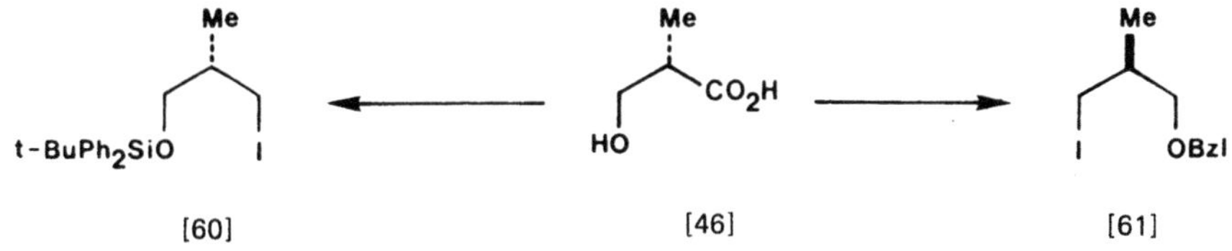

Scheme 21

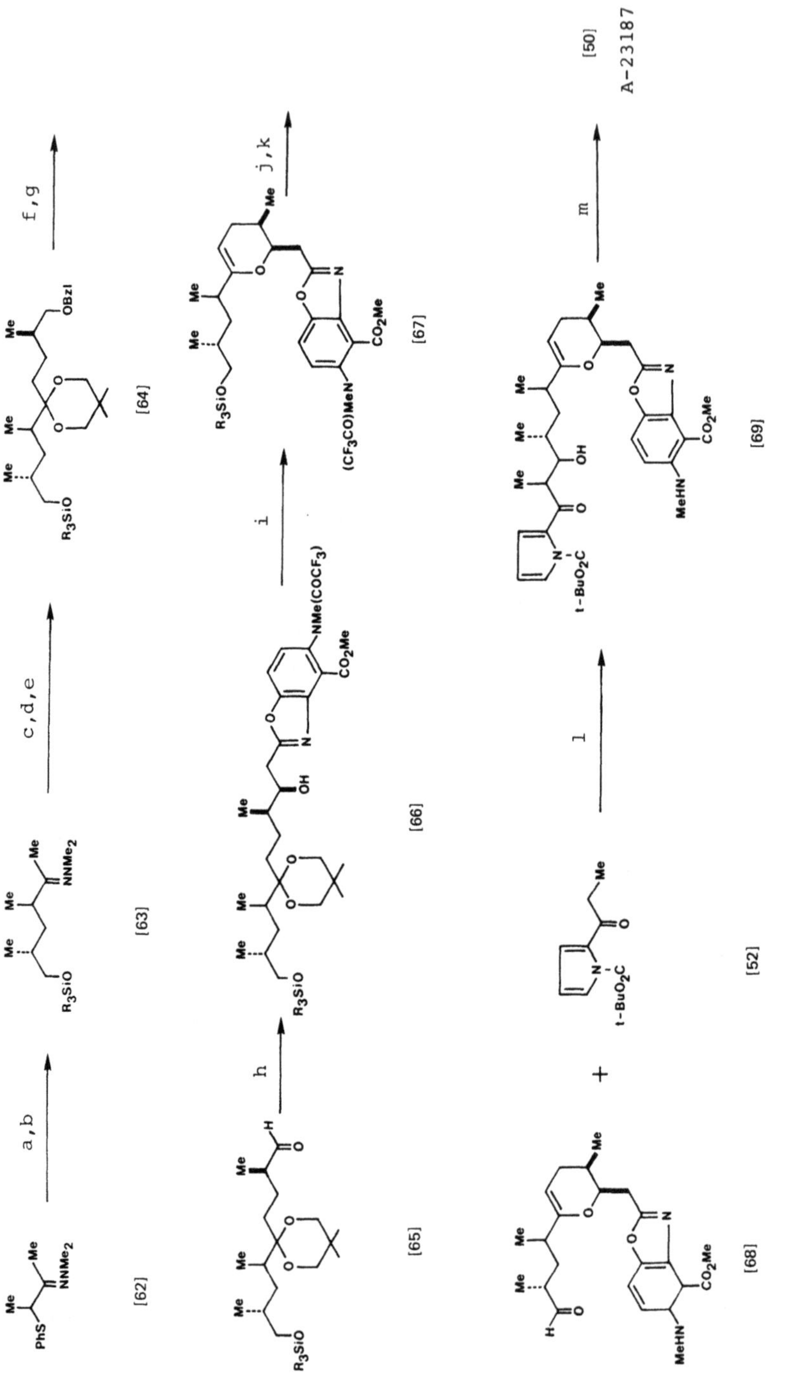

Scheme 22

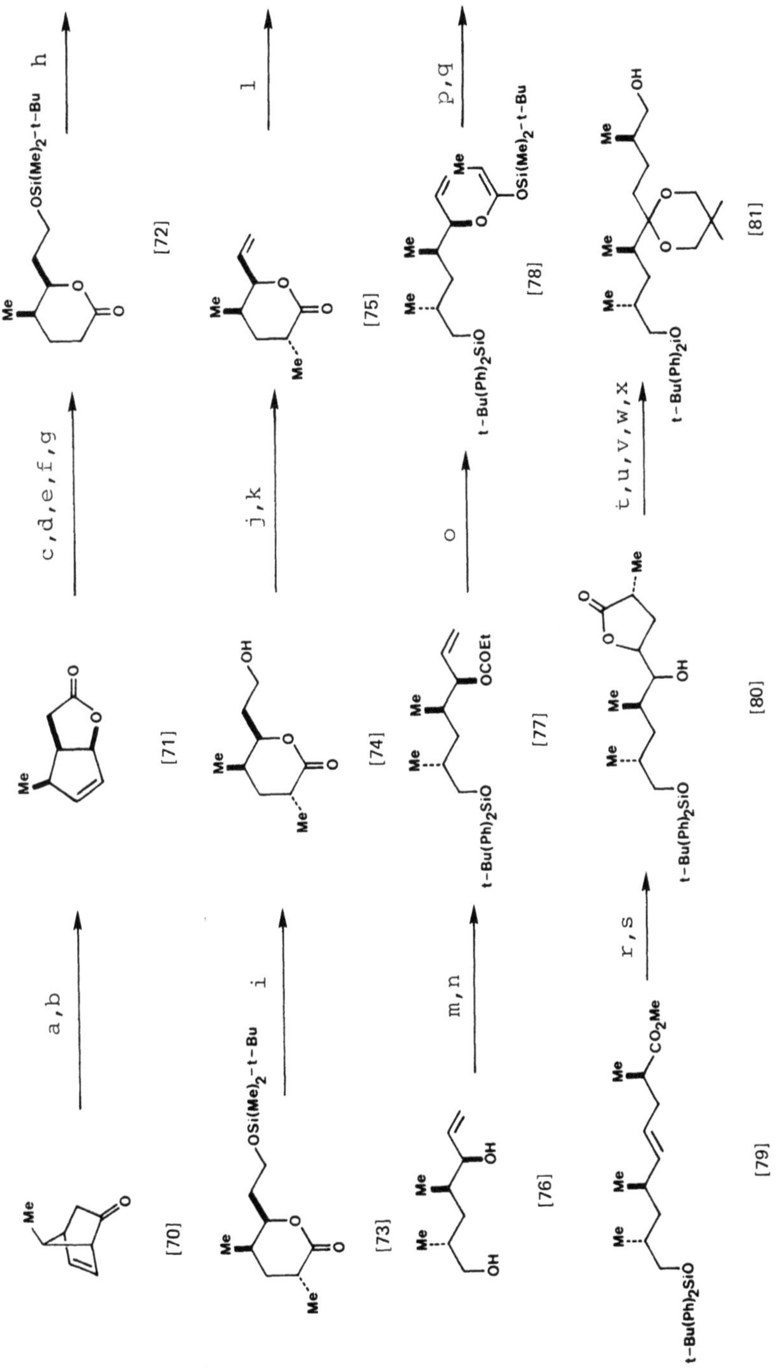

Scheme 23

$Bu^t(Me)_2SiCl/DMF/imidazole$; (f), $CrO_3 \cdot 2Py$; (g), $MCPBA/CH_2Cl_2$;
(h), $LDA/MeI/THF$, (i), 10% HCl/THF; (j), $o-NO_2C_6H_4SeCN/PBu_3/THF$;
(k), 50% H_2O_2/THF; (l), LAH; (m), $Bu^t(Ph)_2SiCl/Et_3N/DMAP/CH_2Cl_2$;
(n), EtCOCl; (o), LDA/THF, $Bu^t(Me)_2SiCl/HMPA$; (p), ester enolate
Claisen rearrang.; (q), CH_2N_2/KOH; (r), OsO_4/Py; (s), CSA/CH_2Cl_2;
(t), $PCC/NaOAc/CH_2Cl_2$; (u), $Al(Hg)/aq$. EtOH-THF; (v), $CH_2N_2/$
Et_2O; (w), $C(Me)_2(CH_2OH)_2/HC(OMe)_3/p-TSA/CH_2Cl_2$; (x), LAH.]

Ester enolate Claisen rearrangement of E-O-silylketene [78], prepared from [77], was used in controlling the relative stereochemistry
of the C-9 and C-15 methyl groups. The ester [79] was then converted to the Evans intermediate [81].

D. Ogawa Synthesis

Ogawa undertook a synthetic route to A23187 from the compound [82]
(Scheme 24), which is available from methyl α-D-glucose in seven
steps. The compound [82] was converted to the iodide [83]. The
compound [82] was also converted to the dithiane [84]. Coupling of
[83] and [84] will provide the C-18 and C-19 segment of A23187.

E. Lasalocid A (X-537A)

The total synthesis of lasalocid A was first achieved by Nakata et al.
(1978) and Nakata and Kishi (1978). Ireland et al. (1980) completed
the total synthesis of lasalocid A by using carbohydrates as precursors.

F. Kishi Synthesis

The key intermediate [95] (Scheme 25) was synthesized by two different routes. The first route used the epoxidation reaction of bishomoallylic alcohols stereoselectively to construct the tetrahydrofurans,
while the second used the lithium aluminum hydride-racemic diamine

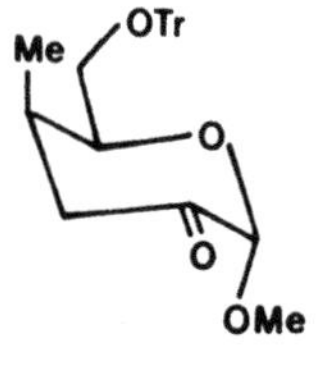

[82] 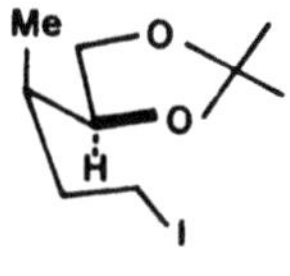   [83] 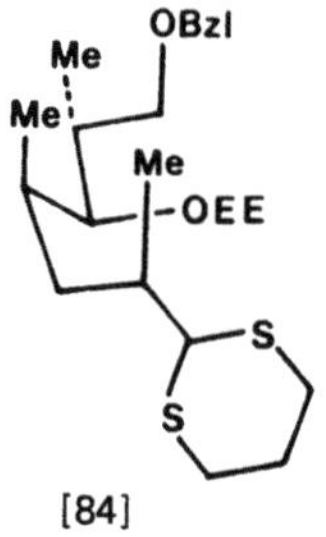   [84]

Scheme 24

[31] reduction of keto epoxides steroselectively to construct tetra-hydrofurans. [The reagents were the following: (a), LAH/Et$_2$O; (b), PCC/CH$_2$Cl$_2$; (c), p-MeOC$_6$H$_4$Br/Et$_2$O; (d), Jones oxid., (e), see Table 4; (f), Bu^{t}O$_2$H/VO(acac)$_2$/NaOAc/C$_6$H$_6$, AcOH; (g), Bu^{t}O$_2$H/VO(acac)$_2$/NaOAc/C$_6$H$_6$; (h), Ac$_2$O/Py; (i), 0.1N H$_2$SO$_4$/aq. acetone/RT; (j), TsCl/Py; (k), K$_2$CO$_3$/MeOH; (l), AcOH; (m), BrCH$_2$OMe/KH/THF; (n), Li/EtOH/liq. NH$_3$; (o), MCPBA/NaHCO$_3$/CH$_2$Cl$_2$; (p), HIO$_4$/aq. dioxane; (q), LAH/THF; (r), TsCl/Py; (s), LAH/Et$_2$O; (t), B$_2$H$_6$/THF, followed by H$_2$O$_2$/NaOH; (u), Jones oxid.; (v), TrBF$_4$/CH$_2$Cl$_2$; (w), NaOH/aq. dioxane.]

1. First route

Ethyl (4E,8E)-2-methyl-4,8-diethyldecadienoate [85], synthesized by adapting Johnson's method, was converted to the ketone [86]. The next step of the synthesis was the reduction of [86] to [87]. Based on Cram's rule, the alcohol [87] was anticipated as the major product. The reduction using recently developed reagents such as L-selectride gave rather disappointing results. However, a highly stereospecific reduction of racemic [86] by the combination of the racemic diamine [31] and lithium aluminum hydride was discovered. The reason for choosing the methyl group as R was purely experimental; various ani-line and napthylamine derivatives were prepared, of which the dia-mine with the methyl group as R was best. The degree of stereospeci-ficity for the *optically active* diamine [31]-LiAlH$_4$ is about half that of the racemic diamine [31]. Thus this is a clear-cut example of double stereodifferentiation. Optical resolution of [87] was achieved by chromatographic separation of its α-methylbenzyl urethane.

Epoxidation of the levorotatory alcohol [87], followed by acetic acid work-up, gave the tetrahydrofuran [89] along with its steroisomer in a ratio of 8:1. Repetition of epoxidation of [89] under the same con-ditions, followed by acetylation, allowed isolation of the epoxide [90], which was transformed to the tetrahydrofuran [92] by four steps. The first three steps were necessary to invert the stereochemistry of the epoxide ring. The overall steroselectivity from [89] to [92] and its steroisomer was 5:1.

The functionalization required for introduction of the ethyl ketone moiety was achieved by eight steps. Deprotection of the C-2 alcoholic group yielded exclusively the ketone [94]. Equilibrium of [94] re-sulted in a 1:1 mixture of [94] and [95], which was well separated by silica gel preparative thin layer chromatography. The recovered ke-tone [94] was recycled.

The ketone [94], belonging to the isolasalocid A series, was stereo-specifically converted to the ketone [2], belonging to the lasalocid series, in two steps; methanesulfonyl chloride-pyridine treatment of [95] afforded the mesylate, whose solvolysis in aqueous acetone in the presence of silver carbonate at room temperature gave a mixture of ketones [2] (65% yield) and [95] (12% yield), which was recycled.

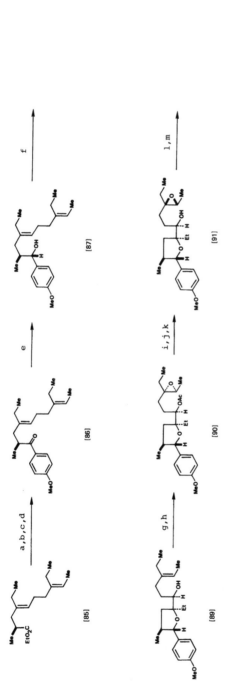

Scheme 25

Table 4

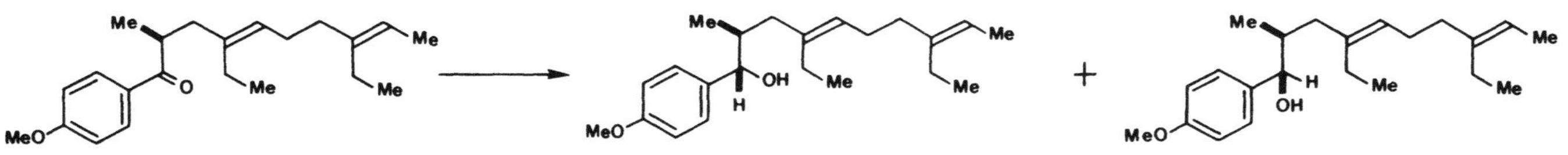

	[87]	[88]
NaBH₄	1	1
L-Selectride	3	1
LiAlH₄	1	1
LiAlH₄-Diamine*		
R = H, * = S	3	1
R = H, * = R,S	6	1
R = CH₃, * = S	6	1
R = CH₃, * = R,S	12	1

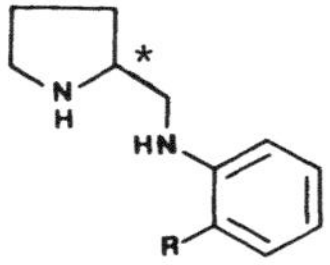

* = Diamine [31]

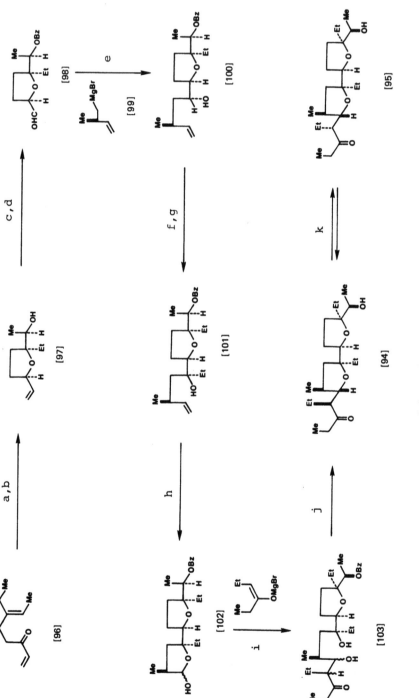

Scheme 26

2. Second route

Application of the synthetic method summarized in Table 3 to the readily available unsaturated ketone [96] (Scheme 26) gave the tetrahydrofuran [97] (65% yield) along with its stereoisomer (6% yield). [The reagents were the following: (a) and (b), see Table 3; (c), BzlBr/KH/THF; (d), O_3/MeOH/$-78°C$; (e), [99]/Et_2O; (f), Jones oxid.; (g), EtMgBr/Et_2O; (h), O_3/MeOH/$-78°C$; (i), the magnesium enolate; (j), p-TSA/C_6H_6/ reflux; (k), NaOH/aq. dioxane.] Optical resolution of [97] was achieved through its hemiphthalate, using strychnine as the resolving reagent. After the secondary alcholic group was protected as its benzyl ether, the levorotatory tetrahydrofuran was oxidized to give the aldehyde [98]. Grignard reaction of [97] with 2-methyl-3-butenyl-magnesium bromide prepared from (+)-1-bromo-2-methyl-3-butene [99] in THF yielded the alcohol [100]. The bromide [99] was synthesized by the method summarized in Scheme 27.

Jones oxidation of [100] followed by treatment with ethylmagnesium bromide in ether gave exclusively the alcohol [101]. The stereochem-istry of [100] and [101] was assigned based on the cyclic model of Cram's rule. Ozonolysis of [101], followed by dimethyl sulfide work-up, afforded the lactol [102]. Treatment of [102] with the magnesium enolate prepared from 4-bromo-3-hexanone gave a mixture of aldols, which was treated with p-TSA in boiling benzene and then deprotected to yield a mixture of the epi-isolasalocid ketone [94] (3 parts) and the isolasalocid ketone [95] (2 parts). Sodium hydroxide treatment of [94] yielded an equilibrium mixture of [95] and [94].

The synthesis of the left half of lasalocid A is summarized in Scheme 28. Treatment of 2-acetoxy-2-methyl-6-carbobenzoxy-7,5-cyclohexa-dien-1-one [109] (Scheme 28) with lithium di(3-methyl-4-pentenyl)cup-rate [110], prepared from (−)-1-bromo-3-methyl-4-pentene [114],

1. $PyH^+CrO_3Cl^-$
2. $CH_2=P(C_6H_5)_3$

[104]   [105]

TFA

1. $MsCl/Et_3N$
2. $LiBr/DMF$

[106]   *Scheme 27*   [107]

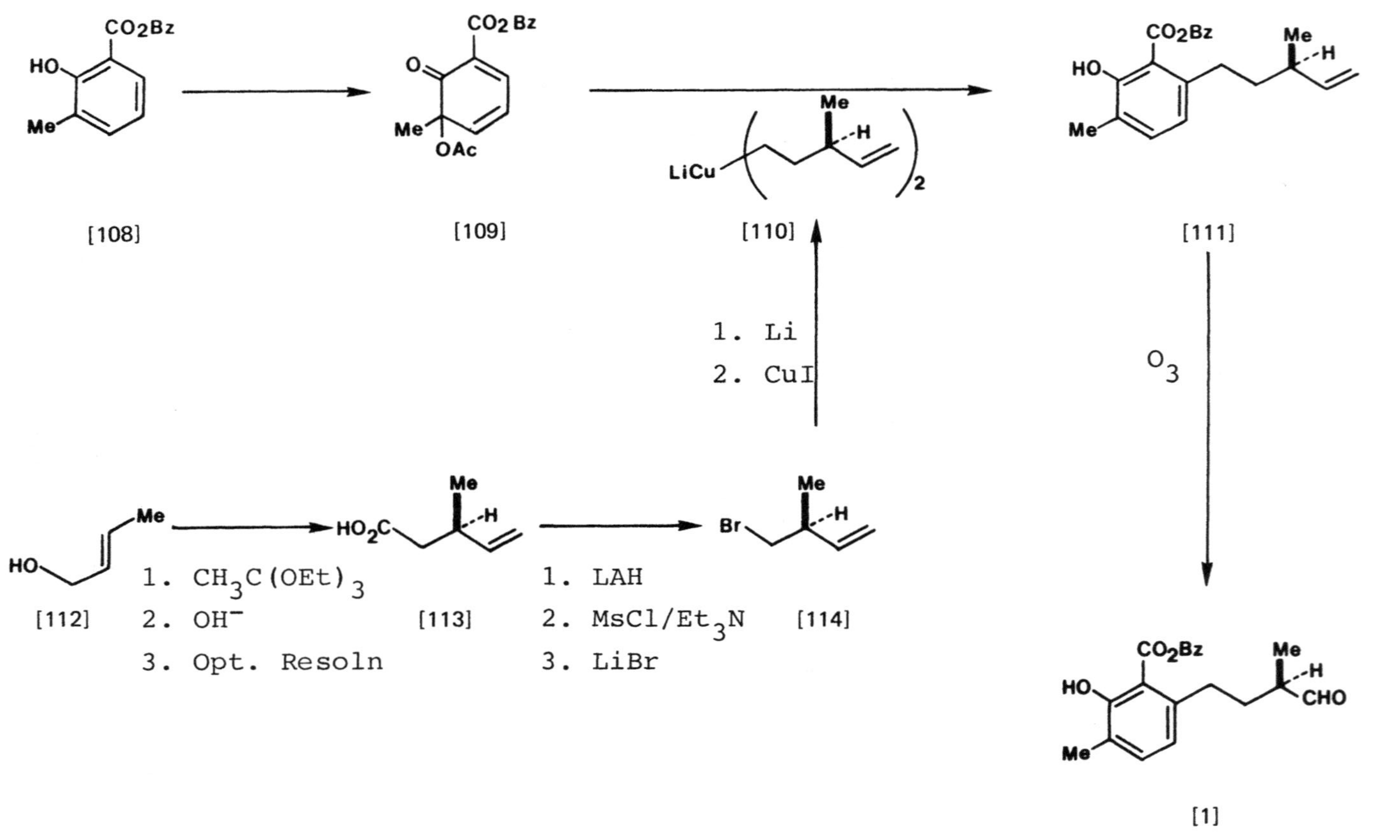
CO2Bz
HO
Me
[108]
CO2 Bz
O
Me
OAc
[109]
LiCu
Me
H
2
[110]
CO2Bz
HO
Me
Me
H
[111]
1. Li
2. CuI
O3
HO
Me
[112]
1. CH3C(OEt)3
2. OH⁻
3. Opt. Resoln
HO2C
Me
H
[113]
1. LAH
2. MsCl/Et3N
3. LiBr
Br
Me
H
[114]
CO2Bz
HO
Me
Me
H
CHO
[1]

Scheme 28

gave the benzyl salicylate [111]. Optically active bromide [114] was prepared by five steps, as shown in Scheme 28. This bromide was also prepared from (S)-β-hydroxyisobutyric acid [46]. Ozonization of [111] in a mixture of methylene chloride and methanol at −78°C afforded the aldehyde [1].

The crossed aldol reaction was originally achieved by using zinc enolate. Later, magnesium dicyclohexylamine was found to be a better base. Debenzylation of [3] was carried out under the standard conditions (H_2/Pd-C/MeOH/RT), and synthetic lasalocid A was quantitatively isolated as its sodium salt.

G. Ireland Synthesis

Ireland envisioned a convergent disconnection of the ketone [2] into three subunits, [116], [117], and [118] (Scheme 29). The plan in-

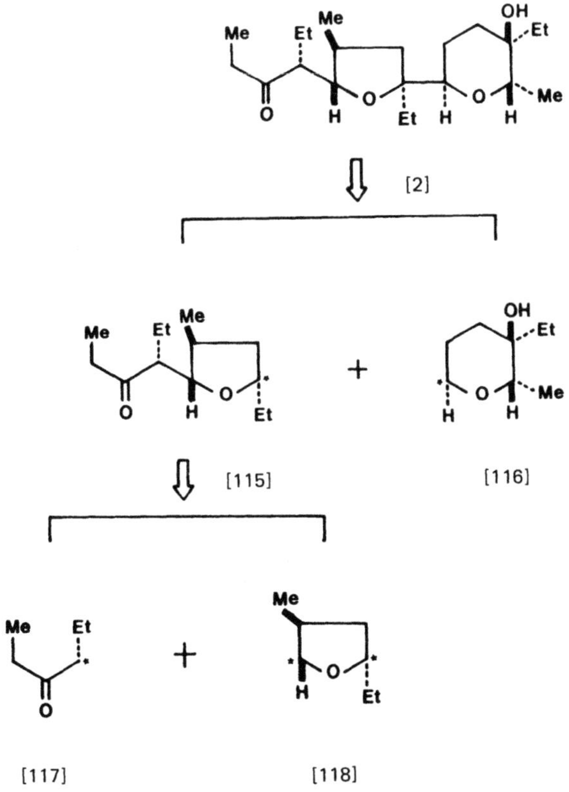

Scheme 29

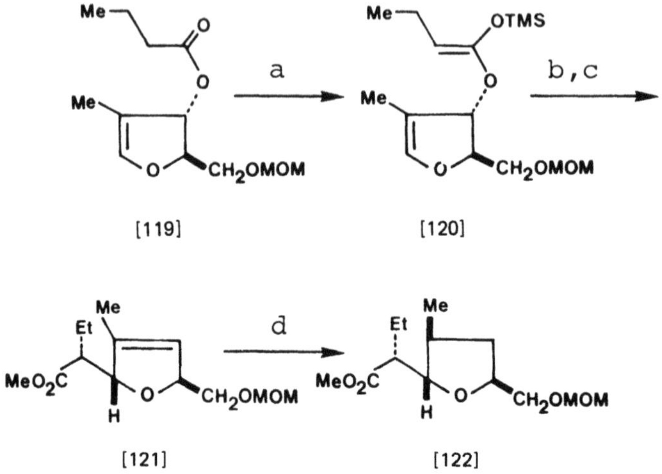

Scheme 30

volved the initial union of [117] and [118], and then subsequent joining of that product with the remaining subunit [116]. These unions
were achieved by using the ester enolate Claison rearrangement reaction investigated by Ireland some years ago. This method is illustrated
by the following example. [3,3] Sigmatropic rearrangement of E-O-
silylketone acetal [120] (Scheme 30), prepared stereoselectively from
the corresponding glycalyl butyrate [119] in 32% HMPA-THF, yielded
the ester [121] after alkaline diazomethane work-up. Hydrogenation
of [121] gave the tetrahydrofuran [122]. The overall stereoselectivity
from [119] to [122] was 75:25. [The reagents were the following: (a),
LDA/23% HMPA-THF, TMSCl; (b), RT; (c), CH_2N_2/aq. NaOH; (d),
H_2/Pd-C/EtOAc.]

   The synthesis of the ketone [2] is summarized in Scheme 31. Notice
that the union of [38] and [39] was achieved again by the ester enolate Claisen rearrangement to give a 76:24 mixture of [40] and its antiepimer. The necessary functionalization at the C-22 position was
achieved via the epoxide [130]; the stereoselectivity of m-chloroperbenzoic acid epoxidation was 78:22. [The reagents were the following:
(a), acetone, H^+; (b), KH, $ClCH_2OMe$; (c), Dibal, Et_2O; (d),
$P(NMe_2)_3$, CCl_4, Li, NH_3; (e), BuLi, n-C_3H_7COCl, LDA, 23% HMPA-
THF, TSMCl, RT, H_2O, OH^-, CH_2N_2; (f), H_2, Pd-C, EtOAc; (g),
$LiAlH_4$, Et_2O; (h), KH, $C_6H_5CH_2Br$; (i), H_3O^+; (j), Pd, O_2, aqueous
$NaHCO_3$; (k), BnOH, HCl; (l), H_2, Pd-C, EtOAc; (m), $(COCl)_2$,
C_6H_6; (n), BuLi, THF, LDA, THF, TMSCl, RT, H_2O, OH^-, CH_2N_2;
(o), H_2, Ni(R), EtOAc; (p), $(C_6H_5)_3$-PCH_2, THF; (q), Me_2SO_4,
$(COCl)_2$, Et_3N; (r), MCPBA, CH_2Cl_2; (s), $Li(Me)_2Cu$, pentane; (t),
Li, NH_3; (u), PCC, CH_2Cl_2; (v), C_2H_5MgBr, THF.]

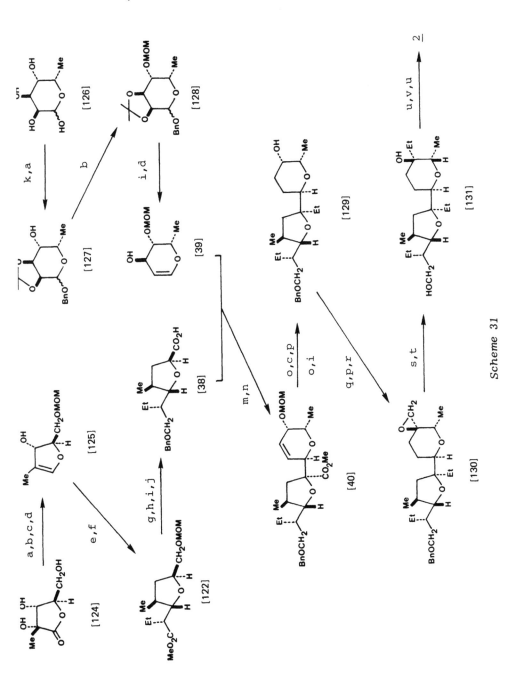

Scheme 31

The union of the left and right halves was achieved by the crossed aldol reaction, but the details as well as the synthesis of the left half have not yet been published [see footnote 5 of Ireland et al. (1980)].

H. Monensin

The total synthesis of monensin was first achieved by Fukuyama et al. (1979b). A crossed aldol reaction was used to join the left and right halves in a stereocontrolled manner. The stereochemistry of the spiro center was controlled by intramolecular ketalization of its open form under thermodynamically controlled conditions.

A highly convergent total synthesis was completed by Collum et al. (1970a, 1980b, 1980c).

I. Kishi Synthesis

Left half. The synthesis of the left half [141] is summarized in Scheme 32. [The reagents were the following: (a), MeC[=P(Ph)$_3$]CO$_2$Et/ C$_6$H$_6$/reflux; (b), LAH/Et$_2$O; (c), C$_6$H$_5$CH$_2$Br/KH/DMF-THF; (d), B$_2$H$_6$/THF/0°C, H$_2$O$_2$/OH$^-$; (e), MeI/KH/DMF-THF/0°C; (f), H$_2$/Pd-C/ MeOH; (g), opt. resoln.; (h), PCC/CH$_2$Cl$_2$; (i), (MeO)$_2$P(O)=C(Me)CO$_2$Me/ THF/−78° to RT; (j), LAH/Et$_2$O; (k), same as step (d); (l), BrCH$_2$ OMe/Me$_2$NC$_6$H$_5$/CH$_2$Cl$_2$/0°C; (m), same as step (c); (n), O$_3$/MeOH/ −78°C; (o), CH$_2$N$_2$/Et$_2$O; (p), conc. HCl/MeOH/reflux; (q), same as step (h).] Hydroboration of [133], followed by alkaline hydrogen perioxide work-up, yielded the alcohol [134] along with its diastereomer in a ratio of 8:1. The origin of the remarkable stereoselectivity observed might be related to the conformation preference of [133]. The preferred conformation of [133] is expected to be [133A], since a considerable steric compression between the two methyl groups or between the methyl and phenyl groups would exist in the alternative two eclipsed conformations. Therefore hydroboration would

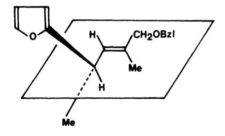

[133A]

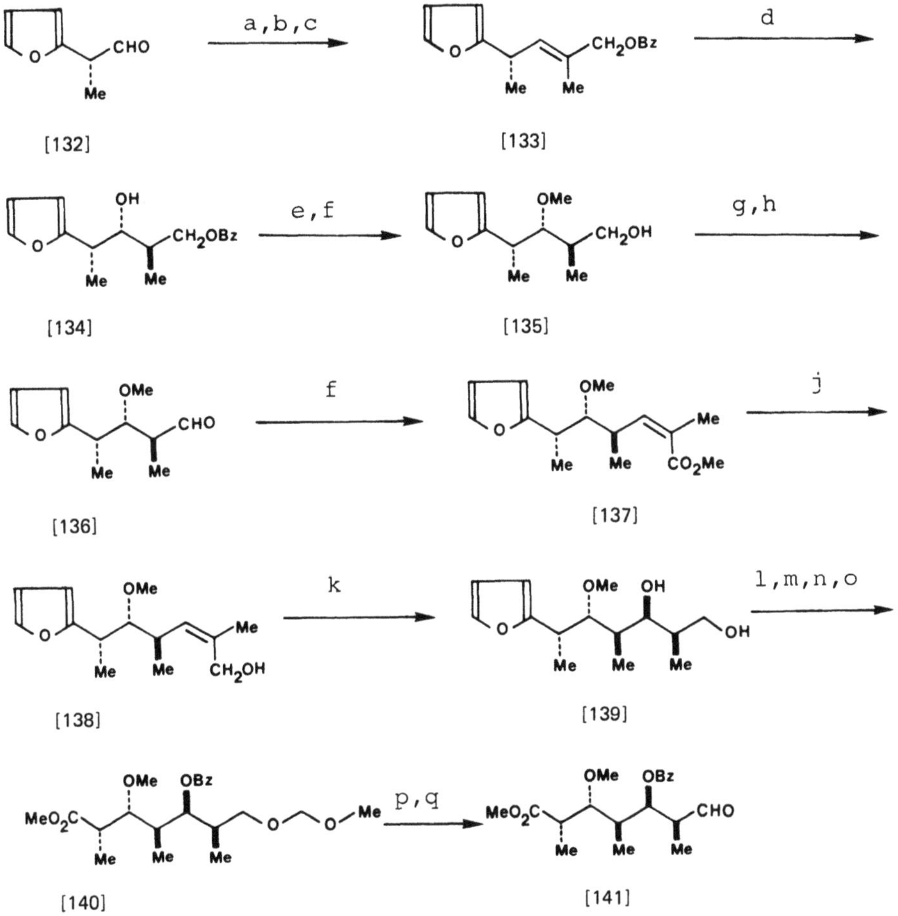

Scheme 32

preferentially take place from the less hindered side to yield the observed major product. To obtain a high degree of stereospecificity it is important to have a substitutent (indicated by an arrow in [133A]) which would make one eclipsed conformation more preferred over the other two.

Optical resolution of [135] was achieved by chromatographic separation of its α-methylbenzyl urethane. The synthesis was continued with the levorotatory alcohol [135]. Cis-allylic alcohol [138] was stereoselectively synthesized by using $(MeO)_2P(O)CHC(CH_3)CO_2Me$ in the Horner-Emmes modification of the Wittig reaction. Hydroboration of [138], followed by alkaline hydrogen peroxide work-up, afforded the alcohol [139] along with its diastereomer in a ratio of 12:1.

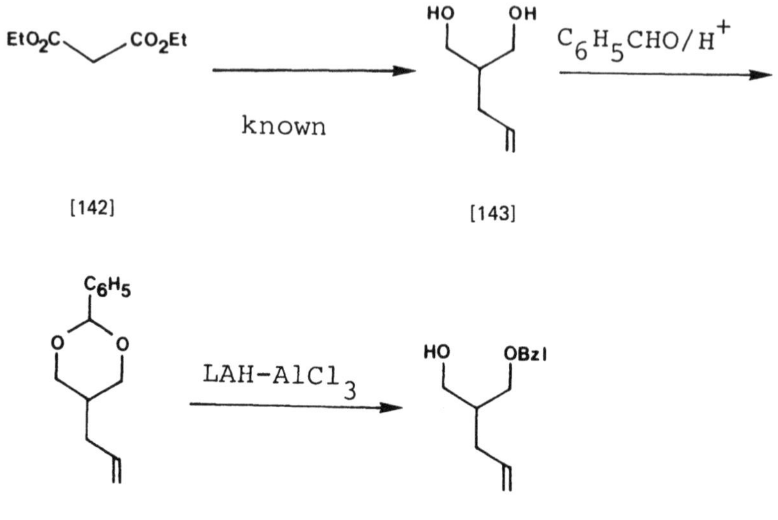

Scheme 33

Right half. The starting material for the synthesis of the right half
was (S)-monobenzyl ether [145] of 2-allyl-1,3-propanediol. The synthesis of this substance is summarized in Scheme 33.

Optical resolution of the monnbenzyl ether [145] was achieved by
chromatographic separation of its α-methyl-α-naphthyl urethane. The
levoratatory monobenzyl ether [145] was converted to the p-methoxy-
acetophenone derivative [148] in eight steps (Scheme 34). [The reagents were the following: (a), PCC/CH_2Cl_2; (b), $MeCH_2(=CH_2)$
$MgBr$/THF/0°C; (c), $MeC(OEt)_3$/$MeCH_2CO_2H$/140°C; (d), LAH/Et_2O;
(e), same as step (a); (f), p-$MeOC_6H_4MgBr$/Et_2O/0°C; (g), Jones
oxid.; (h), BCl_3/CH_2Cl_2; (i), MCPBA/aq. $NaHCO_3$/CH_2Cl_2; (j),
TsCl/Py/0°C; (k), LAH/Et_2O/0°C; (l), CSA/CH_2Cl_2.] The dextrorotatory monobenzyl ether [145] was also transformed to [148] with the
same absolute configuration as that derived from the levorotatory mono-
banzyl ether [148] in 10 steps [(1) $BrCH_2OCH_3$/$(CH_3)_2NC_6H_5$/CH_2Cl_2/
RT, (2) Li/liq. NH_3, (3)-(9) follow steps 1 to 7 for the levorotatory
series, (10) conc. HCl/CH_3OH/60°C] —note the potential symmetry
element of [145].

Epoxidation of [148] was expected to afford the epoxide [149] as the
major product, since the transition state [148A] would experience less
steric hindrance than the alternative transition state [148B] (note the
arrow), assuming this epoxidation involves first a complexation of an
oxidant with the hydroxyl group of [148]. Indeed, m-chloroperbenzoic
acid in methylene chloride-aqueous sodium bicarbonate (two phases) at

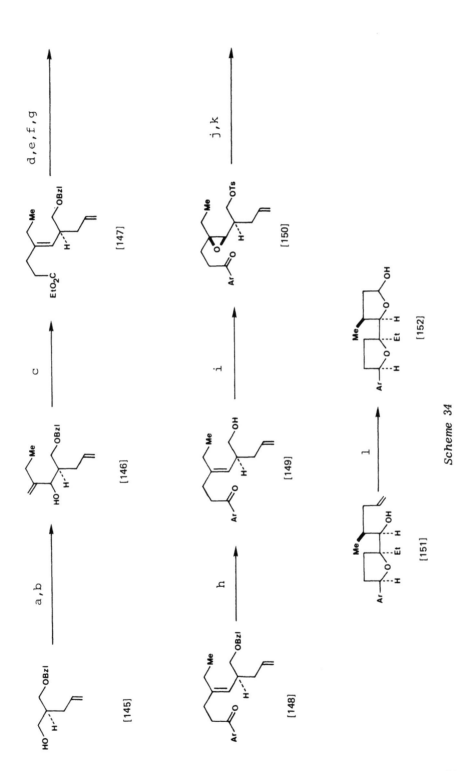

Scheme 34

[149A]   [149B]

[148A,B]

room temperature gave almost quantitatively a single, unstable epoxide [149]. After tosylation [149] was stereospecifically converted to
the tetrahydrofuran [151] by the method described previously. The
ratio of [151] and its diastereomer was 7:2. To have a higher diastereomer ratio the hydroxymethyl group of [149] first had to be reduced
to the corresponding methyl group. This necessary transformation
was possible via the corresponding bromide, followed by treatment
with n-Bu$_3$SnH-AIBN. The reduction of the methyl compound with
lithium aluminum hydride-racemic diamine [31], followed by acid work-
up, gave about an 11:1 ratio of [151] and its diastereomer, but the
overall yield from [149] to [151] was unacceptably low, mainly because
of the practical difficulty encountered as a result of the instability of
[149]. Periodate-osmium tetroxide oxidation of [151] in aqueous dioxane at room temperature yielded the lactol [152].

Baeyer-Villiger oxidation of cis-3,5-dimethylcyclohexanone [153]
(Scheme 35), followed by aqueous potassium hydroxide work-up, gave
the hydroxy acid [155]. Optical resolution of [155] was achieved by
fractional crystallization of its (+)-α-methylbenzylamine salt. The
dextrorotatory hydroxy acid [155] was transformed to the phosphonium
salt [158] in 11 steps. [The reagents were the following: (a),
MCPBA/CH$_2$Cl$_2$; (b), aq. NaOH; (c) opt. resoln., (d), EtOH/H$_2$SO$_4$/
reflux; (e), BrCH$_2$OMe/Me$_2$NC$_6$H$_5$/CH$_2$Cl$_2$, (f), LAH/Et$_2$O; (g),
MsCl/Py/0°C; (h), C$_6$H$_5$SNa/DMF, (i), AcO$_2$H/NaOAc/AcOH-CH$_2$Cl$_2$/
0°C; (j), Δ/CaCO$_3$/decaline; (k), conc. HCl/EtOH/reflux; (l), same
as step (g), (m), LiBr/DMF/100°C; (n), (C$_6$H$_5$)$_3$P/DMF/120°C.]

Wittig reaction of [152] and [158] afforded the cis olefin [159]
(Scheme 36). NBS Bromination of [159] in acetonitrile at room temperature gave a single bromide [160]. Treatment of [160] with superoxide
anion in DMSO containing crown ether gave the alcohol [161]. By-
products of this reaction were olefins formed from elimination of hydrogen bromide.

Functionalization of the p-methoxybenzene ring of [162] was accomplished as summarized in Scheme 37. Magnesium bromide in wet methylene chloride was found most satisfactory to form the enol ether of the

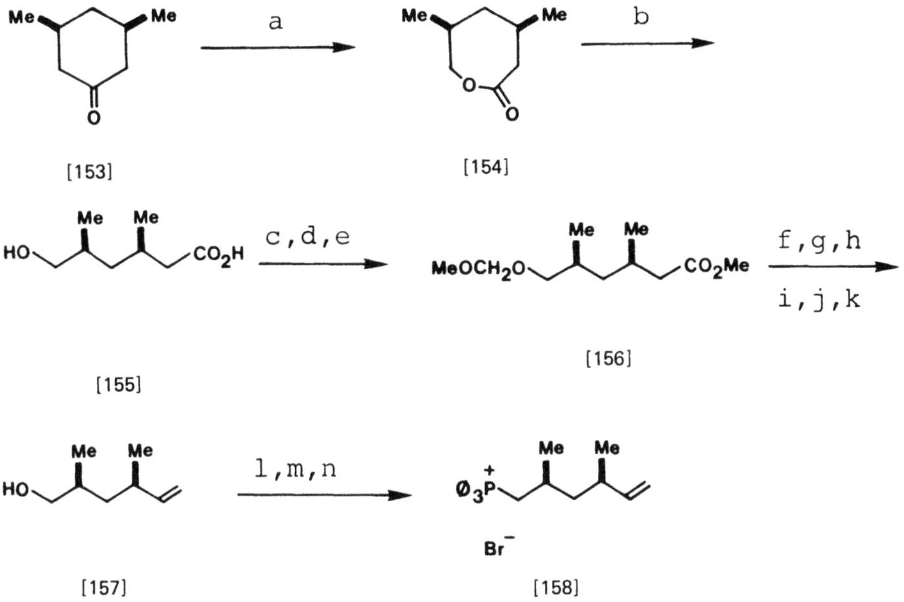

Scheme 35

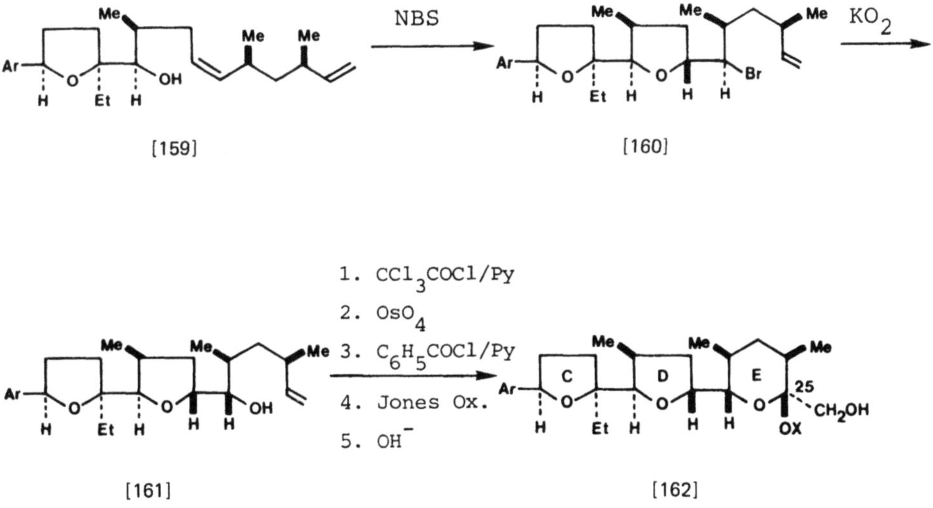

Scheme 36

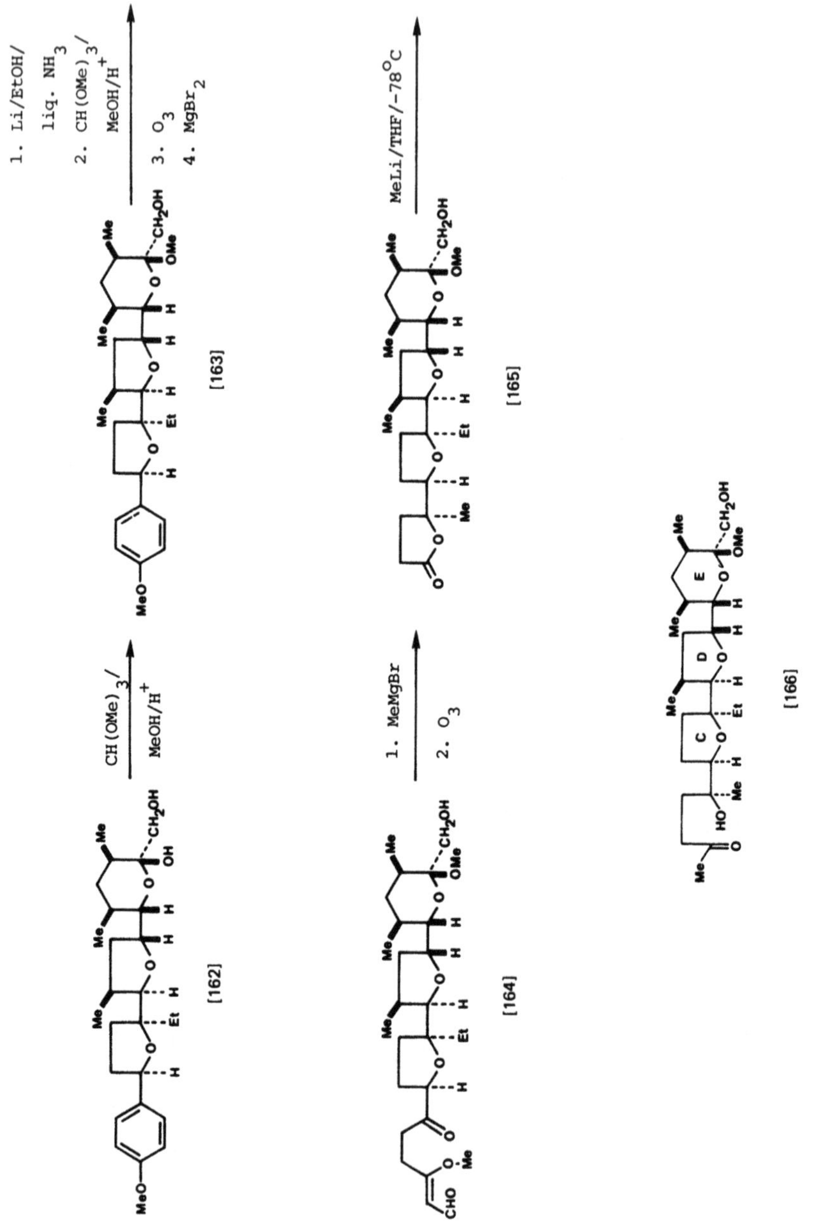

[162]

CH(OMe)$_3$ /
MeOH/H$^+$

[163]

1. Li/EtOH/
   liq. NH$_3$
2. CH(OMe)$_3$ /
   MeOH/H$^+$
3. O$_3$
4. MgBr$_2$

[164]

1. MeMgBr
2. O$_3$

[165]

MeLi/THF/−78°C

[166]

Scheme 37

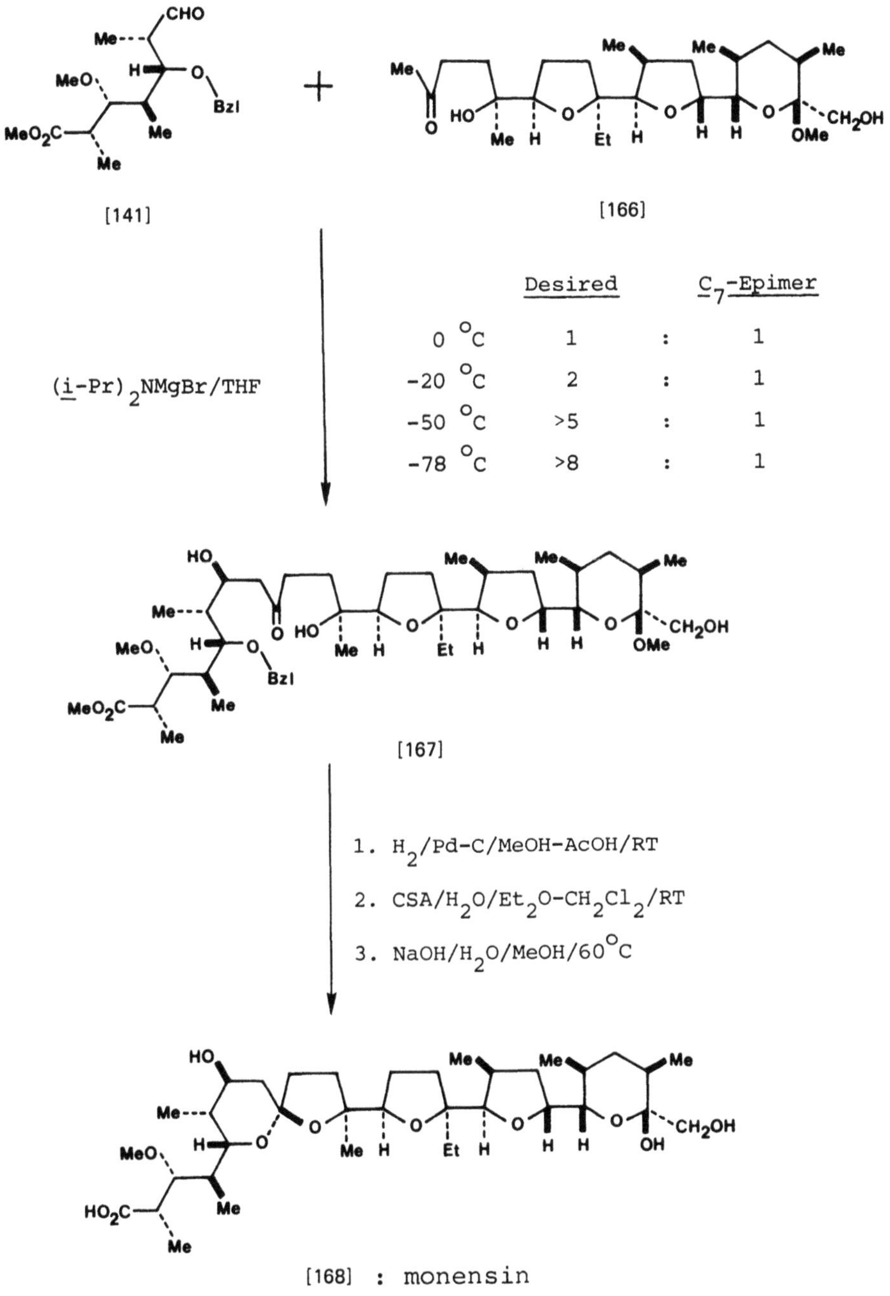

[141]   +   [166]

	Desired		C₇-Epimer
0 °C	1	:	1
-20 °C	2	:	1
-50 °C	>5	:	1
-78 °C	>8	:	1

(i-Pr)₂NMgBr/THF

[167]

1. H₂/Pd-C/MeOH-AcOH/RT

2. CSA/H₂O/Et₂O-CH₂Cl₂/RT

3. NaOH/H₂O/MeOH/60°C

[168] : monensin

Scheme 38

β-ketoaldehyde. Highly stereospecific addition of a Grignard reagent to a ketonic group adjacent to a tetrahydrofuran was demonstrated in the Kishi synthesis of lasalocid A. Transformation of the lactone [165] to the methyl ketone [166] was quantitatively achieved by methyllithium in THF.

The crossed aldol reaction of [141] and [165] was found to be nicely effected by freshly prepared magnesium diisopropylamide in tetrahydrofuran. The ratio of the two diastereomeric aldols was found to be sensitive to the reaction temperature. The diastereomeric aldols were separated by preparative thin layer chromatography to afford the desired aldol [166].

Following the conditions which were established in the model series, the aldol [166] was subjected to the three-step sequence of reactions indicated. Step 2 in this sequence was required to equilibrate the spiroketal center and also to hydrolyze the tertiary methoxy group at the C-25 position. Preparative thin layer chromatography allowed isolation of synthetic monensin [167] as its sodium salt.

L. Still Synthesis

The retrosynthetic analysis of monensin by Still is summarized in Scheme 39. The antibiotic was broken down into four fragments, [169], [171], [173], and [174], three of which contain only vicinal asymmetric centers so that most of the remote stereorelationships may be built up by coupling fragments having the proper absolute configurations. For this reason (−)-malic acid [47], (+)-β-hydroxyisobutyric acid [46], and (R)-citronellic acid [48] were used as the chiral starting materials.

Synthesis of the left-hand fragment [169] of the antibiotic is summarized in Scheme 40. [The reagents were the following: (a), magnesium enolate of 2-methyl-2-trimethylsilyloxy-3-pentanone/THF/−110°C; (b), H_5IO_6/MeOH; (c), KN(TMS)$_2$, Me$_2$SO$_4$; (d), H$_2$/Pd-C/THF; (e), Collins reagent/CH$_2$Cl$_2$; (f), cis-2-butenyldiethylaluminum/THF/−78°C; (g), LiOH/Aq. THF; (h), CH$_2$N$_2$; (i), Et$_3$SiOClO$_3$/MeCN/Py; (j), O$_3$/MeOH/−78°C.] Five chiral centers of the fragment were introduced by two crossed aldol reactions. The stereochemical outcome of the first reaction can be predicted from Cram's cyclic model, while that of the second from the normal Cram's rule. The stereoselectivity observed for for the first reaction was 5:1, and for the second about 3:1.

Synthesis of the central fragment [171] of monensin is summarized in Scheme 41. [The reagents were the following: (a), Me$_2$C(OMe)$_2$/p-TSA; (b), B$_2$H$_6$/THF, H$^+$; (c), C$_6$H$_5$CH$_2$OCH$_2$Cl/Pr$_2$NEt; (d), MeMgBr/THF/−78°C; (e), Bu^{t}Me$_2$SiCl/DMF/imidazole; (f), MeC(=CH$_2$)CH$_2$CH$_2$MgBr/THF; (g), Li/liq. NH$_3$/−78°C; (h), cyclopentanone/p-TSA/CuSO$_4$; (i), NBS/(C$_6$H$_5$)$_3$P.] The key step of this transforma-

[168] : monensin

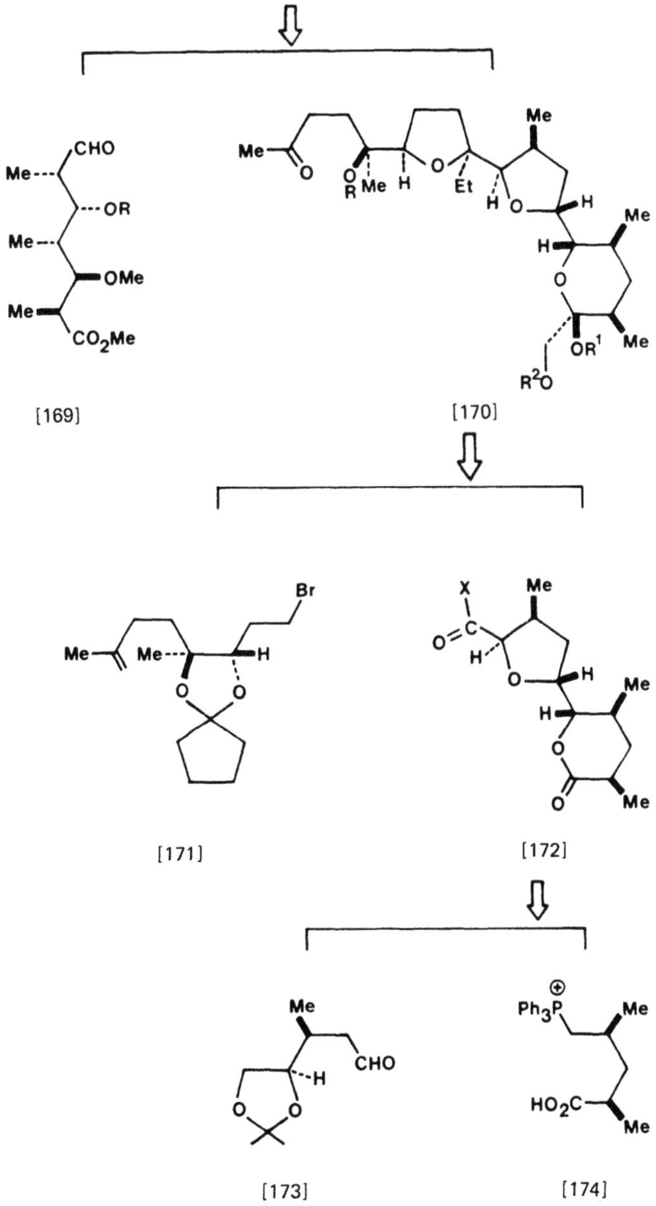

[169]

[170]

[171]

[172]

[173]

[174]

Scheme 39

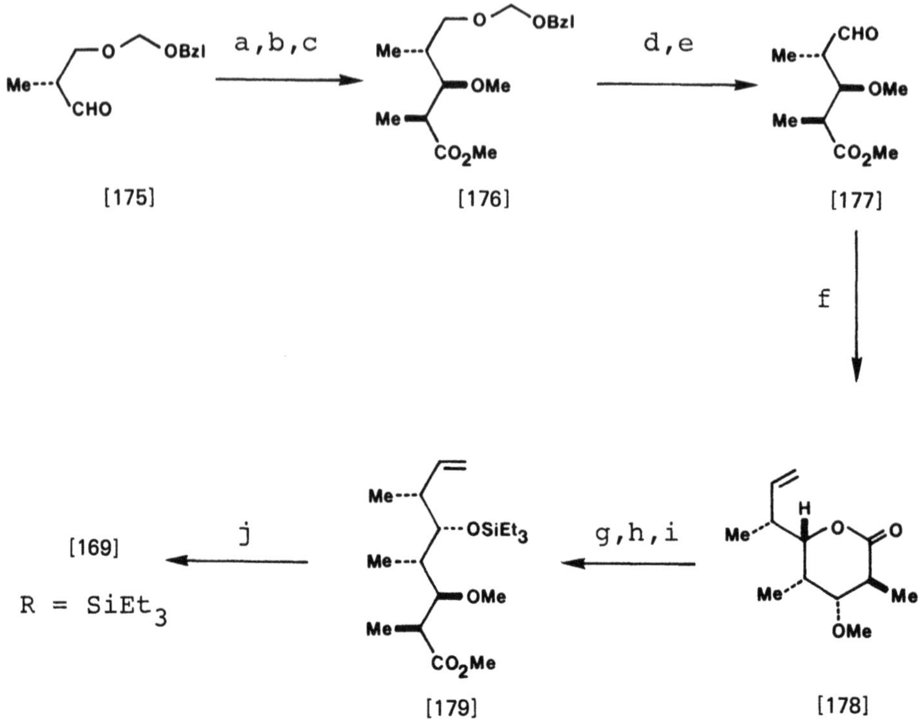

Scheme 40

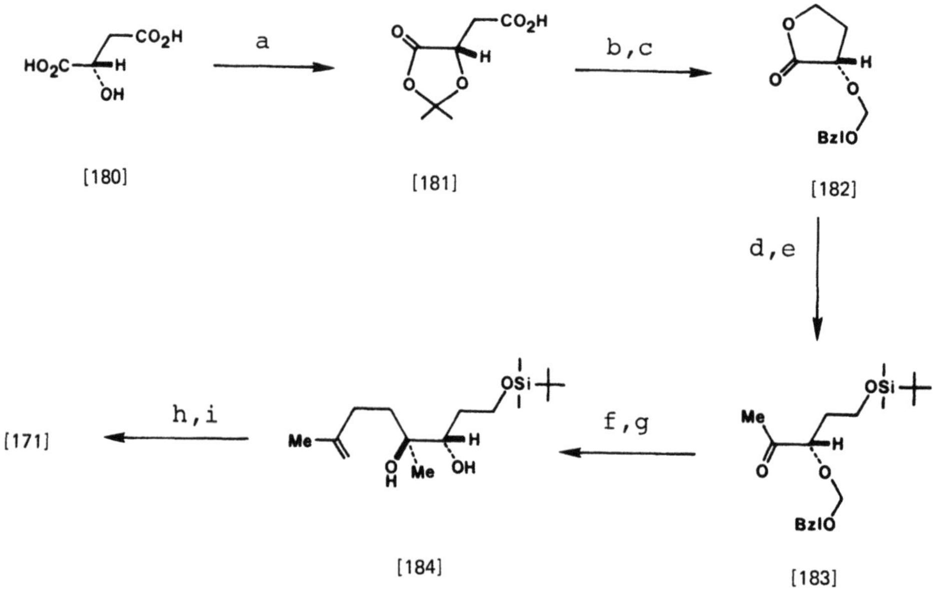

Me···⟨—O⟩—OBzl
ˈCHO
[175]

→ a,b,c →

Me···⟨—O⟩—OBzl
Me···OMe
Me···CO₂Me
[176]

→ d,e →

Me···CHO
Me···OMe
Me···CO₂Me
[177]

↓ f

[178]

→ g,h,i →

[179]

→ j →

[169]
R = SiEt₃

Scheme 40

Scheme 41

HO₂C—⟨OH,H⟩—CO₂H
[180]

→ a →

[181]

→ b,c →

[182]

↓ d,e

[183]

→ f,g →

[184]

→ h,i →

[171]

Scheme 41

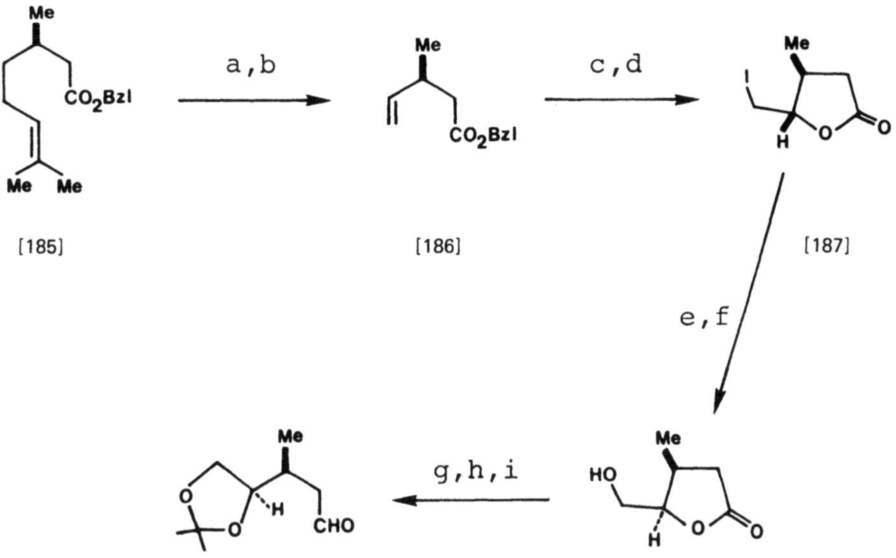

[185] [186] [187]

[189] [188]

Scheme 42

tion is the Grignard reaction of [183] with 3-methyl-3-butenylmagnesium bromide, resulting in [184]. The stereoselectivity in this case was 50:1.

The right-hand fragment [197] (Scheme 44) was constructed from the two fragments [189] and [193]. Synthesis of [189] is summarized in Scheme 42. [The reagents were the following: (a), O_3/acetone/$-78°C$, Jones oxid.; (b), $Pb(OAc)_4$/$Cu(OAc)_2$/C_6H_6/80°C; (c), KOH/aq. MeOH; (d), I_2/MeCN/$-15°C$; (e), $KOCH_2C_6H_5$/THF/$-20°C$; (f), H_2/Pd-C/Et_2O; (g), LAH/Et_2O; (h), acetone/$CuSO_4$/p-TSA; (i), PCC/CH_2Cl_2.] Saponification of [186], followed by iodolactonization, yielded a 20:1 mixture of the lactone [187] and its diastereomer. Inversion at C-17 was then effected by treatment with the potassium salt of benzyl alcohol to produce an intermediate epoxy benzyl ester, which spontaneously cyclized to [188] on hydrogenolysis.

Synthesis of the fragment [193] and the consequent union with [189] are summarized in Scheme 43 and 44, respectively. [The reagents were the following for Scheme 43: (a), lithium enolate of ethyl propionate/THF/$-78°C$; (b), p-TSA/C_6H_6/reflux; (c), H_2/Rh-Al_2O_3/Et_2O/$-10°C$; (d), conc. HI/130°C; (e), $(C_6H_5)_3P$/neat/130°C. The reagents for Scheme 44 were the following: (a), Wittig reaction

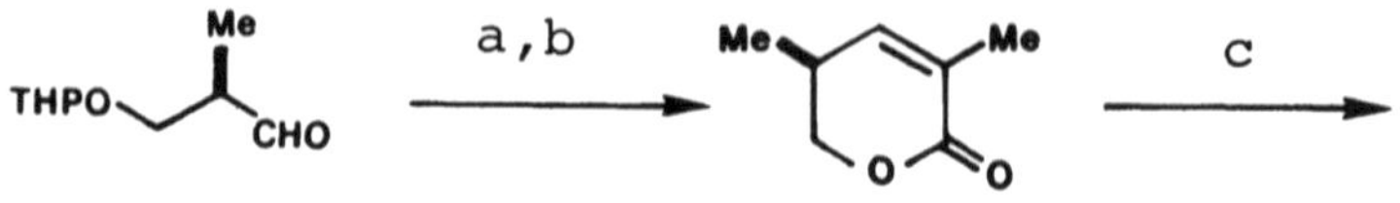

[190]   [191]

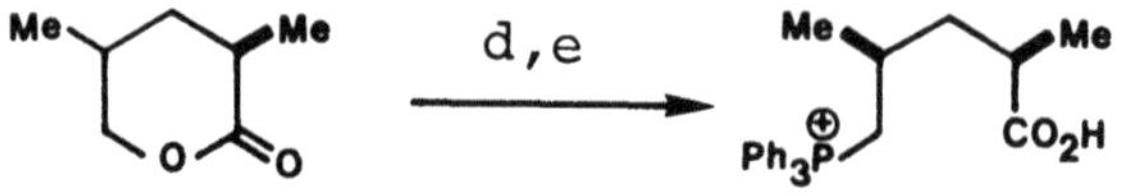

[192]   [193]

Scheme 43

(NaH/DMSO); (b), KIO$_3$/NaHCO$_3$/H$_2$O; (c), AgTFA/CH$_2$Cl$_2$; (d),
Jones oxid.; (e), 2-PyrSH/COCl$_2$/Et$_3$N.] Hydrogenation of [191] with
5% rhodium on alumina gave the valelactone [192] as an 8:1 cis and
trans mixture. Wittig reaction of [189] and [193] yielded the cis olefin [194]. Iodolactonization of [194] gave the lactone [195]. This result was expected from the consideration of the preferred conformation
[194A], of the cis olefin [194].

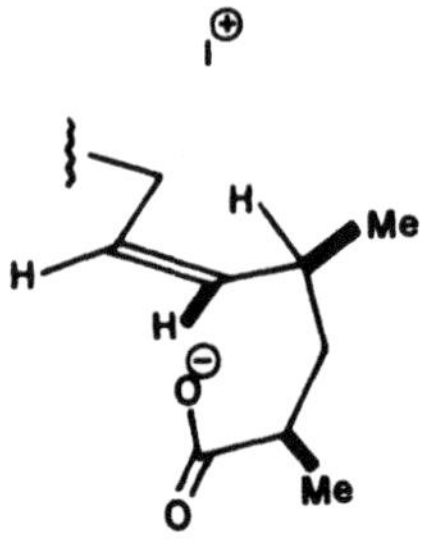

[194A]

Synthesis of the right-hand fragment [203] from [171] and [197] is
summarized in Scheme 45. [The reagents were the following: (a),
Grignard reagent prepared from [171]/CuI Bu$_3$P/THF/−78°C; (b),
EtMgBr/THF/−78°C; (c), NBS/p-TSA/CH$_2$Cl$_2$/0°C; (d), MsCl/Et$_3$N/
CH$_2$Cl$_2$/0°C; (d), NaOAc/60°C; (f), LiCH$_2$OCH$_2$C$_6$H$_5$/THF/−78°C;
(g), HC(OMe)$_3$/p-TSA; (h), Zn(Cu)/NaI/DMF/60°C; (i), Et$_3$SiOClO$_3$/
Py/MeCN; (j), O$_3$/CH$_2$/CH$_2$Cl$_2$/−78°C.] The coupling reaction of [171]
with [197] was well controlled by using cuprous iodide with Grignard
reagent prepared from [171]. The C-16 stereochemistry was again

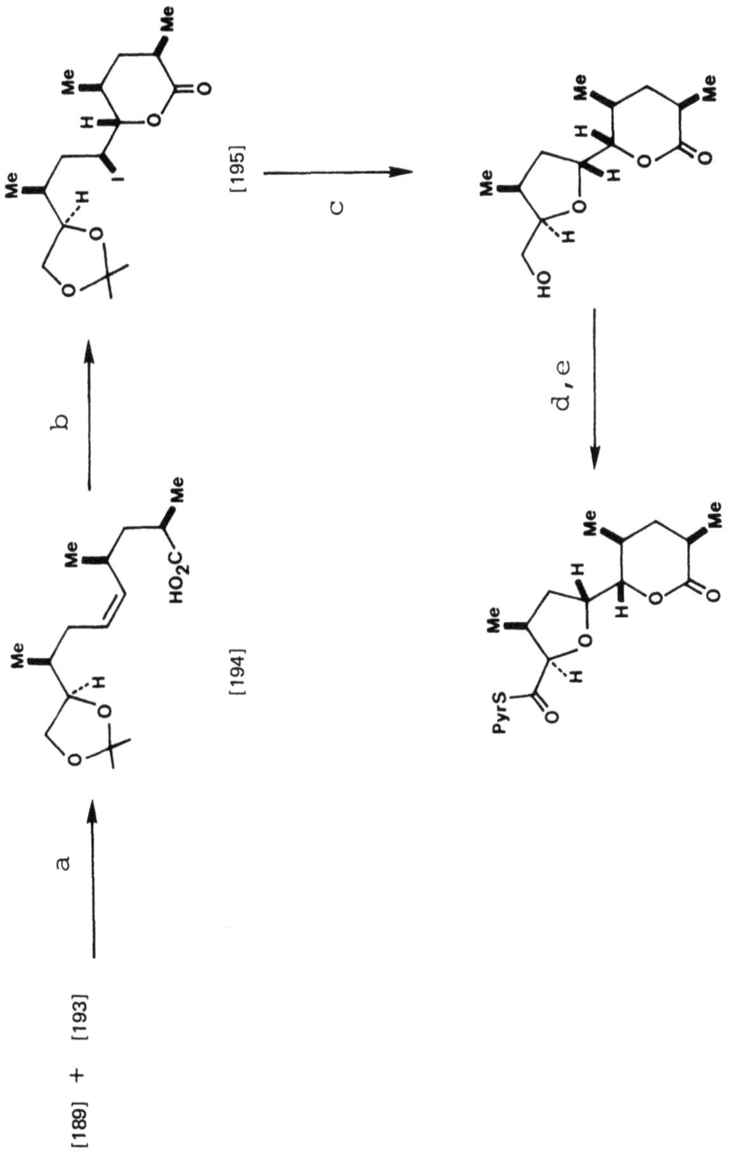

Scheme 44

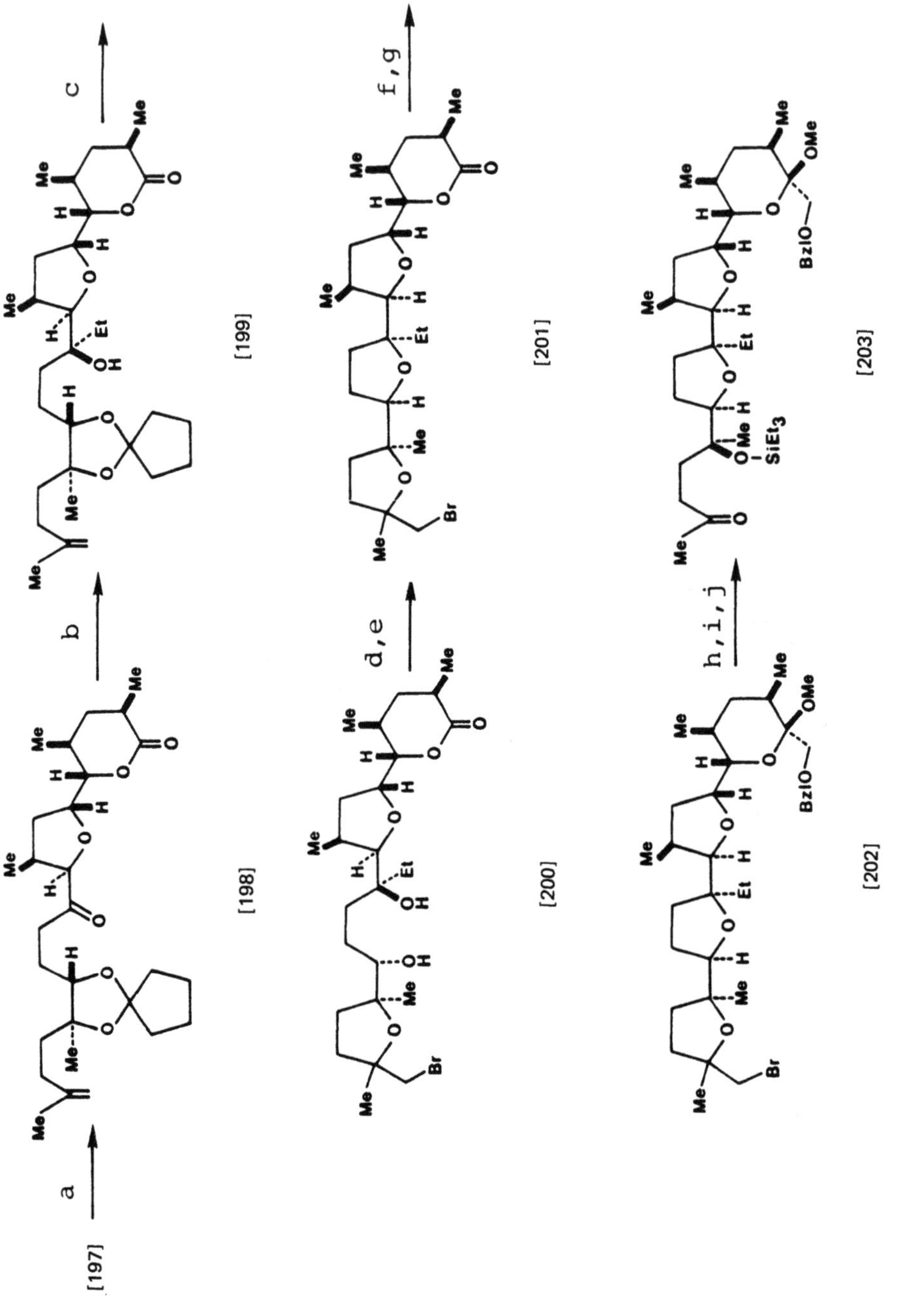

[197]

[198]

[199]

[200]

[201]

[202]

[203]

Scheme 45

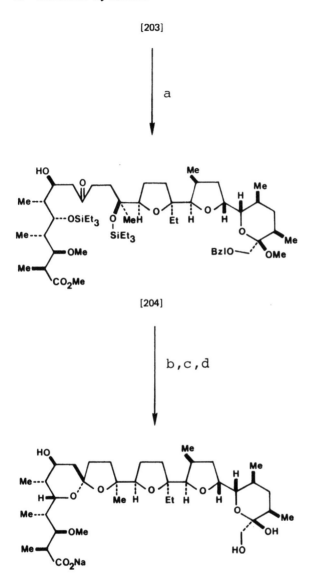

Scheme 46

controlled by the Grignard reaction of [198] with ethylmagnesium bromide. Two tetrahydrofuran rings were constructed by NBS bromination and by cyclization of the mesylate alcohol.

The final coupling and the introduction of the spiroketal (Scheme 46) were the same as the previous synthesis by Kishi. [The reagents were the following: (a), LDA/THF/−78°C, MgBr$_2$, [169]; (b), H$_2$/ Pd-C/Et$_2$O; (c), p-TSA/CH$_2$Cl$_2$/Et$_2$O/H$_2$O; (d), NaOH/aq. MeOH.]

REFERENCES

Baldwin, J. E., Crossley, M. J., Lehtonen, and E. -M. M. (1979). Stereospecificity of oxidative cycloaddition reactions of 1,5-dienes. *J. Chem. Soc. Chem. Commun. 1979*:918.

Collum, D. B., McDonald, J. H., III, and Still, W. C. (1980a). Synthesis of the polyether antibiotic monensin. 1. Strategy and degradations. *J. Am. Chem. Soc. 102*:2117.

Collum, D. B., McDonald, J. H., III, and Still, W. C. (1980b). Synthesis of the polyether antibiotic monensin. 2. Preparation of intermediates. *J. Am. Chem. Soc. 102*:2118.

Collum, D. B., McDonald, J. H. III, and Still, W. C. (1980c). Synthesis of the polyether antibiotic monensin. 3. Coupling of precursors and transformation to monensin. *J. Am. Chem. Soc. 102*:2120.

Crespe, T. M., Probert, C. L., and Sondheimer, F. (1978). An approach to the synthesis of ionophores related to A23187. *Tetrahedron Lett. 1978*:3955.

Descotes, G., and Cottier, L. (1979). Photochemical Synthesis of structural analogs of polyether antibiotics. In *Seventh International Congress of Heterocyclic Chemistry Abstracts*, Tampa, Florida, p. 152 ff.

Evans, D. A., Sacks, C. E., Whitney, R. A., and Mandel, N. G. (1978). Studies directed towards the total synthesis of the ionophone antibiotic A-23187. *Tetrahedron Lett. 1978*:727.

Evans, D. A., Sacks, C. E., Kleschick, W. A., and Taber, T. R. (1979a). Polyether antibiotics synthesis. Total synthesis and absolute configuration of the ionophore A-23187. *J. Am. Chem. Soc. 101*:6789.

Evans, D. A., Vogel, E., and Nelson, J. V. (1979b). Stereoselective aldol condensations via boron enolates. *J. Am. Chem. Soc. 101*:6120.

Fukuyama, T., Vranesic, B., Negri, D. P., and Kishi, Y. (1978). Synthetic studies on polyether antibiotics. II. Stereocontrolled syntheses of epoxides of bishomoallic alcohols. *Tetrahedron Lett. 1978*:2741.

Fukuyama, T., Wang, C.-L, J., and Kishi, Y. (1979a). Total synthesis of monensin. 2. Stereocontrolled synthesis of the right half of monensin. *J. Am. Chem. Soc. 101*:260.

Fukuyama, T., Akasaka, K., Karanewsky, D. S., Wang, C.-L, J., Schmid, G., and Kishi, Y. (1979b). Total synthesis of monensin

3. Stereocontrolled total synthesis of monensin. *J. Am. Chem. Soc. 101*:262.

Grieco, P. A., Williams, E., Tanaka, H., and Gilman, S. (1980). Elaboration of the C(3)-C(12) carbon fragment of calcimycin (A-23187). A formal total synthesis of calcimycin. *J. Org. Chem. 45*:3537.

Hatakeyama, S., Lewis, M. D., and Kishi, Y. (1982). Total synthesis of polyether antiobiotics narasin and salinomycin. In *Frontiers in Chemistry* (28th IUPAC Congress), K. J. Laidler, ed., Pergamon Press, Oxford, p. 287 ff.

Heathcock, C. H., Pirrung, M. C., Buse, C. T., Hagen, J. P., Young, S. D., and Sohn, J. E. (1979). Acyclic stereoselection. 6. A reagent for achieving high 1,2-diastereoselection in the aldol conversion of chiral aldehydes into 3-hydroxy-2-methylcar-boxylic acids. *J. Am. Chem. Soc. 101*:7077, and references cited therein.

House, H. O., Crumrine, D. S., Teranishi, A. Y., and Omstead, H. D. (1973). Chemistry of carbanions. XXIII. Use of metal complexes to control the aldol condensation. *J. Am. Chem. Soc. 95*: 3310.

Ireland, R. E., and Häbach, D. (1980). A convergent scheme for the synthesis of spiroketals and the synthesis of (±)-chalcogran. *Tetrahedron Lett. 1980*:1389.

Ireland, R. E., Thaisrivongs, S., and Wilcox, C. S., (1980). Total synthesis of lasalocid A (X537A). *J. Am. Chem. Soc. 102*:1155.

Kishi, Y. (1980). The total synthesis of monensin. Lect. *Heterocycl. Chem. 5 1980*:5-95.

Masamune, S., Mori, S., Van Horn, D., and Brooks, D. W. (1979). E- and Z-Vinyloxyboranes (alkenyl borinates): Stereoselective formation and aldol condensation. *Tetrahedron Lett. 1979*:1665.

Nakahara, Y., Beppu, K., and Ogawa, T. (1979). Synthesis of physiologically active natural products via carbohydrate synthons. In *22nd Symposium on the Chemistry of Natural Products Abstracts*, Fukoka, Japan, p. 483 ff.

Nakata, T., and Kishi, Y. (1978). Synthetic studies on polyether antibiotics. III. A stereocontrolled synthesis of isolasalocid ketone from acyclic precursors. *Tetrahedron Lett. 1978*:2745.

Nakata, T., Schmid, G., Vranesic, B., Okigawa, M., Smith-Palmer, T., and Kishi, Y. (1978). A total synthesis of lasalocid A. *J. Am. Chem. Soc. 100*:2933.

Petcher, T. J., Weber, H.-P., and Rüegger, A. (1976). Crystal and molecular structure of an iodo-derivative of the cyclic undecapeptide cyclosporin A. *Helv. Chim. Acta 59*:1480.

Schmid, G., Fukuyama, T., Akasaka K., and Kishi, Y. (1979). Total synthesis of monensin. 1. Stereocontrolled synthesis of the left half of monensin. *J. Am. Chem. Soc. 101*:259.

Still, W. C., and McDonald, J. H., III (1980). Chelation-controlled
  nucleophilic additions. 1. A highly effective system for asymmetric induction in the reaction of organometallic with α-alkoxy-
  ketones. *Tetrahedron Lett. 1980*:1031.
Still, W. C., and Schneider, J. A. (1980). Chelation-controlled nucleophilic additions. 2. A highly effective system for asymmetric
  induction in the reaction of organometallic with β-alkoxyalde-
  hydes. *Tetrahedron Lett. 1980*:1035.
Walba, D. M., Wand, M. D., and Wilkes, M. C. (1979). Stereochemistry of the permanganate oxidation of 1,5-dienes. *J. Am. Chem.
  Soc. 101*:4396.

BIBLIOGRAPHY

Since this manuscript was completed a number of important papers
have appeared. Some of these are listed below.

A. Synthetic Methods

1. β-Hydroxy ketone

Crossed aldol reactions currently are a hot research topic. For recent
progress see the following papers and reference papers cited therein.

Heathcock, C. H., Pirrung, M. C., Lampe, J., Buse, C. T., and
  Young, S. D. (1981). Acyclic stereoselection. 12. Double stereodifferentiation with mutual kinetic resolution. A superior class of
  reagents for control of Cram's rule stereoselection in synthesis of
  erythro-α-alkyl-β-hydroxy carboxylic acids from chiral aldehydes.
  J. Org. Chem. 46:2290.
Noyori, R., Nishida, I., and Sakata, J. (1981). Erythro-selective
  aldol reaction via tris(dialkylamino)sulfonium enolates. *J. Am. Chem.
  Soc. 103*:2106.
Masamune, S., Choy, W., Kerdesky, F. A. J., and Imperiali, B.
  (1981). Stereoselective aldol condensation. Use of chiral boron
  enolates. *J. Am. Chem. Soc. 103*:1566.
Evans, D. A., Takacs, J. M., McGee, L. R., Ennis, M. D., Mathre,
  D. J., and Bartroli, J. (1981). Chrial enolate design. *Pure Appl.
  Chem. 53*:1109.

2. *Spiroketal*

Deslongchamps, P., Rowan, D. D., Pothier, N., Sauvé, T., and
  Saunders, J. K. (1981). 1,7-Diosaspiro[5,5]undecanes. An excellent system for the study of stereoelectronic effects (anomeric and
  exo-anomeric effects) in acetals. *Can. J. Chem. 59*:1105.

Hintzer, K., Weber, R., and Schurig, V. (1981). Synthesis of optically active 2S-, and 7S-methyl-1.6-dioxa-spiro[4.5]decane, the pheromone components of *Paravespula vulgaris* (L.), from S-ethyl lactate. *Tetrahedron Lett.* 1981:55.

Phillips, C., Jacobson, R., Abrahams, B., Williams, H., and Smith, L. R. (1980). Useful route to 1,6-dioxaspiro[4.4]nonane and 1,6-dioxaspiro[4.5]decane derivatives. *J. Orig. Chem.* 54:1920.

3. Tetrahydrofurans

Walba, D. M., and Edwards, P. D. (1980). Total synthesis of ionophores. The monensin BC-rings via permanganate promoted stereospecific oxidative cyclization. *Tetrahedron Lett.* 1980:3531.

Wolfe, S., and Ingold, C. F. (1981). Oxidation of olefins by potassium permanganate. ^{18}O-Labeling experiments and mechanism of the oxidation of 1,5-hexadiene. Evidence for a manganese intermediate with coordination number greater than four. *J. Am. Chem. Soc.* 103:940.

Amouroux, R., Folefoc, G., Chastrette, F., and Chastrette, M. (1981). A highly stereoselective route to substituted bis-tetrahydrofurans from 1,5-dienes. *Tetrahedron Lett.* 1981:2259.

B. Total Syntheses

1. A23187 (Calcimycin)

Negri, D. (1980). The total synthesis of polyether antibiotic (−)-A23187. Ph.D. Thesis, Harvard University, Boston, Massachusetts.

Lipshutz, B. H., and Hungate, R. W. (1981). Metalation studies of trisubstituted oxazoles. *J. Org. Chem.* 46:1410.

2. Lasalocid A (X-537A)

Ireland, R. E., McGarvey, G. J., Anderson, R. C., Badoud, R., Fitzsimmons, B., and Thaisrivongs, S. (1980). A chiral synthesis of the left-side aldehyde for lasalocid A synthesis. *J. Am. Chem. Soc.* 102:6178.

3. Narasin

Kishi, Y. (1980). Recent developments in the chemistry of natural products. *Adrichimica Acta* 13:23.

4. Antibiotic X-14547A

Nicolaou, K. C., and Magolda, R. L. (1981). Ionophore antibiotic X-1454A. Degradation studies and stereoselective construction of the "right wing" (C_{11}-C_{25} fragment) by an intramolecular Diels-Alder reaction. *J. Org. Chem.* *46*:1506.

Roush, W. R., and Meyers, A. G. (1981). Antibiotic X-14547A: Total synthesis of the right-hand half. *J. Org. Chem.* *46*:1509.

Edwards, M. P., Ley, S. V., and Lister, S. G. (1981). An intramolecular Diels-Alder approach to the synthesis of the right hand half of the ionophore antibiotic X-14547A. *Tetrahedron Lett.* *1981*:361.

chapter 2

CHEMICAL TRANSFORMATIONS OF POLYETHER ANTIBIOTICS

John W. Westley
Hoffmann-La Roche Inc., Nutley, New Jersey

I. INTRODUCTION

During the period 1967 and 1980 the structures of 60 polyether antibiotics were elucidated by the application of physiochemical techniques, as described in Chapters 3 to 6 of this book. One unfortunate consequence of this modern development has been the almost total abandonment of chemical degradation as a means of structural analysis. Consequently only a quarter of the polyether antiobiotics known in 1980 have been subjected to chemical transformations, and in several of these cases the modifications have been very limited in scope. In this chapter the chemistry of 11 polyether antibiotics will be discussed, and in the cases where data has been published the biological consequences of their chemical transformations will also be presented.

II. LASALOCID

A. Chemical Modifications

The organic chemistry of the lasalocid molecule has been studied in greater detail than any other polyether anbibiotic. The major structural features that influence the chemistry of lasalocid are highlighted in Figure 1. The role that these factors play in the reactions of lasalocid will be revealed in the examples that follow.

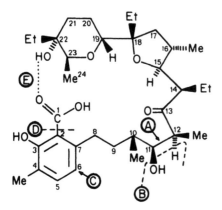

Ⓐ Retroaldol cleavage
Ⓑ Dehydration
Ⓒ Electrophilic substitution
Ⓓ Decarboxylation
Ⓔ Hydrogen bond formation

Figure 1 Structural factors influencing the chemistry of the lasalocid molecule. For a discussion of the numbering system see Chapter 1 of Volume 1.

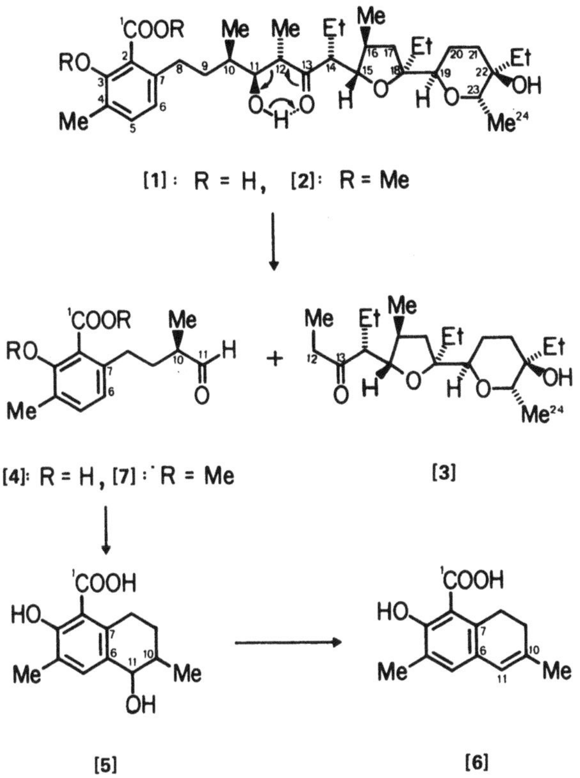

[1]: R = H, [2]: R = Me

[4]: R = H, [7]: R = Me   [3]

[5]   [6]

Scheme 1 Base-catalyzed retroaldol cleavage of lasalocid [1] and the methyl ester methyl ether of the antibiotic [2].

The structure of lasalocid [1] was first published in joint communications by Westley et al. (1970a) and Johnson et al. (1970). In the first of these two papers the presence of a β-ketol system (C-11, C-13) in the molecule was demonstrated (Scheme 1) by the base-catalyzed retrograde-aldol cleavage of lasalocid [1] into 4-[5-ethyl-3-methyl-5-(5-ethyl-5-hydroxy-6-methyl-2-tetrahydropyranyl)-2-tetrahydrofuryl]-3-hexanone [3] and an aldehyde [4] which spontaneously cyclized to 2,5-dihydroxy-3,6-dimethyl-5,67,8-tetrahydro-1-naphtoic acid [5] and a dehydration product of [5], 7,8-dihydro-3,6-dimethyl-2-hydroxy-1-naphthoic acid [6]. Reduction of the ketone moiety in [1] with sodium borohydride gave a compound which was resistent to base attack, confirming the retroaldol mechanism for the cleavage of the β-ketol system present in lasalocid. Methylation of the antibiotic MeI, Ag$_2$O) to the methyl ester methyl ether [2] followed by pyrolysis at 170°C (0.05 mmHg) gave 6-(3-formylbutyl)-2-methoxy-3-methylbenzoic acid, methyl ester

[7], which exhibited a negative Cotton effect. By comparison with S-2-methylbutanal, which has been shown by Djerassi and Geller (1959) to exhibit a positive Cotton effect, [7] must have the R con-figuration.

The second of the two communications (Johnson et al., 1970) sum-marized the x-ray analysis of the barium salt of lasalocid, including the *relative* configuration of the 10 asymmetric centers present in the molecule. In combination with the polarimetric results on [7], the complete structure of lasalocid was defined as 3-methyl-6-(7(R)-ethyl-4(S)-hydroxy-3(R), 5(S)-dimethyl-6-oxo-7-{5(S)-ethyl-3(S)-methyl-5-[5(R)-ethyl-5-hydroxy-6(S)-methyl-2(R)-tetrahydropyranyl]-2(S)-tetrahydrofuryl}-heptyl)salicylic acid.

Subsequent to the work on the structure of the antibiotic, two addi-tional products from the base treatment were isolated and identified as cis- and trans-anhydrolasalocid ([8] and [9], respectively).

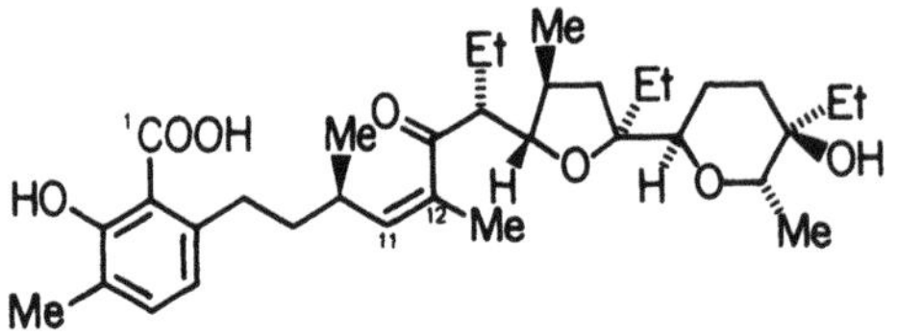

[8]

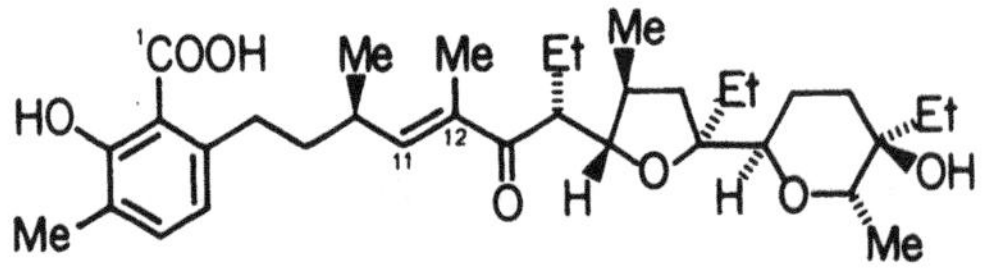

[9]

These compounds arise from dehydration of the β-ketol system (Westley et al., 1973a). Compound [9] was epoxidized to [10] by treatment with 30% H_2O_2 in aqueous methanolic NaOH.

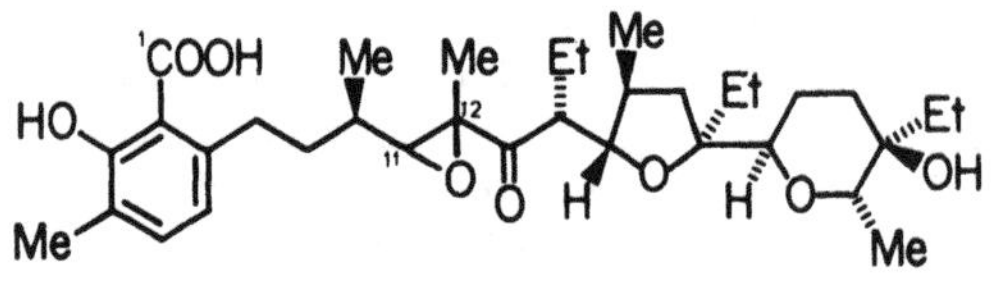

[10]

The base-catalyzed retroaldol cleavage reaction proved useful in biosynthetic studies on [1] (Westley et al., 1970b), but the competing dehydration reaction to the two anhydro-lasalocids [8] and [9] re-

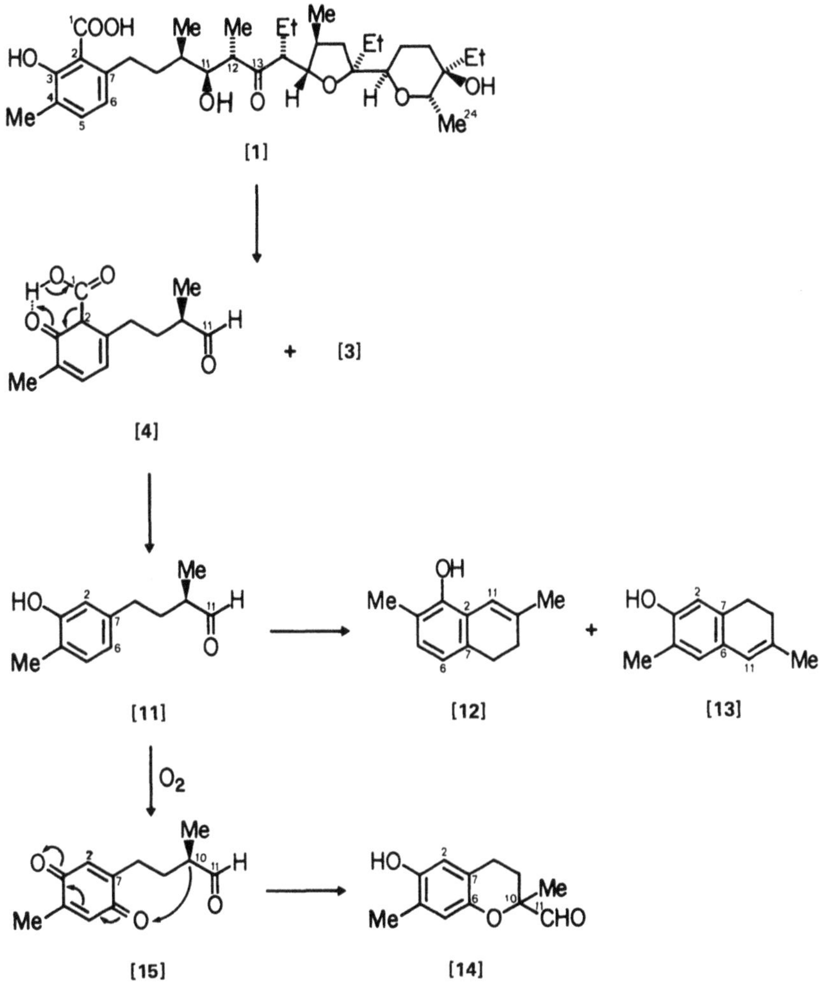

Scheme 2 Pyrolysis of lasalocid.

duced the overall yield of the ketone [3] to approximately 70%. Pyrolysis of lasalocid at 200°C under reduced pressure (0.05 mmHg), however, gave a quantitative yield of [3], indicating that under pyrolytic
conditions [1] is degraded *solely* via the retroaldol *cleavage* route
(Westley et al., 1973b). The other product from the cleavage reaction,
the aldehyde [4], decarboxylates on thermolysis to an intermediate
phenol [11] (Scheme 2) which spontaneously cyclizes with dehydration
to 5,6-dihydro-2,7-dimethyl-1-naphtol [12] and 7,8-dihydro-3,6-di-

methyl-2-napthol [13]. When the antibiotic was heated at 220°C for
1 h in an *open* tube, 3,4-dihydro-2,7-dimethyl-6-hydroxy-2H-1-benzo-
pyran-2-carboxaldehyde [14] was also produced, suggesting that in
the presence of air partial oxidation of the phenol [11] to a quinone
[15] occurred prior to cyclization (Scheme 2).

The quantitative nature of the thermolysis of lasalocid [1] to the
retroaldol ketone [3] led to a gas-liquid chromatographic technique for
determining the level of lasalocid in fermentation broths and the purity
of crystalline samples of the antibiotic (Westley et al., 1974a). This
analytical technique was later developed into an assay for lasalocids A,
B, C, D, and E (Westley et al., 1974b).

The spontaneous cyclizations of the base retroaldol aldehyde [4] to
the tetrahydronaphthoic acid [5] (Scheme 1) and of the pyrolysis
phenol [11] to the two dihydronaphthols [12] and [13] (Scheme 2)
demonstrate the ease of electrophilic substitution of the lasalocid chromophore. Further examples occurred on halogenation of lasalocid to
bromolasalocid [16], chlorolasalocid [17], and iodolasalocid [18]. When
bromination was carried out with N-bromosuccinimide in acetone,
rather than with bromine in methylene chloride, the product was di-
bromodecarboxylasalocid [19], which on hydrogenolysis yielded [20]
the decarboxylated form of lasalocid (Westley et al., 1973a).

[16]: R = Br, [17]: R = Cl, [18]: R = I

[19]: R = Br, [20]: R = H

Pyrolysis of [16] gave a quantitative yield of the retroaldol ketone
[3] together with 3,6-dimethyl-2-naphtol [21] and 4-bromo-5,6-dihy-
dro-2,7-dimethyl-1-naphtol [22]. The conversion of bromolasalocid
into the naphthol [21], in contrast to the 7,8-dihydronaphthol [13]
produced on pyrolysis of the parent antibiotic (Scheme 2), was the result of an additional elimination step (loss of HBr) in the case of the
bromo derivative. In an analagous reaction base-catalyzed retroaldol
cleavage of bromolasalocid gave 3,6-dimethyl-2-hydroxy-1-naphthoic
acid [23].

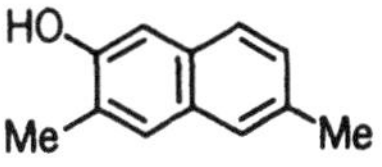

[21] 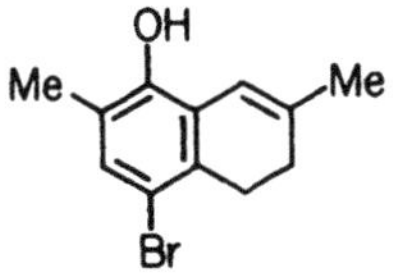 [22] 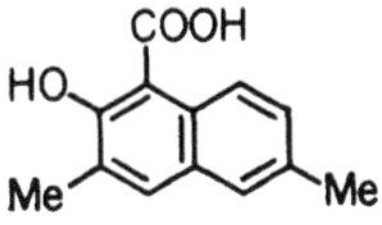 [23]

The retroaldol ketone [3] has been further degraded in connection with our biosynthetic studies (Westley et al., 1970b). In an attempt to isolate the C-methyl group in the terminal tetrahydropyranyl ring, [3] was subjected to Jones oxidation. In addition to the desired aceto-xyketone [25], another ketone [24] was isolated (Scheme 3). Hydrolysis of [25] in base gave the hydroxy ketone [27] and acetic acid. Using ^{14}C-labeled substrates, it was from this set of reactions that we were able to establish that the terminal C-methyl group is biosynthetically derived from acetate, in contrast to the other four C-methyls in lasalocid, which are all propionate derived.

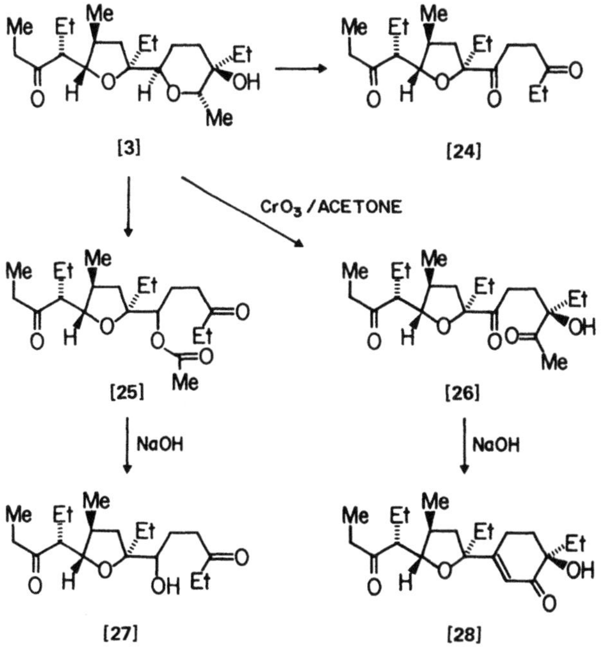

[3] [24]

CrO₃ /ACETONE

[25] [26]

NaOH NaOH

[27] [28]

Scheme 3 Oxidation and hydrolysis of lasalocid retroaldol ketone.

When the base-hydrolysis reaction was carried out on the crude oxidation product from [3], the hydroxy cyclohexenone [28] was also isolated, implying the presence of the hydroxy triketone [26] in the oxidation mixture from [3].

Mass spectrometry was essential in determining the structures of [24], [25], [27], and [28], which, like ketone [3], all had base peaks at m/z 211 due to fragment [29]. This result indicated that Jones oxidation only affected the terminal tetrahydropyranyl ring of the retroaldol ketone [3] (Westley et al., 1973b).

[29]

As part of the investigation into the interaction of electrophilic reagents with lasalocid, the nitration of the antibiotic in glacial acetic acid was attempted (Westley et al., 1971). Treatment with 5 MEq of concentrated nitric acid gave the expected nitrolasalocid [30] (Scheme 4). The major product, however, was shown by base degradation to be dinitrophenol [31], consistent with the observation that nitration of highly substituted benzene derivatives often results in the displacement of substituents meta to the entering group by additional nitro groups.

To confirm the structure of [31], the derivative was treated under basic conditions known to cause cleavage of the antibiotic (Scheme 4). One product was the retroaldol ketone [3] and a second was confirmed by synthesis to be 6-hydroxy-2,7-dimethyl-5-nitroquinoline [33]. A third compound isolated in very low yield was 5-hydroxy-6-methyl-4-nitroindole [34]. The two latter compounds must have arisen from cyclization of the intermediate aldehyde [32]. All of these products were consistent with the proposed dinitrophenol structure [31], as well as with that of a fourth base-degradation product, the α,β-unsaturated ketone [35], which arises from dehydration of the β-ketol system present in [31]. The analogous α,β-unsaturated ketone [36] was isolated from base treatment of nitrolasalocid [30].

The base-catalyzed cyclization of [32] to [33] is a novel type of quinoline synthesis, but the aromatic substituents necessary to cause an ortho-nitrophenylbutyraldehyde to undergo such a reaction were not determined.

Catalytic hydrogenation of nitrolasalocid [30] with Raney nickel yielded aminolasalocid [37], which was acetylated by acetic anhydride in glacial acetic acid to yield the N-acetyl derivative [38]. The IR spectrum exhibited two equal peaks in the N-acetyl region at 1640 and 1660 cm^{-1}, and the NMR spectrum also suggested a mixture of two types of aromatic protons at δ(CDCl$_3$) 7.10 and 6.85 and three methyl peaks at δ 1.86 (S,1,5, CH$_3$CONH), 2.08 (s,1.5, CH$_3$CONH), and 2.17

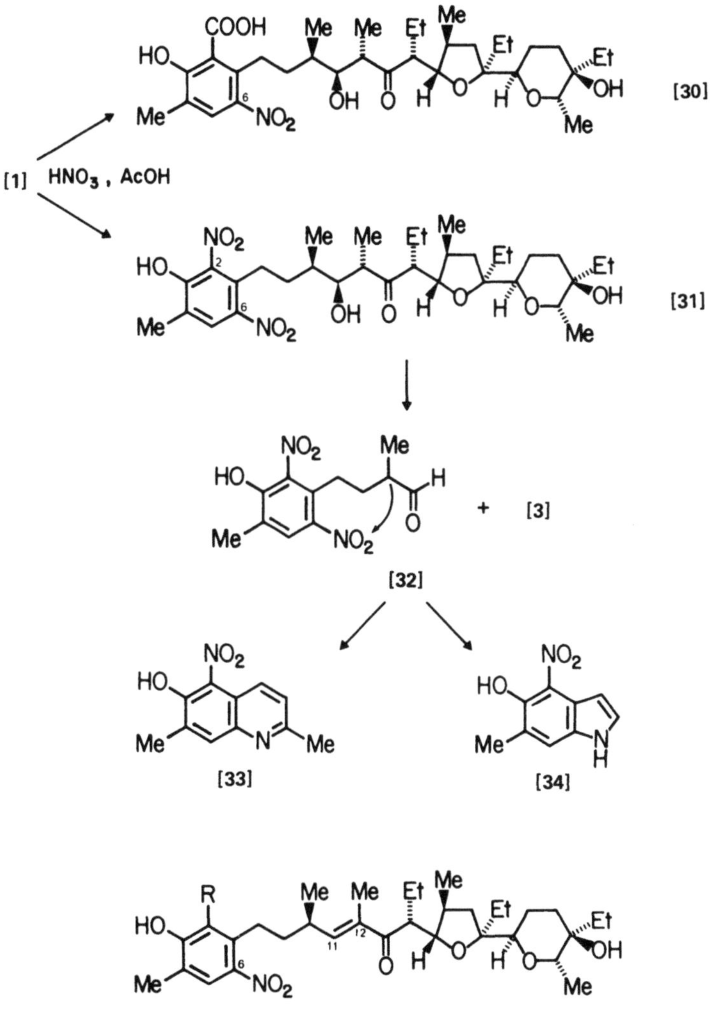

Scheme 4 Nitration of lasolocid.

(S,3,aromatic CH$_3$). These results suggest that N-acetylaminolasalocid exists as an equal mixture of endo-[38a] and exo-[38b] conformers. A similar case has been reported by Garin and Fusman (1964) and probably arises from the restricted rotation about the amide bond.

Refluxing amino lasalocid [37] with benzaldehyde in toluene for 1 h yielded the crystalline benzylideneamino derivative of lasalocid [39].

[37] R = NH$_2$ [38a] R = NH   [38b] R = NH

[39] R = N=CH—⟨benzene⟩

Following the series of reactions involving lasalocid with a variety of electrophilic reagents, a number of the oxygen functions present in the the molecule were modified in order to test the x-ray structure of the barium salt (Figure 2) as a model for the biological action of the antibiotic. Methylation of the antibiotic with methyl iodide in the presence of silver oxide in dimethylformamide (DMF) yielded the methyl ester methyl ether [2] used in the establishment of the absolute configuration of lasalocid as mentioned earlier. When methylene chloride was used as a solvent for this reaction, the simple methyl ester of lasalocid [40] was formed.

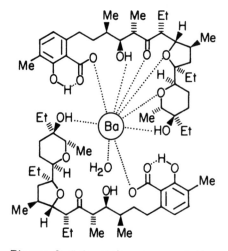

Figure 2 Schematic representation of the barium salt comples of lasalocid exhibiting the oxygen atoms involved in ligand formation with the barium cation.

An alternate route to the ester [40] was the use of ethereal diazomethane; but under these conditions an isomeric methyl ester methyl ether [41] was also formed which was distinct from the earlier dimethoxy derivative [2] formed from MeI/Ag_2O in DMF. Structure [41] was assigned by NMR, which indicated two methoxyl groups in the molecule. Retroaldol cleavage of [41] gave a derivative of ketone [3] in which the teritary alcohol was shown by NMR and mass spectrometry to be methylated. Diazomethane treatment of the methyl ester [40] or the retroaldol ketone [3], however, failed to cause methylation of the tertiary alcohol. These results suggest a mechanism in which, at least partially, the intermediate cation $[CH_3N]^+$ is complexed (Smith, 1966) and reacts with the tertiary alcohol prior to methylation of the carboxyl group of lasalocid by a second diazomethane molecule to form [41]. Methylation of the tertiary alcohol in lasalocid, which usually requires acidic catalysts such as boron trifluoride etherate (Muller and Rundell, 1958) or fluoroboric acid (Caserio et al. 1958), supports the hypothesis that intramolecular catalysis is involved in the hydrogen-bound carboxyl and hydroxyl groups, as illustrated in Figure 1 (E).

[40] R_1 = Me R_2 = R_3 = H

[41] R_1 = R_3 = Me R_2 = H

[42] R_1 = R_3 = H R_2 = Me

[43] R_1 = CH_2—⟨⟩ R_2 = R_3 = H

[44] R_1 = R_3 = CH_2—⟨⟩

The phenolic methyl ether [42] of lasalocid was prepared from a mixture of the benzyl ester [43] and the benzyl ester benzyl ether [44], which were synthesized in turn by treatment of the antibiotic with phenyldiazomethane (Sarin and Fusman, 1964). This mixture was reacted with MeI/Ag_2O in DMF followed by hydrogenation in ethanol with 10% Pd on charcoal to yield [42].

A number of synthesized phenolic esters of lasalocid include the acetate, propionate, butyrate, pentanoate, hexanoate, heptanoate, octanoate, decanoate, and p-bromobenzoate (structures [45] to [53], respectively). Esterification was achieved by treating a solution of the sodium salt of lasalocid in pyridine with the appropriate acid anhydride or acid chloride. Acylation of lasalocid with trifluoroacetic anhydride in pyridine gave a bis(trifluoroacetyl) derivative [54] in which the secondary

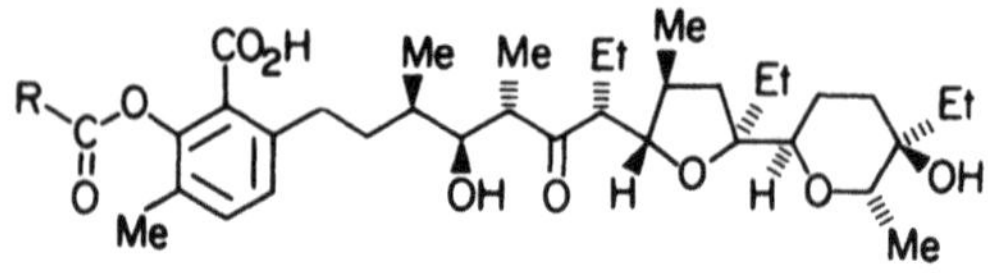

[45] R = Me

[46] R = Et

[47] R = C₃H₇

[48] R = C₄H₉

[49] R = C₅H₁₁

[50] R = C₆H₁₃

[51] R = C₇H₁₅

[52] R = C₉H₁₇

[53] R = BrC₆H₄

alcohol, as well as the phenolic group, was esterified. A desoxy derivative of lasalocid in which the secondary alcohol was missing [55] was
prepared by hydrogenation of the trans-anhydro-lasalocid [9] in ethanol, using 10% Pd on charcoal.

The other modifications of lasalocid reported in the nonpatent literature involve the ketone function. As mentioned in the paper describing the structure of the antibiotic (Westley et al., 1970a), treatment of
lasalocid with sodium borohydride in ethanol yielded a dihydro derivative [56] which, unlike the parent antibiotic, was stable to base, confirming the reduction of the carbonyl group. Refluxing lasalocid in
ethanol for 60 hr with hydroxylamine yielded isomeric oximes of the
antibiotic [57] and [58] which were separable by fractional crystallization.

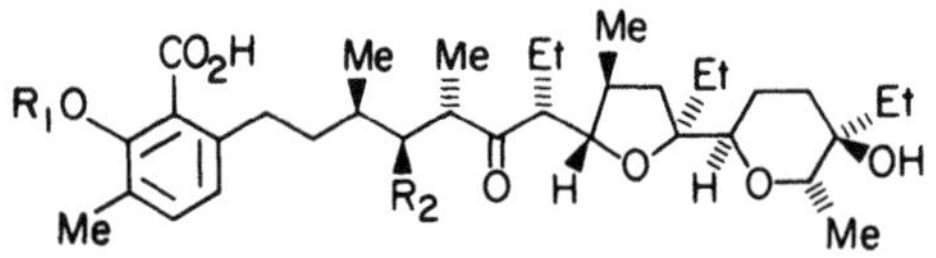

[54] R₁ = CF₃CO, R₂ = CF₃CO.O

[55] R₁ = R₂ = H

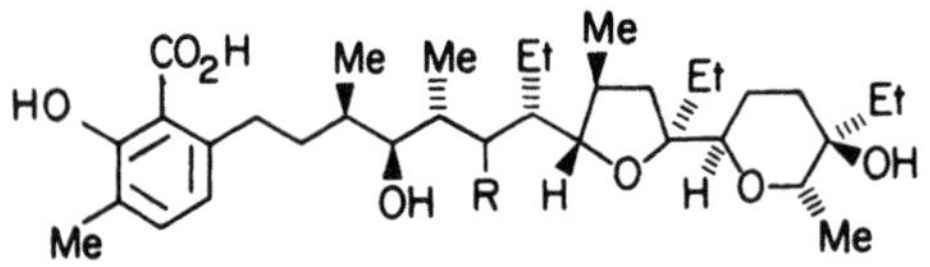

[56] R = OH

[57] R = HO-N⫽

[58] R = HO-N⫽

[59] $R_1 = CO_2^-$, $R_2 = N_2^+$

[60] $R_1 = CO_2H$, $R_2 = -N=N-$

In addition to the 60 derivatives discussed so far from the scientific literature, in particular from Westley, et al. (1973a), other derivatives have appeared in the patent literature (Stempel and Westley, 1974, 1976). In particular, two additional aromatic derivatives, diazolasalocid [59] and phenylazolasalocid [60], have also been described.

B. Biological Activity

Under normal conditions both procaryotic and eucaryotic cells extrude Ca^{2+} and Na^+ cations while accumulating Mg^{2+} and K^+ cations. The cells achieve this by the utilization of specific transport proteins embedded in the cytoplasmic membrane of the cell. The ionophore antibiotics owe their biological activity to their ability to interfere with this natural transport system.

According to the most popular model (Bakker, 1979, and references therein), the transport proteins form a fluid mosaic structure with the lipids of the cytoplasmic membrane in the form of a bimolecular layer. The polar heads of the lipids face the two aqueous solutions and their lipophilic tails form the inner core of the membrane. The transport of cations across this hydrophobic core requires extremely high activation energies, but the ionophores possess the ability to lower this energy barrier and consequently abolish the gradients of Ca^{2+}, Mg^{2+}, K^+, and Na^+ cations and protons across the membrane.

Both gram-positive bacteria and animal cells are sensitive to this effect resulting from the presence of ionophores, but the cell walls of gram-negative bacteria do not allow the permeation of hydrophobic molecules with molecular weights of 600 and above (Nikaido, 1976). Similarly, the pore size of the polysaccharide layer surrounding the cytoplasmic membrane of fungi determines whether or not a particular species of fungi is sensitive to ionophores.

The distinguishing characteristic of the polyether antibiotics compared to other ionophores is the presence of a carboxylic acid moiety. By virtue of this functional group they are able to replace the water mantle which normally surrounds alkaline or alkaline earth cations and then transport them as neutral hydrophobic complexes across the membrane. The structures of these neutral complexes have been studied extensively in the crystalline state by x-ray analysis (see Chapter 3).

By adopting a conformation in which all the oxygens of the molecule are concentrated at the center around the cation and all the lipophilic branched alkyl groups are spread over the outer surface of the complex, the polyether antibiotics catalyze an electroneutral cation-proton exchange across the membrane, moving as undissociated acids in one direction and neutral complexes in the other.

In the case of lasalocid this type of complexation is illustrated in a schematic manner for the barium salt in Figure 2. From this illustration it would appear that all the oxygens, with the possible exception of the phenolic hydroxyl group, are necessary for complexation of the barium cation. In an attempt to determine more precisely whether this represents the sole criterion for the biological activity of the lasalocid molecule, all the degradation and transformation products of lasalocid described in the preceding section have been tested in vitro for antibacterial activity against *Bacillus* E (ATCC 27859) and in most cases against *Bacillus* TA (ATCC 27860) also. Of these derivatives 20 retained significant in vitro activity (Table 1). Table 1 lists their pKa' values in 60% aqueous methanol and their partition coefficients in 1-octanol:water in the cases where these physical constants were determined. From Table 1, the most interesting compounds in terms of in vitro antibacterial activity are the aromatic derivatives substituted para to the phenolic group of lasalocid ([16] to [39]), [59], and [60] and the phenolic ether and ester derivatives ([42] to [53]).

As expected, the nature of the para substituent has a profound effect on the pKa' of the salicylic acid moiety in lasalocid. Nitration to [30] causes a drop in pKa' from 4.4 to 2.4, whereas aminolasalocid [37] and the diazo derivative [59] have pKa' values of 6.0 and 6.6, respectively. The relative in vitro activities of these three derivatives ranged from 2 to 15% of lasalocid activity versus *Bacillus* E and from 1 to 24% versus *Bacillus* TA, indicating that any deviation in the acidity of the carboxyl group in lasalocid has a detrimental effect on the antibacterial activity of the antibiotic.

When lasalocid is partitioned between n-octanol and water, the fraction of antibiotic in the lipidlike organic phase is more than 700 times the amount found in the aqueous phase. This kind of partition is entirely consistent with the mechanism of action discussed earlier in this section. Halogenation of lasalocid to bromolasalocid, chlorolasalocid, and iodolasalocid ([16] to [18], respectively) approximately doubles this partition coefficient, whereas conversion to nitrolasalocid [30] more than halves the value, and reduction of [30] gave a compound (aminolasalocid [37]) with a partition coefficient of only 1.9. In terms of in vitro antimicrobial activity the three halogenated derivatives are considerably more active than the nitrogen-containing derivatives [30] and [37] to [39], suggesting at least a qualitative correlation between activity and the partition coefficient for the derivatives of lasalocid substituted para to the phenolic hydroxyl.

Table 1 Comparison of the Apparent pKa', Partition Coefficient, and Relative in Vitro Activity of Lasalocid and 20 Derivatives

Compound	pKa' in 60% aqueous methanol[a]	Partition coefficient[b]	Relative in vitro activity[c] versus		Compound number
			Bacillus E (ATCC 27859)	Bacillus TA (ATCC 27860)	
Lasalocid	4.4	705	100	100	[1]
Bromolasalocid	3.9	1775	67	124	[16]
Chlorolasalocid	4.0	1330	73	140	[17]
Iodolasalocid	3.9	1556	55	112	[18]
Nitrolasalocid	2.4	291	16	24	[30]
Aminolasalocid	6.0	1.9	2	1	[37]
N-Acetylaminolasalocid	4.3	11	2	1	[38]
Benzylideneaminolasalocid		7.3	2	1	[39]
Lasalocid methyl ether		349	2	1	[42]
Lasalocid acetate	4.15	9	2	1	[45]
Lasalocid propionate			2	1	[46]
Lasalocid butyrate			4	1	[47]
Lasalocid penatoate		120	9	1	[48]
Lasalocid hexanote			23		[49]
Lasalocid heptanoate			19		[50]
Lasalocid octanoate		163	14	35	[51]
Lasalocid decanoate		557	4	16	[52]
Lasalocid bromobenzoate		3031	10	28	[53]
Lasalocid oxime			10		[57]
Diazolasalocid	6.6		12		[59]
Phenylazolasalocid			17	45	[60]

[a]Calculated from UV spectral data at various pH values (Albert and Serjeant, 1962).
[b]Concentration in 1-octanol:concentration in water.
[c]Cup plate (12-min) agar diffusion assay.

For the phenolic ether and esters of lasalocid, however, there appears to be no correlation between in vitro activity and the partition coefficient. The least active of these derivatives are the methyl ether [42], the acetate [45], and the propionate [46]. One possible explanation for this diminished activity is that the longer-chain esters are more susceptible to esterases and lipases and that their relatively higher activities are simply a measure of the more rapid hydrolytic release of lasalocid than from, for instance, the hexanoate [49], heptanoate [50], octanoate [51], and decanoate [52].

In conclusion, with the possible exception of the phenolic hydroxyl group, any modification of the oxygen functionalities of lasaslocid results in the loss of virtually all in vitro antibacterial activity. Similarly, any fragmentation of the molecule is equally effective in destroying activity. The only compounds in which the activity is retained and in some cases enhanced are the halogenated derivatives. For the latter three derivatives their higher activity may be linked to enhanced lipophilicity.

III. MONENSIN AND DIANEMYCIN

The structure of monensin was shown by x-ray crystallographic analysis of the silver salt to be [61] (Scheme 5) (Agtarap et al., 1967).

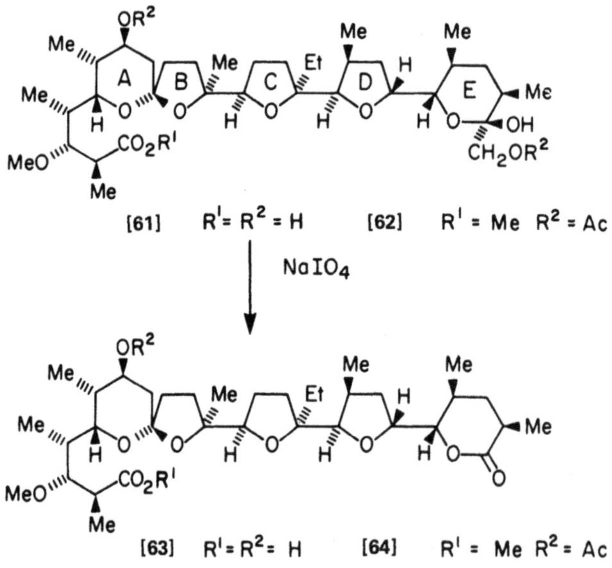

Scheme 5 Acetylation, methylation, and periodate oxidation of monensin.

Acetylation of [61] with acetic anhydride-pyridine followed by treatment with diazomethane (Scheme 5) gave the crystalline methyl ester diacetate [62]. Treatment of monensin with 1 mol of periodate yielded formaldehyde and dehydroxymethylmonensin [63], which upon acetylation and treatment with diazomethane yielded a crystalline monoacetyl methyl ester [64]. These results were consistent with the presence of vicinal primary and tertiary hydroxyl groups (ring E) and an isolated secondary hydroxyl group (ring A) in monesin [61].

Monensin is stable in basic solution but is quite sensitive to acid. This acid instability is due primarily to the presence of a spiroketal group (rings A and B), according to Agtarap and Chamberlin (1968). They found that treatment of the antibiotic with aqueous acid in dioxane yielded an amorphous compound which absorbed in the ultraviolet at 281 μm. By analogy with the antibiotic tylosin (Morin and Gorman, 1964), this UV absorption was interpreted as indicating the presence of an $\alpha,\beta,\gamma,\delta$-unsaturated ketone substituted by a methyl group in the γ position, as illustrated in structure [65].

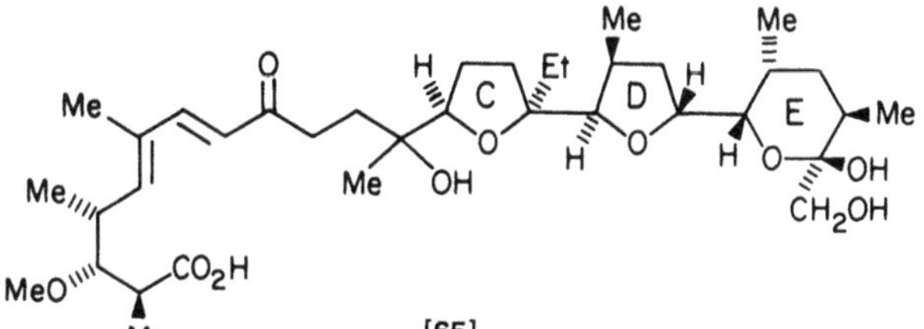

[65]

Oxidation of [65] with a mixture of periodate and permanganate (Edward et al., 1961) yielded an aldehydo-acid, which was esterified to [66] with diazomethane, and a dilactone [67].

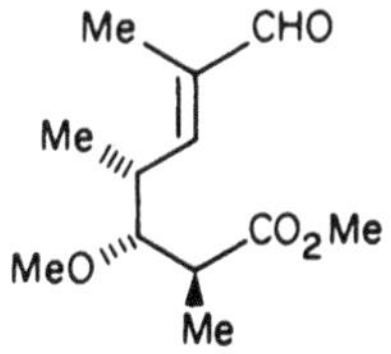

[66] 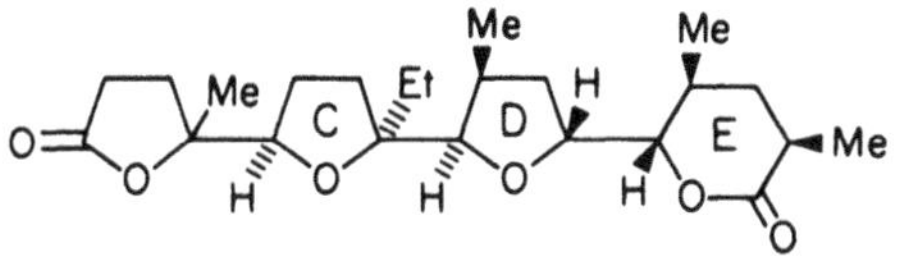   [67]

Oxidation of the diacetate methyl ester of monensin [62] with chromic acid in aqueous acetic acid at room temperature gave a mixture of neutral and acidic fragments. The acidic fraction was treated with diazomethane, and the resulting mixture of methyl esters resolved by column chromatography to yield [68] to [71]. Under the same conditions monensin was found to yield the dilactone [67] and the monolactone [71].

Me,,,,—CO$_2$Me
MeO''''—*CO$_2$Me
Me

[68]

Me,—CO$_2$Me
Me,,,,
MeO''''—*CO$_2$Me
Me

[69]

Me,—CO$_2$Me
Me,,,,
O—C—Me
MeO''''—*CO$_2$Me
Me

[70]

Me,—CO$_2$Me
Me,,,,
MeO''''
Me

[71]

By degrading the *trideutero*methyl ester of diacetylmonensin with the same procedure, the carboxyl carbon of monensin (marked with an asterisk in [68] to [70]) was shown to be present in at least three degradation products from the chromic acid oxidation. The structures of the degradation products suggest that they are derived by the oxidation of intermediates such as the dienone [65].

The presence of a 1,2-glycol in dianemycin was demonstrated by an analogous periodate oxidation to that illustrated for monensin in Scheme 5 (Hamill et al, 1969), with the production of formaldenhyde and a δ-lactone.

VI. NIGERICIN AND X-206

Together with lasalocid, nigericin and antibiotic X-206 were the first polyether antibiotics to be reported in the literature (Berger et al., 1951). However, 17 years elapsed before the structure of nigericin [72] (Scheme 6) was published independently by Steinrauf et al. (1968) and as polyetherin A, by Kubota et al. (1968). In the second of these papers the periodate oxidation of nigericin to a δ-lactone and formaldehyde was reported in reaction analogous to that discussed for monensin and dianemycin in the previous section. Chromic acid oxidation of the δ-lactone afforded [73] to [75], all shown to contain the A ring of nigericin, as illustrated in Scheme 6.

The structure of antibiotic X-206 [76] was not finally deduced until 1975 (Blount and Westley, 1965). Jones oxidation of antibiotic X-206 yielded a dicarboxylic acid [77] derived from the A' ring of the antibiotic, which was an isomer (at C-3) of the dicarboxylic acid [73] obtained from the A ring of nigericin. In addition to [77], oxidation of antibiotic X-206 produced a compound [78] containing three carbonly

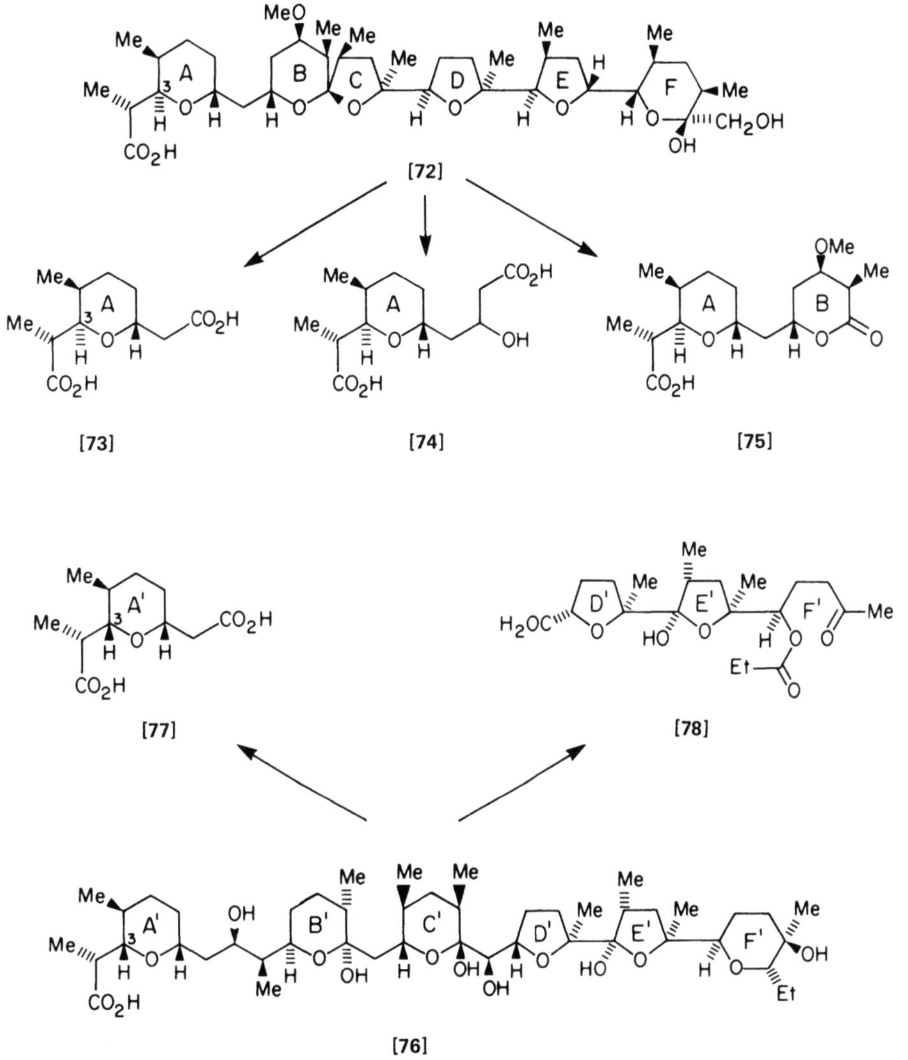

Scheme 6 Chromic acid oxidation of nigericin and X-206.

functionalities (a carboxylic acid, a methyl ketone, and a propionate ester) which were derived from rings D', E', and F' of antibiotic X-206 (Scheme 6).

V. ANTIBIOTIC A204

A. Chemical Modifications

In an excellent review by Hamill and Crandall (1978), the chemistry, biology, and a detailed description of the isolation procedures for six of the most important polyether antibiotics were reported. One of the antibiotics reviewed was A204A, whose structure had been determined earlier as [79] by Jones et al. (1973).

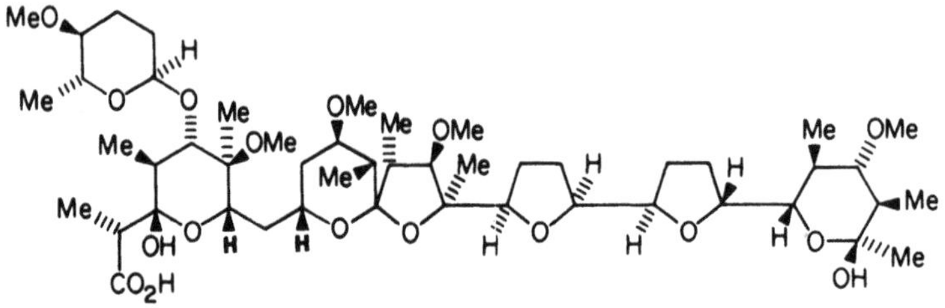

[79]

Like monensin and lasalocid A, antibiotic A204A is the major component of an antibiotic complex which also includes A204B and A204C. In the patent literature (Hamill, 1975, 1976, Chamberlin, 1976) A204A is referred to as A204I.

The A204 complex is isolated by first extracting the filter cake from the fermentation with aqueous methanol, followed by evaporation for methanol removal and extraction of the resulting aqueous slurry with ethyl acetate. This process yields a crude mixture of the sodium and potassium salts of the complex. If, however, the aqueous slurry is acidified to pH 3 prior to ethyl acetate extraction in an attempt to isolate the free acid of the A204 complex, considerable degradation occurs and subsequent crystallization from methanol results in the formation of the methyl ether [80].

The facile formation of [80] led to the synthesis of a number of related alkyl ethers and thioethers such as the ethyl, n-propyl, iso-

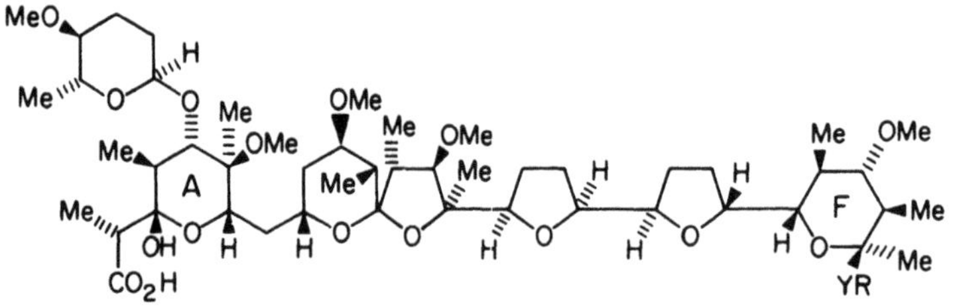

[80] Y = O , R = Me   [83] Y = O , R = iso-C_3H_7
[81] Y = O , R = Et   [84] Y = O , R = n-C_4H_9
[82] Y = O , R = n-C_3H_7 [85] Y = S , R = Me

propyl, and n-butyl ethers and the methyl thioether [81] to [85],
respectively).

Although in the patent literature cited earlier in this section the
alkyl group (R) is attached incorrectly to the hemiketal in ring A of
A204A, subsequent studies (R. L. Hamill, personal communication,
1979) show that the hemiketal in *ring F* is the site of alkylation as
illustrated in formulas [80] to [85]. The derivatives are prepared
from the antibiotic with the corresponding alcohol or thiol, with the
assistance of an acid catalyst at room temperature.

Treatment of antibiotic A204A with sodium borohydride in aqueous
dioxane produces a dihydro derivative whose structure has not been
rigorously established. Chamberlin (1976) suggests that dihydro-
A204A is most likely formed by opening the A ring of [79] to give the
triol corresponding to structure [86].

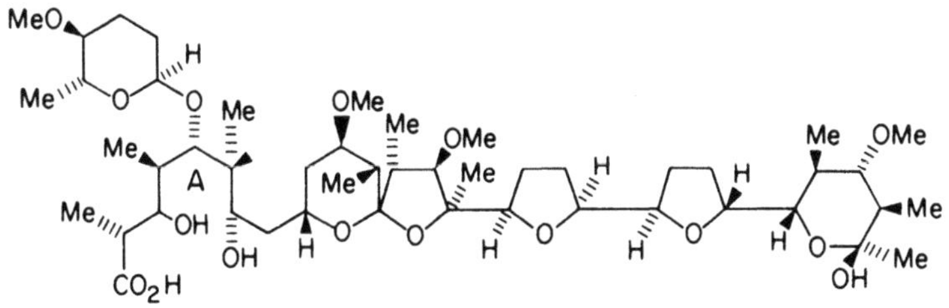

[86]

B. Biological Activity

The biological activity of the monoether and dihydro derivatives of
A204A have been described in the patent literature (Hamill, 1975;
Chamberlin, 1976). Both the methyl and ethyl ethers [80] and [81]

Table 2 Comparison of the Acute Toxicities Orally in Mice of A204A
and derivatives

Compound	LD_{50}(mg/kg) ranges	Compound number
Antibiotic A204A	8.3 - 12.3	[79]
A204A methyl ether	35 - 80	[80]
A204A ethyl ether	35 - 195	[81]
A204A n-propyl ether	32 - 44	[82]
A204A iso-propyl ether	20 - 36	[83]
Dihydro-A204	28	[86]

Table 3 Efficacy of A204A Derivatives Against *E. tenella* in Brolier Cockerels

Compound	Percentage in diet	Percentage mortality	Percentage weight gain	Percentage reduction in lesion score	Compound number
A204A methyl ether	0.005	0	98	98	[80]
A204A ethyl ether	0.005	5	95	95	[81]
A204A n-propyl ether	0.005	0	96	100	[82]
	0.0025	0	87	50	
A204A iso-propyl ether	0.0025	0	95	< 40	[83]
Infected controls	0	45	83	0	
Dihydro-A204A	0.0044	0	92	60	[86]
Infected controls	0	26	42	0	

inhibit the growth of *Bacillus subtilis* and *Mycobacterium avium* at levels as low as 1.25 µg/ml, and anaerobic bacteria at levels as low as 0.5 µg/ml.

All of the derivatives are less toxic than the parent antibiotic, as indicated in Table 2.

The only other biological activities reported in the patent literature of the A204A derivatives refer to their anticoccidial activities and their effect on feed utilization efficiency in ruminants, subjects dealt with in detail in Chapter 6 of Volume 1.

Briefly, for the coccidiostat testing, weak-old chicks were fed a diet containing the drug for 48 hr and then each bird was inoculated with sporulated oocysts of *Eimeria tenella*. The results, which were evaluated 7 days after inoculation, are summarized in Table 3.

The derivatives of A204A were also reported in the cited patent literature to have increased the ratio of propionate production relative to acetate and butyrate when added in vitro to rumen fluid obtained from a fistulated steer. This has been shown to be related to an improvement in feed utilization efficiency in ruminants (see Chapter 6 of Volume 1).

VI. GRISORIXIN AND ALBORIXIN

The molecular structure of grisorixin was determined to be [87] by Alléaume and Hickel in 1970 from the x-ray crystallographic analysis of the silver salt. Comparison of [87] with the structure of nigericin [72] revealed only one difference. Whereas the nigericin molecule terminates at C-30 with a hydroxymethyl group, in the case of grisorixin the terminal methyl group is not hydroxylated. In all other respects, including the absolute configuration of their 19 asymmetric centers, the two antibiotics are identical.

Accompanying the report of the x-ray analysis of grisorixin was a second communication by Gachon et al. (1970) in which some chemical transformations of the antibiotic were reported. Methylation of grisorixin with diazomethane yielded the ester [88] which on treatment with methanolic sulfuric acid was further transformed into the methyl ester methyl ether [89] in a reaction analogous to the formation of the methyl ether of A204A [80] as discussed earlier. Acetylation of the methyl ester with acetic anhydride-pyridine affords an acetate [90] in which the hemiketal ring F of the antibiotic has been opened. The opening of ring F was also achieved reductively using $LiAlH_4$ in ether to give [91], which on acetylation yielded the triacetate [92]. Oxidation of the methyl ester of grisorixin [88] with chromic acid in aqueous acetic acid yielded both neutral and acidic fractions (Gachon and Kergomard, 1975).

The methylated acid fraction was resolved into five components. Two of these, the dimethyl esters of [73] and [74] obtained by oxidation of nigericin, confirmed the identity of the A rings of both anti-

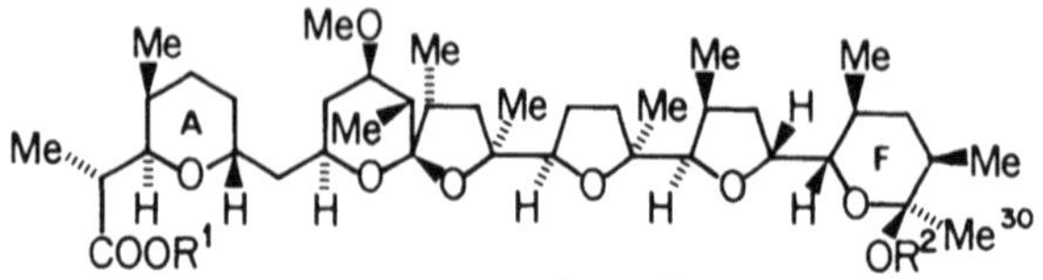

[87] :   R^1 = R^2 = H
[88] :   R^1 = Me, R^2 = H
[89] :   R^1 = R^2 = Me

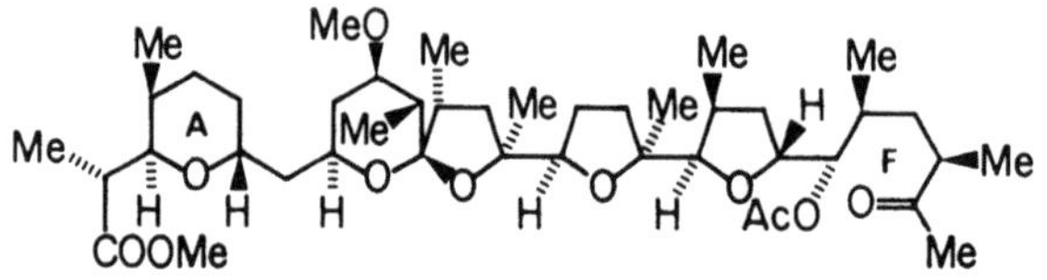

[90]

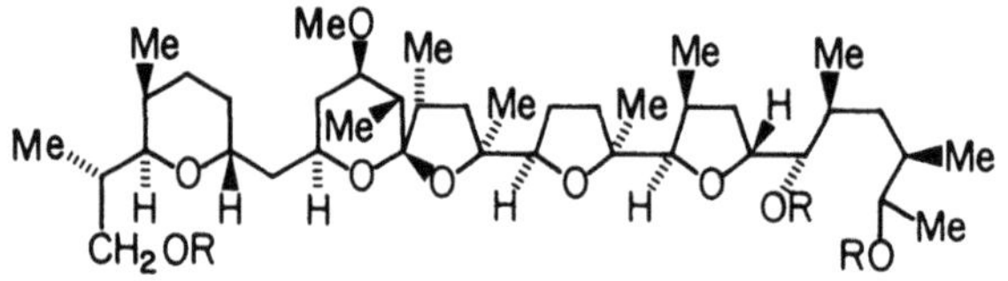

[91] :   R = H
[92] :   R = Ac

biotics. The other three dimethyl esters were shown by mass spectrometry and proton NMR to be [93], [95], and [96], in agreement with the x-ray analysis (Scheme 7). From the neutral fraction, two compounds were characterized as [94] and [97] (Scheme 7). The largest of the characterized fragments [97] was the methyl ester of the δ-lactone obtained by periodate oxidation of nigericin.

The structure of alborixin was first described in 1976 by Gachon et al. and later revised by Seto et al. (1979). The error in the original publication arose from a simple notational mistake in translating the three-dimensional structure to the planar one. The revised structure [98] differed from that of antibiotic X-206 [76] by a single extra methyl group on the A ring at C-6.

In the report by Gachon et al. (1976) some chemical transformations of alborixin were described. These included methylation with diazomethane to [99], formation of a triacetate of unknown structure, and reduction with sodium borohydride in ethanol to yield the tetrahydro and hexahydro derivatives ([100] and [101], respectively) based on mass-spectral fragmentation patterns and the nature of the oxidation products from periodate treatment of [101].

The only report comparing the relative activity of alborixin, grisorixin, and their derivatives described their comparative effects on K$^+$ and [^{3}H]glutamate efflux from rat liver mitochondria by Chapel et al.

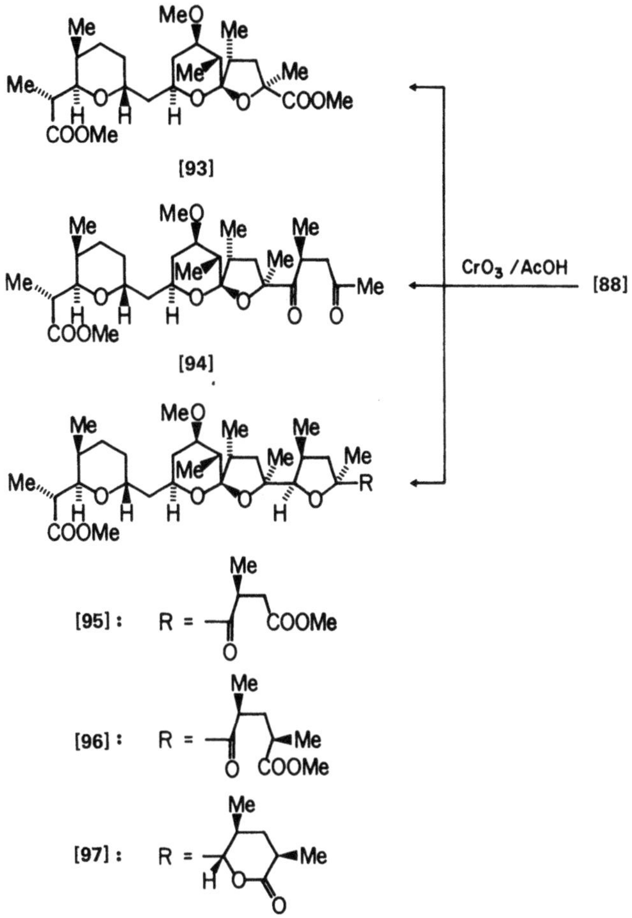

[93]

[94]

CrO₃ /AcOH [88]

[95]: R =

[96]: R =

[97]: R =

Scheme 7 Grisorixin oxidation products.

(1979). In this study the alkali cation selectivities of grisorixin [87], dihydrogrisorixin [91], alborixin [98], and hexahydroalborixin [101] were first determined using a liquid-membrane electrode. Both anti-biotics [87] and [98] had the same order of affinities: $K^+ > Rb^+ > Na^+ > Cs^+ > Li^+$, whereas dihydrogrisorixin was slightly different ($K^+ > Na^+ > Rb^+ > Cs^+ > Li^+$), and in particular the preference for K^+ was much diminished. Hexahydroalborixin had no complexing activity.

The four compounds were then tested for their effects on rat liver mitochondria already enlarged by the uptake of K^+ and [³H]glutamate in the presence of valinomycin. The contraction of the mitochondria on addition of each polyether was monitored by absorbance changes due to

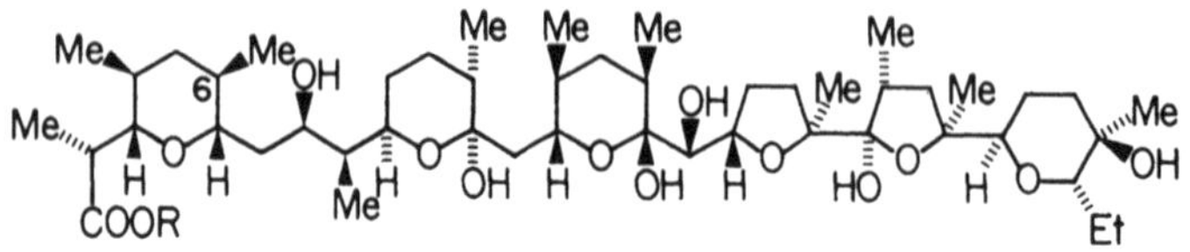

[98] :   R = H
[99] :   R = Me

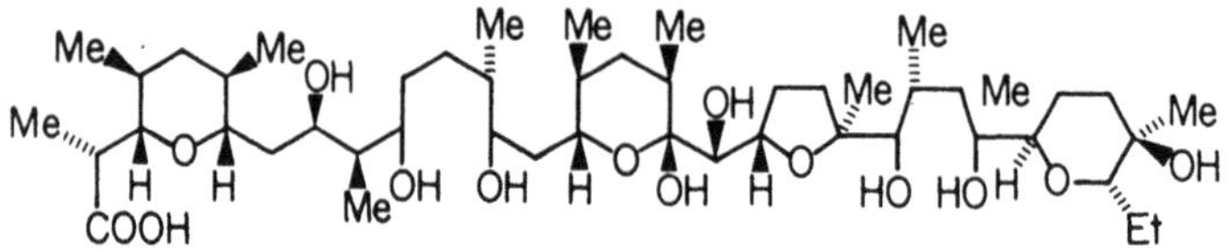

[100]

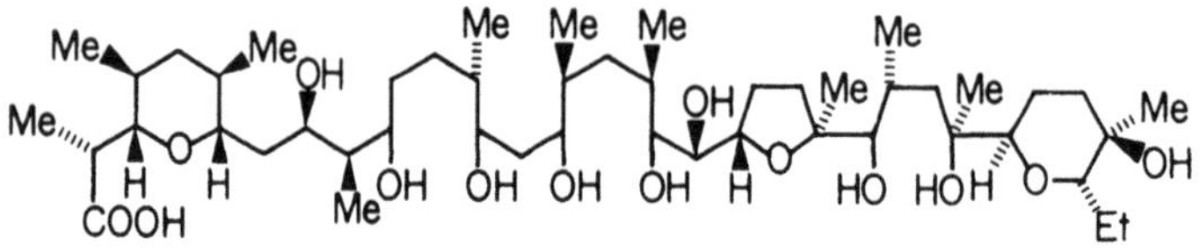

[101]

light scattering, and then the levels of K^+ and [^{3}H]glutamate remaining in the mitochondria were determined. Both antibiotics [87] and [98] caused rapid contraction in the size of the mitochondrial particles and loss of K^+ ions and glutamate. Dihydrogrisorixin [91] did induce a slight loss of K^+ ion, but not of glutamate, and had no effect on the particle size of the mitochondria. Hexahydroalborixin [101] was devoid of any activity.

The conclusion of this study was that although the reduction of the hemiketal moieties in alborixin and grisorixin increases the number of hydroxyl groups as potential cation ligands, the disruption in the conformation of the antibiotic caused by the ring openings virtually destroyed their ionophore character and in particular their affinity for K^+.

VII. LYSOCELLIN

A. Chemical Modifications

The structure of lysocellin was determined to be [102] by x-ray analysis of the silver salt by Otake et al. (1975b). In the course of a search for minor metabolites in the lysocellin fermentation Koenuma and Otake (1977) discovered two structural analogs of [102] designated L_1 and M_1. Attempts to detect the presence of these analogs in the fermentation broth prior to extraction were unsuccessful, suggesting that the compounds were in fact artifacts produced during the

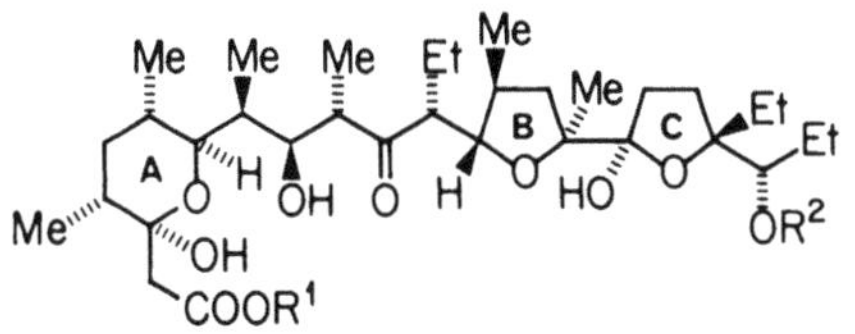

Me Me Me Et Me
Me
B
C
Et
Et
A ''H OH O H O HO O
Me''' ''OH ÒR²
COOR¹

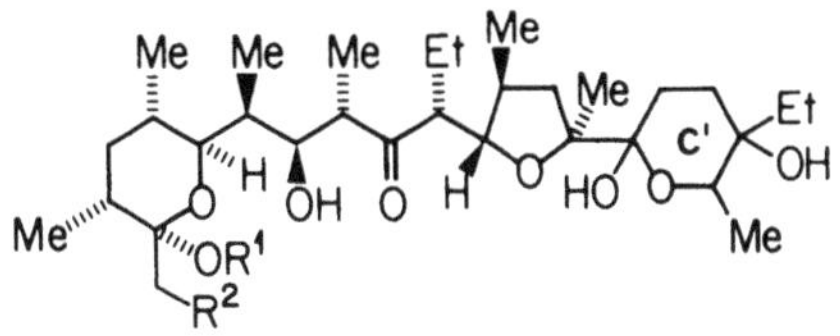

[102] : R¹ = H,   [105] : R¹ = Me,   [108]: R¹ = Me,
R² = H   R² = H   R² = Ac

Me Me Me Et Me
Me
C'
Et
OH
''H OH O H O HO O Me
Me''' ''OR¹
R²

[103] : R¹ = H,   [104] : R¹ = Me,
R² = COOMe   R² = H

Me Et Me   Me Et Me
Me   Me
Me   Me
C
Et Et   C'
Et
O H O ÒH O   ⇌   O H O HO O OH
ÒH   Me

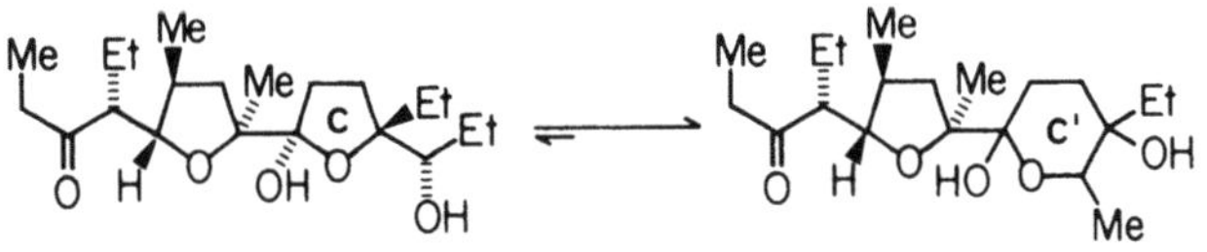

[106]   [107]

Me Me Me Et Me
Me
C
Et Et
''H OR OR H O HO O
Me''' ''OH ÒR
CH₂OR

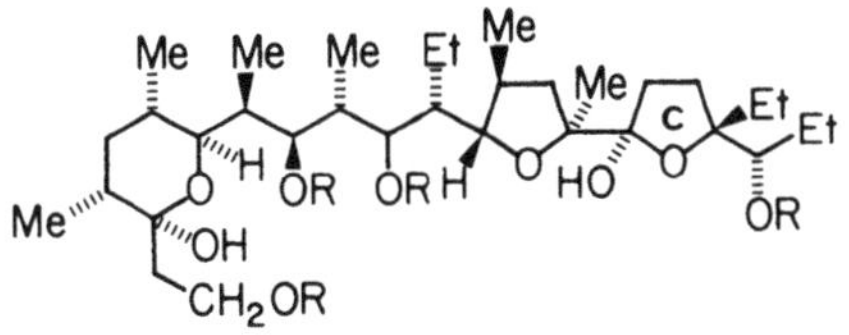

[109] : R = H   [110]: R = Ac

workup of the crude extract. This was confirmed when the two compounds were produced simply by refluxing [102] in methanol containing acetic acid. The structures of L_1 and M_1 were shown to be [103]
and [104], respectively, by a combination of mass spectrometry and
proton NMR. A major structural change between the artifacts and the
parent antibiotic is the transformation of the tetrahydrofuranyl ring C
in [102] into a tetrahydropyranyl ring C' in [103] and [104]. The
methyl ester of lysocellin (isomeric with [103]) prepared from [102] by
diazomethane treatment retained the tetrahydrofuranyl ring C [105].

In a reaction analogous to the retroaldol cleavage of lasalocid discussed in the first section of this chapter, base treatment of lysocellin
causes a retrograde-aldol cleavage of the β-ketol system in [102] from

Table 4 Relative Antibacterial Activity[a] of Lysocellin and Seven
Derivatives Against *Bacillus subtilis* PCI 209P

Compound	Relative antibacterial activity (%)	Compound number
Lysocellin	100	[102]
Artifact L_1	0.56	[103]
Artifact M_1	3.3	[104]
Lysocellin methyl ester	2.8	[105]
Retroaldol ketone (ring C)	—[b]	[106]
Retroaldol ketone (ring C')	—	[107]
Lysocellin methyl ester acetate	—	[108]
Lysocellin hexol	3.3	[109]

[a]Antibacterial activity was measured by the agar disk method.
[b]Inactive at a concentration of 200 µg/ml.

which just the neutral ketone fragment [106] was isolated and characterized. On standing, [106] was reported to slowly equilibrate to the
tetrahydropyranyl ring C' analog [107]. Using the same technique
employed to distinguish lasalocid from iso-laslocid retroaldol ketone
(Westley et al. 1974c), Koenuma and Ōtake (1977) took advantage of
the acetylation reaction to discriminate between [106], which was
acetylated, and [107], which was unaffected. This simple test was
also utilized to distinguish lysocellin methyl ester [105], which on
acetylation yielded the monoacetate [108] from the isomeric methyl
ester (L_1) [103], which did not acetylate.

Reduction of lysocellin methyl ester [105] with sodium borohydride
yielded the hexol [109], which on treatment with acetic anhydride in
pyridine formed a tetraacetate [110].

B. Biological Activity

In the report by Koenuma and Ōtake (1977) the relative activity of the
analogs and degradation products of lysocellin were compared with the
parent antibiotic against *Bacillus subtilis* PCI 209P. The results are
presented in Table 4.

From the results in Table 4, all of the chemical transformations of
lysocellin described by Koenuma and Ōtake caused considerable losses
in activity. While the complete inactivity noted for the retroaldol
ketones was consistent with the inactivity of lasalocid degradation
products, the slight activity still retained by the methyl esters [104]

[105] was inconsistent with the antimicrobial results for lasalocid where the methyl ester was completely inactive. The slight activity of the hexol [109] is an interesting observation, as it suggests, along with the results for [104] and [103], that the carboxyl group of lyso-cellin may not be essential for at least part of the antibacterial activity of the antibiotic.

VIII. LONOMYCIN

A. Chemical Modifications

Some chemical reactions of lonomycin were reported in the patent liter-ature (Yamagishi et al, 1980) as part of a claim for a variety of bio-logical activities for lonomycin derivatives.

The structure of the antibiotic was established as [111] by x-ray crystallography in 1975 (Ōtake et al., 1975a) and in the following year identified with DE-3936 (Oshima et al., 1976).

Reduction of lonomycin with borohydride yielded a mixture of dihy-drolonomycins [112] and [113] in which the F ring had been opened as reported for the LiAlH$_4$ reduction of grisorixin. In the case of lono-mycin, however, the two optical isomers were separated into dihydro-lonomonycins I [112] and II [113], identical in all respects eccept for the configuration at C-29.

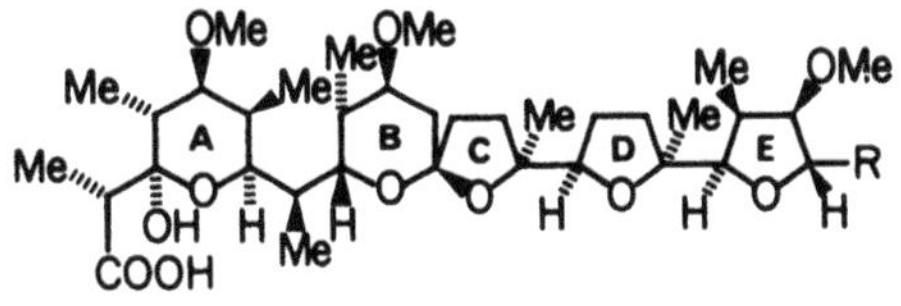

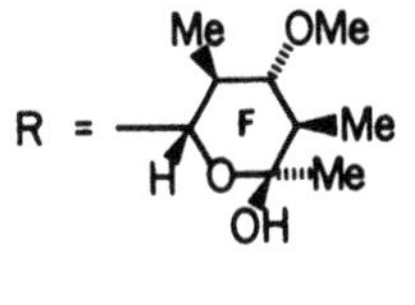

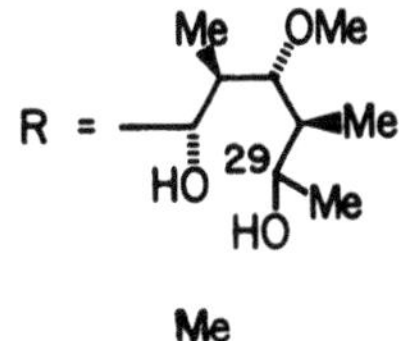

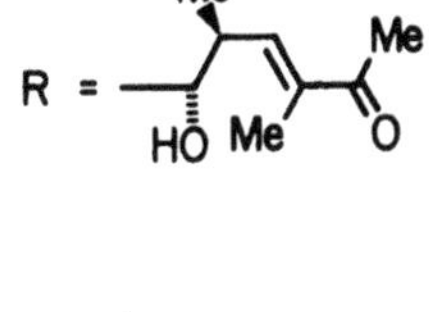

Table 5 Mouse Acute Toxicities of Lonomycin and Three Derivatives

Compound	LD_{50} (mg/kg)		Compound number
	Intraperitoneal	Per os	
Lonomycin	8.3	4.9	[111]
Dihydrolonomycin I	11.3	6.0	[112]
Dihydrolonomycin II	15.2	10.8	[113]
Oxolonomycin	117		[114]

In a second type of chemical modification lonomycin was treated with sodium hydroxide in aqueous acetone at room temperature for 30 hr. The site of reaction was again the F ring in [111]. The base-catalyzed ring opening was accompanied by a concomitant elimination of methanol to yield an α, β-unsaturated ketone which was designated oxolonomycin [114].

B. Biological Activity

The acute toxicities in mice of the two dihydrolonomycins were only marginally less than lonomycin, but the LD_{50} i.p. of oxolonomycin was more than 10 times higher than that of the parent antibiotic (Table 5).

Table 6 Antibacterial Activity[a] of Lonomycin Derivatives as Determined by the Agar Dilution Test

	Compound number		
	[112]	[113]	[114]
1. Anaerobic bacteria			
Peptostreptococcus anaerobis	25	6.75	3.13
Peptococcus magmus	1.56	1.56	1.56
Eubacterium lentum	25	25	12.5
Clostridium tetani	6.29	6.25	1.56
2. Aerobic bacteria			
Staphylococcus aureus	100	50	50
Bacillus subtilis	100	100	100

[a]MIC (μg/ml).

Oxolonomycin was found active at 500 ppm against *Eimeria tenella* in chickens. All three derivatives are active against *Taxoplasma tachy-zoites* at the 0.1-μg level. Another activity exhibited by all of the derivatives was against Newcastle disease virus, with a minimal inhibitory concentration (MIC) of 3.1 μg/ml for the dihydrolonomycins and 0.8 μg/ml for [114].

The final claim for these versatile derivatives was as antibacterial agents, particularly against anaerobic bacteria. The MIC values of the derivatives in vitro for various bacteria selected from the patent are summarized in Table 6.

IX. SALINOMYCIN

The final example of the reactions of polyether antibiotics to be discussed here involves salinomycin [115] (Scheme 8). As in virtually every case in the class, the structure was assigned by x-ray crystallography (Kinashi et al., 1973). Chemical degradation of the antibiotic was only attempted as part of a study which led to the complete assignment of the ^{13}C NMR spectrum of salinomycin (Seto et al., 1977). Noting the presence of the same β-ketol system as in lasalocid and lysocellin, the antibiotic was treated with base in the expectation that the retrograde-aldol reaction would provide a ketone with the loss of the A ring as observed for the other polyethers. In the case of salinomycin, however, a cleavage reaction different (Scheme 8) from the retrograde aldol predominated to yield a γ-lactone [116].

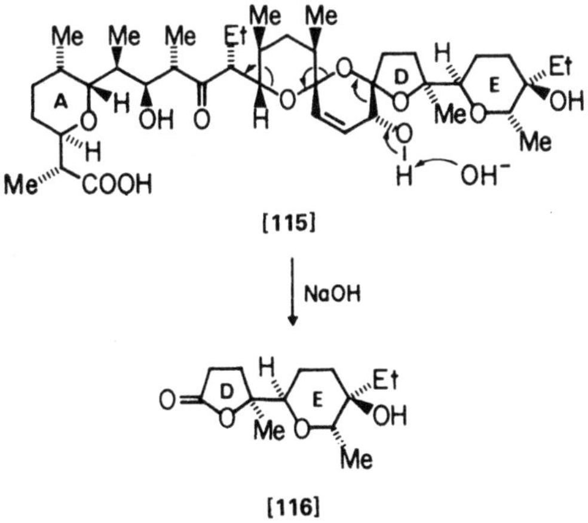

Scheme 8 Base cleavage of salinomycins.

X. CONCLUSIONS

Due in part to the outstanding successes of x-ray crystallography in determining the structure of polyether antibiotics, the chemistry of these compounds has been rather slow to emerge. This chapter, however, has not only attempted to show that a growing number of reactions are being reported for the polyether antibiotics, but also to compile this information as a foundation for future progress in the field.

Part of the chemistry described in this chapter has been synthetic in nature and has derived from the traditional search of the medicinal chemist for an active but less toxic analog. The degradative chemistry of polyether antibiotics has come mostly from biosynthetic studies. In the earlier work with ^{14}C-labeled antibiotics fragmentation was used to help assign the labeling pattern for each precursor. More recently, the tool of choice has been ^{13}C NMR, and well-characterized degradation products are excellent models to help assign the complete spectrum of an antibiotic prior to the use of labeled precursors.

The reactions summarized in this chapter can be classified according to the specific molecular sites at which they take place. One or more of these sites are found in all polyether antibiotics. The conclusion drawn from this is that virtually all the known polyether antibiotics are potentially amenable to one or more reactions already reported in the literature. One of the first such reactions was the conversion of monensin and dianemycin to their δ-lactone analogs with periodate. Another early example was the retrograde-aldol cleavage of the β-ketol system in lasalocid to yield fragments essential to the determination of both the absolute configuration and the biosynthesis of that antibiotic. The moiety which has since provided the greatest variety of chemical transformations is the ketal, or masked ketone, present in one form or another in the majority of polyether antibiotics. For instance, in the case of monensin the spiroketal system accounts for the acid instability of that antibiotic, whereas the substituted bis-spiroketal in salinomycin can be cleaved by base. In other antibiotics cyclic hemiketals have provided a source of semisynthetic ethers as well as a site for ring opening by hydride reduction, acetylation, or base hydrolysis, and even a site for ring expansion in the case of lysocellin. In addition, ketals are often the first point of attack in the most popular method used to degrade polyether antibiotic molecules, chromic acid oxidation, which yields complex mixtures of neutral and acidic fragments ranging in size from seven carbons up to just one carbon short of the complete antibiotic molecule.

Unfortunately, the published data on structure-activity relationships for the semisynthetic analogs of polyether antibiotics are for the most part extremely limited. From all that has been reported, it would appear that any fragmentation of the molecule results in complete loss of activity. Nevertheless, the most promising semisynthetic polyethers until now are the halogenated derivatives of lasalocid and the alkyl ethers of A204A; they are less toxic than their parent antibiotics while still retaining their biological activity. Unfortunately, in several cases in the patent literature the relative activity of the derivatives compared to the parent antibiotic is impossible to assess, as the activity of the antibiotic is not included as a control.

One of the advantages of the polyether antibiotics that has not yet been fully exploited is the detailed knowledge gained by x-ray of the conformation and ligand binding sites in these molecules. Perhaps chemical modifications based on a systematic analysis of these factors will produce analogs of greater biological interest in the future.

REFERENCES

Agtarap, A., and Chamberlin, J. W. (1968). Monensin, a new biologically active compound. IV. Chemistry. *Antimicrob. Agents Chemother.* *1967*:359-362.

Agtarap, A., Chamberlin, J. W., Pinkerton, M., and Steinrauf, L. (1967). The structure of monensic acid. *J. Am. Chem. Soc. 89*: 5737-5739.

Albert, A., and Serjeant, E. P. (1962). *Ionization Constants of Acids and Bases.* Methuen, London.

Alléaume, M., and Hickel, D. (1970). The crystal structure of grisorixin silver salt. *Chem. Commun. 1970*:1422-1423.

Bakker, E. P. (1979). Ionophore antibiotics. In *Antibiotics Vol. 5,* Part 1, F. E. Hahn (Ed.). Springer-Verlag, Berlin, pp. 67-95.

Berger, J., Rachlin, A. I., Scott, W. E., Sternbach, L. H., and Goldberg, M. W. (1951). The isolation of three new crystalline antibiotics from Streptomyces. *J. Am. Chem. Soc. 73*:5295-5298.

Blount, J. F., and Westley, J. W. (1975). X-ray crystal and molecular structure of antibiotic X-206. *Chem. Commun. 1975*:533.

Caserio, M. C., Roberts, J. D., Neeman, M., and Johnson, W. S. (1958). Methylation of alcohols with diazomethane. *J. Am. Chem. Soc. 80*:2584-2585.

Chamberlin, J. W. (1976). Dihydro-A204. U.S. Patent 3,985,872.

Chapel, M., Jeminet, F., Gachon, P., Debise, R., and Durand, R. (1979). Comparative effects of ionophores grisorixin, alborixin and two derivatives on K$^+$ glutamate efflux in rat liver mitochondria. *J. Antibiot. 32*:740-745.

Djerassi, C., and Geller, L. E. (1959). Optical rotatory dispersion XXIV. *J. Am. Chem. Soc. 81*:2789-2794.

Edward, J. T., Holder, D., Lunn, W. H., and Puskas, I. (1961). Oxidation of cholest-4-en-3-one with periodate. *Can. J. Chem. 39*:599-600.

Gachon, P., and Kergomard, A. (1975). Grisorixin, an ionophorous antibiotic of the nigericin group. II. Chemical and structural study of girsoroxin and some derivatives. *J. Antibiot. 28*:351-357.

Gachon, P., Kergomard, A., Veschambre, H., Esteve, C., and
 Staron, T. (1970). Grisorixin, a new antibiotic related to nigeri-
 cin. *Chem. Commun. 1970*:1421-1422.
Gachon, P., Farges, C., and Kergomard, A. (1976). Alborixin, a
 new antibiotic ionophore: Isolation, structure, physical and chemi-
 cal properties. *J. Antibiot. 29*:603-610.
Hamill, R. L. (1975). A204I derivatives. U.S. Patent 3,807,832.
Hamill, R. L. (1976). A204I derivatives. U.S. Patent 3,953,474.
Hamill, R. L., and Crandall, L. W. (1978). Polyether antibiotics.
 In *Antibiotics: isolation, separation and purification.* M. J. Wein-
 stein and G. H. Wagman (Eds.). Elsevier, New York, pp. 481-
 519.
Hamill, R. L., Hoehn, M. M., Pittenger, G. E., Chamberlin, J. W.,
 and Gorman, M. (1969). Dianemycin, an antibiotic of the group
 affecting ion transport. *J. Antibiot. 22*:161-164.
Johnson, S. M., Liu, S. J., Herrin, J., and Paul, I. C. (1970).
 The crystal and molecular structure of the barium salt of an antibiotic containing a high proportion of oxygen. *J. Am. Chem. Sco.
 92*:4428-4435.
Jones, N. D., Chaney, M. O., Chamberlin, J. W., Hamill, R. L.,
 and Chen, S. (1973). Structure of A204A, a new polyether antibiotic. *J. Am. Chem. Soc. 95*:3399-3400.
Kinashi, H., Otake, N., Yonehara, H., Sato, S., and Saito, Y.
 (1973). The structure of salinomycin, a new member of the poly-
 ether antibiotics._ *Tetrahedron Lett. 1973*:4955-4958.
Koenuma, M., and Otake, N. (1977). Studies on ionophorous anti-
 biotics. XI. The artifacts and degradation products of lysocellin.
 J. Antibiot. 30:819-828.
Kubota, T., Matsutani, S., Shiro, M., and Koyama, H. (1968).
 The structure of polyetherin A. *Chem. Commun. 1968*:1541-1543.
Morin, R. B., and Gorman, M. (1964). The partial structure of
 tylosin, a macrolide antibiotic. *Tetrahedron Lett. 1964*:2339-2345.
Muller, E., and Rundell, W. (1958). Preparation of ethers from
 alcohols with diazomethane and boron trifluoride etherate. *Angew.
 Chem. 70*:105.
Nikaido, H. (1976). Outer membrane of *Salmonella typhimurim.*
 Transmembrane diffusion of hydrophobic substances. *Biochem.
 Biophys. Acta 433*:118-132.
Oshima, M., Ishizaki, N., Abe, K., Ukawa, M., Marumoto, Y.,
 Nakatsuka, K., Horiuchi, T., Tonooka, Y., Yoshino, S., and
 Kanda, N. (1976). Antibiotic DE-3936, a polyether antibiotic
 identical with lonomycin. *J. Antibiot. 29*:354-365.
Ōtake, N., Koenuma, M., Miyamae, H., Sato, S., and Saito, Y.
 (1975). Studies on the ionophorous antibiotics. Part III. The
 structure of lonomycin, a polyether antibiotic. *Tetrahedron Lett.
 1975*:4147-4150.

Ōtake, N., Koenuma, M., Kinashi, H., Sato, S., and Saito, Y. (1975b). The crystal and molecular structure of the silver salt of lysocellin, a new polyether antibiotic. *Chem. Commun.* 1975:92-93.

Sarin, E. S., and Fusman, G. D. (1964). A convenient preparation of benzylesters of N-benzyloxycarbonylamino acids. *Biochem. Biophys. Acta 82*:175-178.

Seto, H., Miyazaki, Y., Fujita, K., and Ōtake, N. (1977). Studies on ionophorous antibiotics X. The assignment of ^{13}C-NMR spectrum of salinomycin. *Tetrahedron Lett.* 1977:2417-2420.

Seto, H., Mizoue, K., Ōtake, N., Gachon, P., Kergomard, A., and Westley, J. W. (1979). The revised structure of alborixin. *J. Antibiot. 32*:970-971.

Smith, P. A. S. (1966). Azides and diazo compounds. In *Open Chain Nitrogen Compounds*. vol. 2. Benjamin, New York, p. 229.

Steinrauf, L. K., Pinderton, M., and Chamberlin, J. W. (1968). The structure of nigericin. *Biochem. Biophys. Res. Commun. 33*: 29-31.

Stempel, A., and Westley, J. W. (1974). Diazo derivatives of lasalocid. U.S. Patent 3,836,516.

Stempel, A., and Westley, J. W. (1976). Phenylazo derivatives of lasalocid. U.S. Patent 3,950,320.

Westley, J. W., Evans, R. H., Williams T., and Stempel, A. (1970a). Structure of antibiotic X-537A. *Chem. Commun.* 1970:71-72.

Westley, J. W., Evans, R. H., Pruess, D. L., and Stempel, A. (1970b). Biosynthesis of antibiotic X-537A. *Chem. Commun.* 1970:1467-1468.

Westley, J. W., Schneider, J., Evans, R. H., Williams, T. H., Batcho, A. D., and Stempel, A. (1971). Nitration of lasalocid and facile conversion to 6-hydroxy-2,7-dimethyl-5-nitroquinoline, *J. Org. Chem. 36*:3621-3624.

Westley, J. W., Oliveto, E. P., Berger, J., Evans, R. H., Glass, R., Stempel, A., Toome, V., and Williams, T. H. (1973). Chemical transformations of lasalocid and their effect on biological activity. *J. Med. Chem. 16*:397-403.

Westley, J. W., Evans, R. H., Williams, T. H., and Stempel, A. (1973b). Pyrolytic cleavage of lasalocid and related reactions. *J. Org. Chem. 38*:3431-3433.

Westley, J. W., Evans, R. H., and Stempel, A. (1974a). Gas liquid chromatographic determination of antibiotic X-537A, lasalocid. *Anal. Biochem. 59*:574-582.

Westley, J. W., Benz, W., Donahue, J., Evans, R. H., Scott, C. G., Stempel, A., and Berger, J. (1974b). Biosynthesis of lasalocid III: Isolation and structure determination of four homologs of lasalocid A. *J. Antibiot. 27*:744-753.

Westley, J. W., Blount, J. F., Evans, R. H., Stempel, A., and

Berger, J. (1974c). Biosynthesis of lasalocid II: X-ray analysis of a naturally occurring isomer of lasalocid A. *J. Antibiot. 27:* 597-604.

Yamagishi, M., Mizoue, K., Hara, H., Omura, S., Seto, H., and Ōtake, N. (1980). Novel Ionomycin derivatives. U.S. Patent 4,199,515.

chapter 3

X-RAY STRUCTURES OF THE POLYETHER ANTIBIOTICS

Eileen N. Duesler* and Iain C. Paul
School of Chemical Sciences, University of Illinois, Urbana, Illinois

I. INTRODUCTION

X-ray structure analysis has been the single most powerful technique
in unraveling the structures of the polyether ionophores. These
compounds, often with built-in heavy atoms, generally form crystals
of good quality from nonpolar solvents. Since the pioneering study
(Agtarap et al., 1967) of the silver salt of monensin that revealed a
new structural class in 1967, x-ray analyses have been carried out on
19 distinct acid ionophores. In some cases different derivatives or
salts have been studied. In other situations so great has been the
interest in this class of compound that the same antibiotic, often as the
same derivative, has been examined more or less simultaneously by
different groups. Such parallel studies have often led to confusion in
nomenclature. A listing of the acid ionophores studied by x-ray methods and the form in which they have been studied is given in Table I.
While the primary objective of most of the x-ray work has been the establishment of constitution and stereochemistry, a few of the polyether
ionophores have been examined more extensively in order to provide
information on their function.

---

*Present affiliation: The University of New Mexico, Albuquerque, New
Mexico

Table 1 Cell Data for Polyether Antibiotics and Derivatives[a]

Compound name	Formula	Crystal system	a
A-130A (Ro21-6150 lenoremycin silver salt[b] (ethanol)	$C_{47}H_{77}O_{13} \cdot Ag$	Orthorhombic	28.179(5)
A-204A			
Silver salt:acetonate	$C_{49}H_{83}O_{17} \cdot Ag \cdot C_3H_6O$	Monoclinic	26.971(4)
Sodium salt:acetonate (acetone-water)	$C_{49}H_{83}O_{17} \cdot Na \cdot C_3H_6O$	Monoclinic	27.539(4)
Free acid:hydrate: acetonate (acetone-water)	$C_{49}H_{84}O_{17} \cdot H_2O \cdot C_3H_6O$	Monoclinic	27.576(2)
A-23187			
Free acid (from acetone)	$C_{29}H_{37}N_3O_6$	Monoclinic	15.759(4)
Calcium salt:dihydrate (95% ethanol)	$(C_{29}H_{36}N_3O_6)_2 \cdot Ca \cdot 2H_2O$	Monoclinic	23.715(7)
Calcium salt:diethanolate[c] (50% ethanol)	$(C_{29}H_{36}N_3O_6)_2 \cdot Ca \cdot 2C_2H_5OH$	Orthorhombic	24.120(8)
Alborixin			
Potassium salt (aq. ethanol)	$C_{48}H_{83}O_{14} \cdot K$	Monoclinic	12.202(4)
Antibiotic-6016			
Thallium salt (—)	$C_{46}H_{77}O_{16} \cdot Tl$	Orthorhombic	18.767
Carriomycin			
Thallium salt	$C_{47}H_{79}O_{15} \cdot Tl$	Monoclinic	15.416
Dianemycin			
Potassium salt hydrate (Sodium and thallium salts isomorphous) (isopropanol:water 1:1)	$C_{47}H_{77}O_{14} \cdot K \cdot H_2O$	Orthorhombic	9.59
Grixorixin			
Silver salt (aq. acetone)	$C_{40}H_{67}O_{10} \cdot Ag$	Orthorhombic	20.011
Thallium salt:hydrate	$C_{40}H_{67}O_{10} \cdot Tl \cdot H_2O$	Monoclinic	11.626
Free acid:hydrate	$C_{40}H_{68}O_{10} \cdot H_2O$	Orthorhombic	24.438

Å		Angle (°)			Z	Space group	References
b	c	α	β	γ			
9.582(2)	18.096(3)	90	90	90	4	$P2_12_12_1$*	1,2
14.517(2)	14.419(2)	90	91.94(1)	90	4	C2*	3
14.515(2)	14.406(2)	90	92.36(1)	90	4	C2	3
14.711(1)	14.348(1)	90	92.57(4)	90	4	C2	4
10.377(4)	8.592(3)	90	95.97(2)	90	2	$P2_1$	5
15.130(4)	17.841(6)	90	90.67(4)	90	4	C2	6
17.608(9)	14.930(9)	90	90	90	4	$P2_12_12_1$	7
16.087(5)	13.471(5)	90	102.43	90	2	$P2_1$	8
22.671	12.402	90	90	90	4	$P2_12_12_1$*	9
12.325	14.442	90	105.42	90	2	$P2_1$*	10
18.54	28.75	90	90	90	4	$P2_12_12_1$*	11
17.266	13.330	90	90	90	4	$P2_12_12_1$*	12
16.766	11.799	90	109°36'	90	2	$P2_1$*	13
12.040	14.452	90	90	90	4	$P2_12_12_1$	14

Table 1 (Continued)

Compound name	Formula	Crystal system	a
Ionomycin			
Ca²⁺ salt (n-heptane:methylene dichloride)	$C_{41}H_{70}O_9 \cdot Ca \cdot \frac{1}{2}C_7H_{16}$	Orthorhombic	12.12(2)
Cd²⁺ salt (n-heptane:methylene dichloride)	$C_{41}H_{70}O_9 \cdot Cd \cdot \frac{1}{2}C_7H_{16}$	Orthorhombic	12.152(5)
Cd²⁺ salt (n-hexane:methylene dichloride)	$C_{41}H_{70}O_9 \cdot Cd \cdot \frac{1}{2}C_6H_{14}$	Monoclinic	12.132(2)
K-41			
Sodium salt of p-I benzoate (water:n-hexane)	$C_{55}H_{84}O_9I \cdot Na \cdot H_2O \cdot C_6H_{14}$ ($C_{48}H_{82}O_8$-acid)	Orthorhombic	36.330(4)
Sodium salt of p-Br benzoate (water:n-hexane)	$C_{55}H_{84}O_9Br \cdot Na \cdot H_2O \cdot C_6H_{14}$	Orthorhombic	33.963(3)
Lasalocid			
Barium salt·hydrate (ethanol-water)	$(C_{34}H_{53}O_8)_2 \cdot Ba \cdot H_2O$	Monoclinic	14.59(4)
Silver salt·acetonate (acetone-water)	$(C_{34}H_{53}O_8 \cdot Ag)_2 \cdot 2CH_3COCH_3$	Monoclinic	12.25(3)
Silver salt of 5-NO₂ derivative·methanolate (methanol-water)	$(C_{34}H_{52}O_{10}N \cdot Ag)_2 \cdot 2CH_3OH$	Monoclinic	13.333(3)
Sodium salt of 5-bromo derivative·form I (CCl₄)	$(C_{34}H_{52}O_8Br \cdot Na)_2$	Orthorhombic	16.92(2)
Sodium salt of 5-bromo derivative·Form II (acetone or ethyl acetate)	$(C_{34}H_{52}O_8Br \cdot Na)_2$	Orthorhombic	20.67(1)
Sodium salt hydrate (95% ethanol)	$(C_{34}H_{53}O_8 \cdot Na \cdot H_2O)_2$	Monoclinic	12.148(2)
Sodium salt·methanolate (methanol)	$C_{34}H_{53}O_8 \cdot Na \cdot CH_3OH$	Orthorhombic	20.202(2)
Cesium salt (dichloromethane: hexane)	$C_{34}H_{53}O_8 \cdot Cs$	Orthorhombic	13.612(1)
R(+)-1-Amino-1-(4-bromophenyl)-ethane salt (−)	$C_{34}H_{53}O_8 \cdot C_8H_{11}NBr$	Orthorhombic	14.098(1)

| Å | | Angle (°) | | | | | | |
b	c	α	β	γ	Z	Space group	References
18.85(1)	12.11(1)	90	90	90	4	$P2_12_12$	15
18.688(3)	12.079(1)	90	90	90	4	$P2_12_12$*	15
33.991(14)	13.191(3)	90	116.0(0)	90	4	$P2_1$	15
15.321(4)	12.790(1)	90	90	90	4	$P2_12_12$*	
15.407(2)	12.943(1)	90	90	90	4	$P2_12_12_1$	16
17.95(5)	13.99(4)	90	105°17'(15')	90	2	$P2_1$	17,18
16.81(3)	19.82(4)	90	97°39'(1')	90	2	$P2_1$	19
19.825(5)	14.526(4)	90	107.15(2)	90	2	$P2_1$	20
23.90(3)	18.55(1)	90	90	90	4	$P2_12_12_1$	21
16.05(1)	43.39(1)	90	90	90	8	$C222_1$	21
27.589(3)	11.802(3)	90	110.25(1)	90	2	$P2_1$	22
17.678(2)	10.221(1)	90	90	90	4	$P2_12_12_1$	23
20.247(4)	12.837(1)	90	90	90	4	$P2_12_12_1$	24
16.573(6)	20.373(8)	90	90	90	4	$P2_12_12_1$	25

Table 1 (Continued)

Compound name	Formula	Crystal system	a
Lasalocid (cont.)			
5-Bromolasalocid· hemihydrate (hexane:methylene dichloride)	$(C_{34}H_{53}O_8Br)_2 \cdot H_2O$	Monoclinic	14.622(7)
5-Bromolasalocid: ethanolate (ethanol)	$C_{34}H_{53}O_8Br \cdot C_2H_5OH$	Orthorhombic	26.811(7)
Lasalocid:methanolate Form I (methanol)	$C_{34}H_{54}O_8 \cdot CH_3OH$	Orthorhombic	26.628(10)
Form II (methanol)	$C_{34}H_{54}O_8 \cdot CH_3OH$	Orthorhombic	10.056(2)
Isolasalocid			
5-Bromoisolasalocid	$C_{34}H_{53}O_8Br$	Orthorhombic	11.772(6)
Lonomycin			
(DE-3936;emericid) Silver salt (−)	$C_{44}H_{75}O_{14} \cdot Ag$	Monoclinic	15.011
Sodium salt (nearly isomorphous) (−)	$C_{44}H_{75}O_{14} \cdot Na$	Monoclinic	14.768
Silver salt dimethanoleate (methanol-water)	$C_{44}H_{75}O_{14} \cdot Ag \cdot 2CH_3OH$	Orthorhombic	15.818
Thallium salt (methanol-water)	$C_{44}H_{75}O_{14} \cdot Tl$	Orthorhombic	16.257
Lysocellin			
Silver salt hemihydrate (−)	$C_{34}H_{59}O_{10} \cdot Ag \cdot \frac{1}{2}H_2O$	Orthorhombic	16.259 16.283(7)
Monensin			
Sodium salt dihydrate [acetone(ethanol): water]	$C_{36}H_{61}O_{11} \cdot Na \cdot 2H_2O$	Monoclinic	16.3 (1)
Sodium salt dihydrate	$C_{36}H_{61}O_{11} \cdot Na \cdot 2H_2O$	Orthorhombic	16.387(4)
Sodium salt anhydrous	$C_{36}H_{61}O_{11} \cdot Na$	Monoclinic	9.238(5)
Silver salt·dihydrate [acetone(ethanol): water]			
Form I	$C_{36}H_{61}O_{11} \cdot Ag \cdot 2H_2O$	Monoclinic	16.4 (1)
Form II	$C_{36}H_{61}O_{11} \cdot Ag \cdot 2H_2O$	Orthorhombic	16.46(2)
Potassium salt·dihydrate [ethanol-(acetone):water]	$C_{36}H_{61}O_{11} \cdot K \cdot 2H_2O$	Orthorhombic	16.39(2)
Thallium salt·dihydrate [ethanol-(acetone):water]	$C_{36}H_{61}O_{11} \cdot Tl \cdot 2H_2O$	Orthorhombic	16.35(6)

Å		Angle (°)					
b	c	α	β	γ	Z	Space group	References
17.096(9)	14.693(8)	90	95.73(5)	90	2	$P2_1$	26
13.243(3)	10.745(2)	90	90	90	4	$P2_12_12_1$	27
13.014(5)	10.609(3)	90	90	90	4	$P2_12_12_1$	28
18.893(4)	19.442(3)	90	90	90	4	$P2_12_12_1$	28
13.013(3)	24.039(9)	90	90	90	4	$P2_12_12_1$	29
13.402	12.789	90	111.3	90	2	$P2_1$*	30
13.507	12.775	90	110.7	90	2	$P2_1$	30
25.821	12.776	90	90	90	4	$P2_12_12_1$*	31
25.731	12.502	90	90	90	4	$P2_12_12_1$*	32
26.460	8.916	90	90	90	4	$P2_12_12_1$*	33,34
26.519(16)	8.930(5)	90	90	90	4		
9.3 (05)	12.7 (05)	90	86.0(1)	90	2	$P2_1$	35
18.684(4)	12.792(2)	90	90	90	4	$P2_12_12_1$	36
12.702(1)	16.274(7)	90	101.0	90	2	$P2_1$	36
9.4 (05)	12.7 (05)	90	85.5(1)	90	2	$P2_1$	35
18.81(2)	12.73(2)	90	90	90	4	$P2_12_12_1$*	35,37
18.92(2)	12.74(2)	90	90	90	4	$P2_12_12_1$	35
19.57(6)	12.59(6)	90	90	90	4	$P2_12_12_1$	35

Table 1 (Continued)

Compound name	Formula	Crystal system	a
Monensin (continued)			
Free acid hydrate (abs. ethanol)	$C_{36}H_{62}O_{11} \cdot H_2O$	Orthorhombic	15.15
Free acid·NaBr complex (chloroform:methanol and ethylether-pet. ether)	$C_{36}H_{62}O_{11} \cdot NaBr$	Orthorhombic	16.618(4)
Nigericin (Polyetherin A) Silver salt[d] (ethanol) (ethanol-water)	$C_{40}H_{67}O_{11} \cdot Ag$	Orthorhombic	23.762(4)
Salinomycon p-Iodophenacyl ester (ethanol)	$C_{50}H_{75}O_{12}I$ ($C_{40}H_{70}O_{11}$)	Orthorhombic	20.981(2)
Septamycin p-Bromophenacyl ester:hydrate (−)	$C_{56}H_{87}O_{17}Br \cdot H_2O$ ($C_{48}H_{82}O_{16}$)	Orthorhombic	12.728(3)
X-206 Silver salt	$C_{47}H_{81}O_{14} \cdot Ag^{e}$ ($C_{45}H_{77}O_{13} \cdot Ag$)	Hexagonal	22.90
Free acid·hydrate	$C_{47}H_{82}O_{14} \cdot H_2O$	Orthorhombic	12.465
X-14547A R(+)-1-Amino-1-(4-bromophenyl)-ethane salt (−)	$[C_{31}H_{48}NO_4]_2 \cdot C_8H_{10}NBr$	Tetragonal	15.456(2)

[a] *indicates that the absolute configuration was deterimined by x-ray methods.
[b] Reference is made to a sodium salt in the paper by Blount et al. (1975), but x-ray data are only given for the silver salt.
[c] Reference is made to a "nearly isomorphous" manganese salt in the paper by Chaney et al. (1976), but no cell data were given.
[d] A sodium salt, isomorphous with the silver salt, was reported by Steinrauf, et al. (1968), but no details were given.
[e] The molecular formula given by Blount and Westley (1971) was revised by them (1975).

1. Koyama and Utsumi-Oda (1977).
2. Blount et al. (1975).
3. Jones et al. (1973).
4. Smith et al. (1978b).
5. Chaney et al. (1974).
6. Smith and Duax (1976).
7. Chaney et al. (1976).
8. Alléaume et al. (1975).
9. Ōtake et al. (1978).
10. Ōtake et al. (1977).
11. Czerwinski and Steinrauf (1971).
12. Alléaume and Hickel (1970).
13. Alléaume and Hickel (1972).
14. Alléaume (1974).
15. Toeplitz et al. (1979).
16. Shiro et al. (1978).

Å		Angle (°)			Z	Space group	References
b	c	α	β	γ			
23.61	10.65	90	90	90	4	$P2_12_12_1$	38
18.702(4)	12.923(3)	90	90	90	4	$P2_12_12_1$*	39
14.591(2)	12.080(2)	90	90	90	4	$P2_12_12_1$*	40,41,42
22.761(2)	10.493(1)	90	90	90	4	$P2_12_12_1$*	43,44
9.909(2)	48.708(7)	90	90	90	4	$P2_12_12_1$*	45
22.90	17.44	90	90	120	6	$P6_3$*	46
16.402	25.122	90	90	90	4	$P2_12_12_1$	47
15.456(2)	20.526(8)Å	90	90	90	4	$P4_32_12$*	48

17. Johnson et al. (1970a).
18. Johnson et al. (1970b).
19. Maier and Paul (1971).
20. C. I. Hejna, E. N. Duesler, and I. C. Paul, unpublished data (1972).
21. Schmidt et al. (1974).
22. Smith et al. (1978a).
23. Chiang and Paul (1977).
24. W. F. Paton and I. C. Paul, unpublished data (1978).
25. Westley et al. (1977).
26. Bissell and Paul (1972).
27. C. C. Chiang and I. C. Paul, unpublished data (1976).
28. Friedman et al. (1979).
29. Westley et al. (1974).
30. Riche and Pascard-Billy (1975).
31. Yamazaki et al. (1976).
32. Ōtake et al. (1975b).
33. Ōtake et al. (1975a).
34. Koenuma et al. (1976).
35. Pinkerton and Steinrauf (1970).
36. Smith and Duax (1979).
37. Agtarap et al. (1967).
38. Lutz et al. (1971).
39. Ward et al. (1978).
40. Kubota et al. (1968).
41. Steinrauf et al. (1968).
42. Shiro and Koyame (1970).
43. Kinashi et al. (1973).
44. Kinashi et al. (1975).
45. Pletcher and Weber (1974).
46. Blount and Westley (1971).
47. Blount and Westley (1975).
48. Westley et al. (1979).

Apart from the original papers, there has been relatively little in the way of classification or review of the three-dimensional structures. Among the most notable exceptions are a review by Truter (1976), in which she discussed the structures of the Ca^{2+} ionophores, and Westley (1977, 1978) has reviewed a number of aspects of the polyether antibiotics, including their structures. However, a more detailed discussion of the structures of the ionophores as revealed by x-ray analysis is certainly overdue. Unfortunately, full details of many of the structures have not been published and in many cases the atomic coordinates resulting from the x-ray analyses were not available. Nevertheless, a great deal of structural information is available and we hope that the present chapter will contribute to our knowledge of the polyether antibiotics and provide a fairly comprehensive account of what is known up to the late fall of 1979.

In the following sections the polyether antibiotics are discussed individually in alphabetic order, with most space being given to those for which coordinate data are accessible and to those which have been most extensively studied. At the conclusion of these descriptions there is a brief section discussing several general features of structural interest and how these features may relate to the biological functions of the acid ionophores.

II. POLYETHER ANTIBIOTICS

1. A-130 (Lenoremycin)

The crystal structure of the silver salt of this ionophore has been studied by two groups. The ionophore was named A-130 by Koyama and Utsumi-Oda (1977), while it was named Ro-21-6150 by Blount et al. (1975); this terminology was subsequently changed to lenoremycin. As the paper by Koyama and Utsumi-Oda (1977) contains much more crystallographic detail, including the atomic coordinates, most of the geometrical information contained in this section is based on that paper. However, as pointed out by these authors, the coordinates presented in their paper correspond to the absolute configuration opposite from that of the naturally occurring ionophore. All drawings and data in this section correspond to the true absolute configuration as determined by both groups. The atom numbering used in this section is shown on the structural formula (Figure 1). While a sodium salt is mentioned in one of the papers, the only derivative for which x-ray data are available is the silver salt. Two views of the molecular structure are shown in Figures 2 and 3. The anion of the ionophore is wrapped around the Ag^+ ion in the fashion typical of all complexed ionophores. The main chain, i.e., C(1)——C(47) is elliptical, with

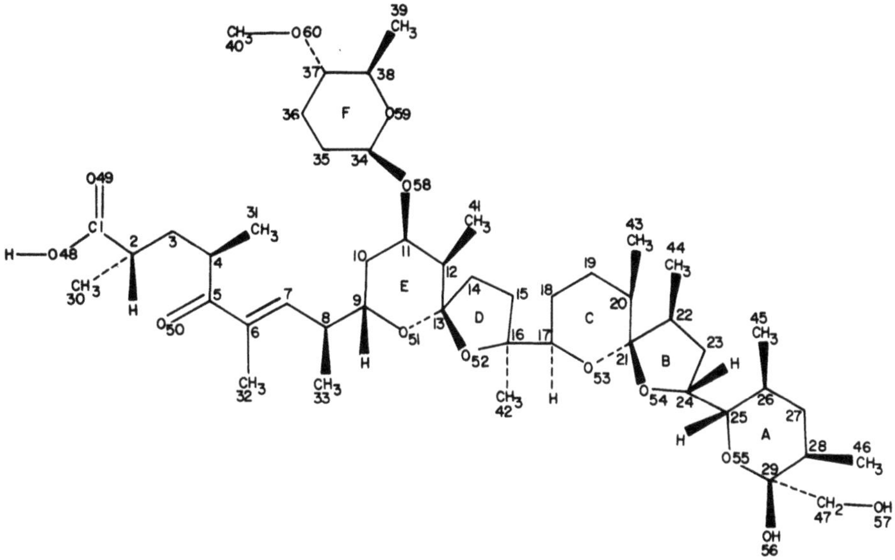

Figure 1 The structural formula of A-130 showing the atom numbering used in this discussion.

most of the oxygen atoms which are part of or directly attached to the main chain pointing to the interior of the ellipse; the exceptions are one of the carboxyl atoms, O(48), the ketone oxygen, O(50), and an ether oxygen O(51). The ellipse is stabilized by two essentially parallel hydrogen bonds involving the two hydroxyl groups attached to ring A and the two carboxylate oxygen atoms (Table 2). One face of the hydrophilic elliptical cavity is capped by ring F such that O(58) and O(59) are both coordinated to the Ag$^+$ ion; the methoxyl oxygen O(60) is not part of the interior of the structure.

Table 2 The O---O Distances (Å) Involved in the Hydrogen Bonds in A-130

O(56)——H---O(48)	2.673(9)
O(57)——H---O(49)	2.604(9)

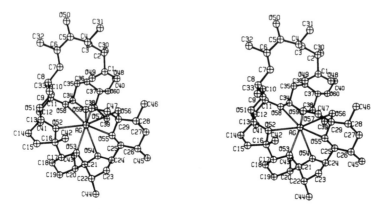

Figure 2   Stereoscopic view of the Ag⁺ salt of A-130. The Ag⁺——O coordination is represented by unshaded bonds.

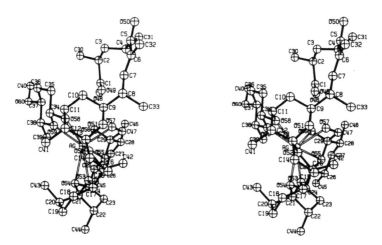

Figure 3   Another view of the Ag⁺ salt of A-130 at right angles to the view in Figure 2.

Table 3 Ag$^+$——O Coordination Distances (Å) in A-130

Ag$^+$——O(52)	2.751(6)	Ag$^+$——O(56)	3.006(7)
Ag$^+$——O(53)	2.483(5)	Ag$^+$——O(57)	2.375(7)
Ag$^+$——O(54)	2.875(6)	Ag$^+$——O(58)	2.672(6)
Ag$^+$——O(55)	2.636(6)	Ag$^+$——O(59)	2.461(6)

Source: Koyama and Utsumi-Oda, 1977.

The silver ion is eight coordinated, i.e., there are eight Ag$^+$——O distances in the range 2.375 to 3.006 Å (Table 3). It is interesting to note that neither of the carboxylate oxygen atoms is directly coordinated to the Ag$^+$ ion; the shorter Ag$^+$——O (carboxylate) distance is 3.990(6) Å. The coordination sphere of the Ag$^+$ is quite irregular, with the C(42)-methyl group filling what appears to be a gap in the coordinate sphere.

In general, the bond lengths and angles have normal values. Of interest is the geometry at the apiro ring junctions. At C(13), the junction between rings D and E, two of the angles, C(14)-C(13)-O(52) and C(14)-C(13)-O(51), are significantly less than tetrahedral,

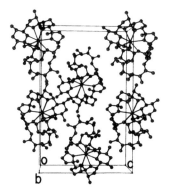 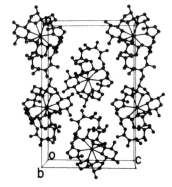

Figure 4 The arrangement of molecules in the crystal for A-130. The reference molecule, i.e. that for which coordinates are given, is the central molecule to the upper, back part of the unit cell.

102.4(7) and 104.9(9)°, while C(12)-C(13)-C(14) is considerably greater, 116.7(9)°. At C(21), the junction between rings B and C, another
unsymmetrical set of angles is found. However, while the corresponding angle C(20)-C(21)-C(22) is greatest [118.6(8)°], the two smaller
ones in this case are O(53)-C(21)-O(54) [104.0(6)°] and C(22)-C(21)-
O(54) [104.4(8)°].

The arrangement of molecules of A-130 in the unit cell is shown in
Figure 4. The packing is dominated by contacts between nonpolar
groups. None of the four oxygen atoms, O(48), O(50), O(51), and
O(60), that lie somewhat to the outside of the molecule appear to
play a significant role in the organization of the molecules in the
crystal.

The melting points of the Na⁺ salt (235°C) and Ag⁺ salt (157-
160°C) are comparable to those of organic molecules and are not typical of metal salts. As the crystal is dominated by nonpolar van der-
Waals contacts, this is not unexpected.

2. A 204A

In the case of A204A, x-ray structures have been reported on "nearly isomorphous" silver and sodium salts as 1:1 acetonates (Na salt;
mp 144 to 145°C) by Jones et al. (1973) and on the free acid as a 1:1:1
complex of ionophore:water:acetone (mp 96-98°C) by Smith et al.
(1978b). Coordinates have been published for both the salts and the
free acid. In the present discussion we shall adopt the numbering
scheme (Figure 5) used by Smith et al. (1978b).

The overall conformations of the two salts and the free acid are
very similar (see Figure 6 and 7). In the subsequent discussion we
shall describe only the structure of the sodium salt, as the structure
of the silver salt appears to be essentially identical to it (Jones et al.,
1973). In the sodium salt the conformation of the backbone of the
molecule is stabilized by "head-to-tail" hydrogen bonding between
O(14)——H---O(1) (carboxyl); the O(14)---O(1) distance is 2.69 Å.
The tertiary hydroxyl O(3)——H also forms a hydrogen bond to O(1);
O(3)---O(1) is 2.60 Å. The Na⁺ ion is complexed to six oxygen atoms,
both carboxyl oxygens, and four ether oxygens at distances of less
than 3.0 Å (Table 4). The molecular backbone has a rather complex
shape which rather resembles those of the metal cryptates (Dieterich
et al., 1973). Rings A to E are almost circular, providing a "basket"
lined with oxygen atoms in which the ion can sit. The rest of the main
chain loops above the basket to provide further complexing opportunities for the metal. Ring G is not involved in metal coordination and
does not appear to serve any functional role in the coordination. Several oxygen atoms [O(9), O(13), O((6), O(5), O(16), and O(17)],
all lie to the outside of the complex, making it appear more polar than

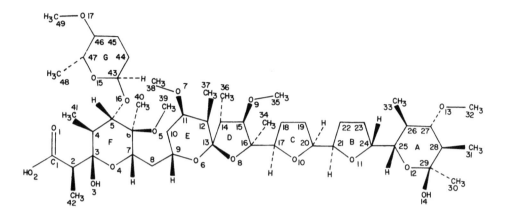

Figure 5 The structure of A204A showing the atom numbering.

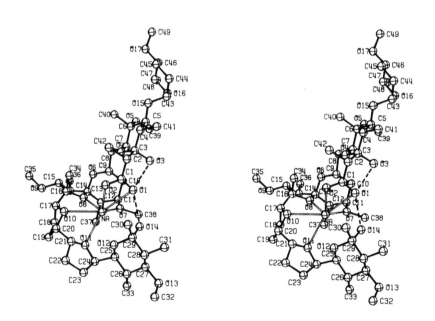

Figure 6 The structure of the Na$^+$ salt of A204A. Hydrogen bonds are shown by discontinuous lines.

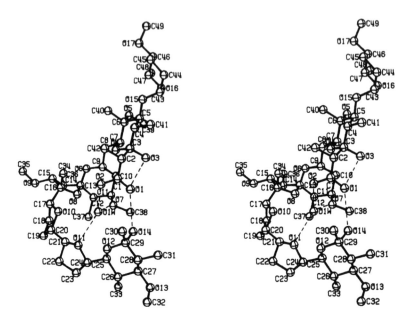

Figure 7   The structure of the free acid of A204A showing the enclosed
water molecule. Hydrogen bonds are indicated by discontinuous lines.

Table 4   Na$^+$—O Distances (Å) in the Na$^+$-A204A Complex Compared
with O(W)---O Distances (Å) in the Free Acid[a]

	Na$^+$	O(W)		Na$^+$	O(W)
O(1)	2.97	3.09(1)	O(8)	2.74	2.92(1)
O(2)	2.71	2.56(1)	O(10)	2.85	3.02(1)
O(7)	2.72	2.73(1)	O(11)	2.75	2.85(1)

[a]No standard deviations were given for the atomic coordinates of the
Na+ salt of A204A, hence deviations cannot be calculated for bond
distances of lengths.
Source: Smith et al., 1978.

the complexes of many other ionophores. The cavity for the metal
ions is from 5 to 6 Å in diameter.

Considering the opportunities for rotational freedom, especially in
the ring F to G region, the overall shape of the free acid is remarkably
similar to that of the salt. The changes in torsion angles in the backbone of the molecule are all less than 8° and those for all but four of
the 19 angles are less than 4° (Smith et al., 1978). In the free acid
the central cavity is occupied by the water molecule. Many hydrogen
atoms were located in this structure determination, allowing the hydrogen-bonding pattern to be established. The head-to-tail hydrogen
bond between $O(14)$——H and $O(1)$ is much longer (possibly as a result of the lack of charge on the carboxyl group), with a length of
2.99(1) Å, while the $O(3)$——H---$O(1)$ distance is 2.64(1) Å. The
water molecule acts as an acceptor forming an $O(2)$——H---(W) hydrogen bond of length 2.56(1) Å and as a donor of two hydrogen bonds
to the ether oxygen atoms $O(7)$ and $O(11)$. The $O(W)$---$O(7)$ and
$O(W)$---$O(11)$ lengths are 2.73(1) and 2.85(1) Å, respectively, and
the $O(7)$---$O(W)$---$O(11)$ angle is 110.6(3)°. The role of the $O(3)$——H
---$O(1)$ hydrogen bond in the structure of both Na⁺ salt and free acid
may be to lock the carboxyl group in an orientation where it can have
maximum interaction with both the ion and the water molecule. The
$C(42)$-$C(2)$-$C(1)$-$O(2)$ torsion angles in the salt and the acid are -5.7
and 4.7°, values that are close to an eclipsing position. The distances
of the enclosed water molecule from the oxygen atoms that coordinate
to the Na⁺ salt are also given in Table 4.

There are changes in the distribution of the bond angles at the
spiro ring junction, $C(13)$, between the acid and the salt. In both
compounds the smallest angle is $C(14)$-$C(13)$-$O(8)$; it is 102.8° in the
acid and 103.4° in the salt. However, $O(6)$-$C(13)$-$O(8)$ is the largest
angle in the acid (113.5°), while $C(14)$-$C(13)$-$C(12)$ is the largest
angle in the salt (118.9°).

The same groups of the salt and the acid are C2 and the cell dimensions are almost the same, and the crystal structures are likewise very
similar. A view of the crystal packing for the free acid of A204A is
shown in Figure 8. Both salts and the acid crystallize as 1:1 acetonates. The positions of the atoms in the acetone molecules were located. The acetone molecule is positioned to the $O(1)$——$O(3)$ region
of the ionophore; however, the distances are quite long [$O(1)$---$C(25)$
is 3.81 Å in the free acid)]. The acetone molecules, as pairs, are
trapped in cages in the crystal that are formed by eight ionophore
species (Figure 8).

3. A23187

This ionophore is rather unusual in that it complexes only divalent cations and also in that it contains three nitrogen atoms. It is a relative-

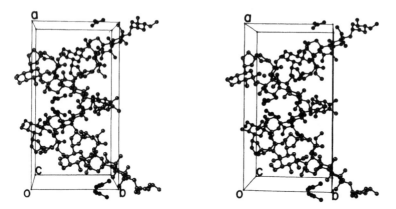

Figure 8 A view of the packing in the crystal of the free acid of
A 204A. The atoms and bonds of the acetone molecules have been
blackened. The reference molecule is the one to the upper, right corner of the unit cell. The "pocket" for the two acetone molecules and
part of its surroundings can be seen both to the left of the drawing
and to the lower right.

ly small molecule, $C_{29}H_{37}N_3O_6$, mol wt = 523.6, as ionophores go. In
the following discussion we have adopted the numbering system, shown
in Figure 9, used by Smith and Duax (1976) in their description of
the hydrated Ca^{2+} salt.

The crystal structures have been determined for the free acid of
A23187 (mp 181-182°C) as crystallized from acetone (Chaney et al.,
1974), and for two solvated calcium salts a dihydrate (Smith and Duax,
1976) and a diethanolate (Chaney et al., 1976). Reference is also made
by Chaney et al. (1976) to an unpublished structure of a manganese-
A23187 complex that is "nearly isomorphous" with the calcium diethanolate. There has apparently been no experimental determination of the
absolute configuration, it being assumed on the basis of the chiralities
found in other polyether ionophores with spiro six-membered rings.

A stereoscopic view of the free acid is shown in Figure 10. Here we
see the familiar circular shape with the polar atoms mainly directed
toward the interior and the exterior consisting of hydrocarbon
groups. The circular conformation is stabilized by three apparent
hydrogen bonds: N(25)——H---O(1C), N(2A)——H---O(1B), and
probably O(1C)——H---N(8) (Table 5); the latter hydrogen bond would
require an antiplanar configuration for the carboxyl group, which

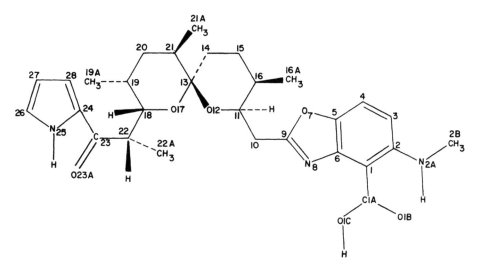

Figure 9 The structural formula of A23187 showing the atom numbering used in the present discussion.

would be quite unusual (Leiserowitz, 1976). However, the dimensions O(1C)---N(8) of 2.65(1) Å and C(1A)——O(1C)---N(8) of 92.9(5)° are consistent with such a hydrogen bond.

The structures of the two solvated calcium salts have many similarities but several interesting differences (Figure 11). Crystals of the dihydrate were obtained from a 95% ethanol solution, while the diethanolate was obtained from 50% ethanol; the exact conditions and de-

Table 5 Hydrogen-Bonding Dimensions in the Free Acid of A-23187

	Distance (Å)		Angle (°)
N(2A)---O(1B)	2.72(1)	C(2)-N(2A)---O(1B)	86.4(5)
N(25)---O(1C)	3.04(1)	C(24)-N(25)---O(1C)	121.1(6)
O(1C)---N(8)	2.65(1)	C(1A)-O(1C)---N(8)	92.9(5)

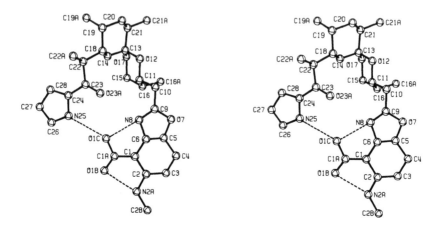

Figure 10 Stereoscopic view of the free acid of A23187. Hydrogen bonds are shown by discontinuous lines.

tails of the crystallization procedure were not published, but they presumably account for the incorporation of different solvents. The cell data for the two solvates are quite similar (Table 1), but the space groups are different; they are C2 in the case of dihydrate and $P2_12_12_1$ in the case of diethanolate. In both complexes the calcium ion is co-ordinated to two A23187 anions and the structures of the two complexes possess pseudo twofold rotational symmetry. In each case the Ca^{2+} ion is coordinated to O(1C), O(23A), and N(8) in both anions. However, while in the diethanolate the metal ion is six-coordinated, in the dihydrate one of the solvent water molecules fills a seventh coordination site along the pseudo twofold axis (Figure 11b). In the diethanolate the coordination sphere is a fairly regular octahedron, with the O—Ca^{2+}—O, O—Ca^{2+}—N, and N—Ca^{2+}—N angles falling into the ranges 83.5(8) to 99.7(9)° and 171.2(9) to 176.2(9)° (Table 6), the Ca^{2+}—O distances range from 1.93(2) to 2.10(2) Å, while the Ca^{2+}—N distances are 2.21(2) and 2.22(2) Å. In the dihydrate one of the two water molecules enters the coordination sphere of the calcium ion, causing considerable distortion. This water molecule O(1S) lies along the pseudo twofold axis. Most of the distortion of the octahedral arrangement arises from a mutual displacement of the two anions rather than from any conformational change in the anions between the two salts. There is also a significant increase in the Ca^{2+}—— ligand

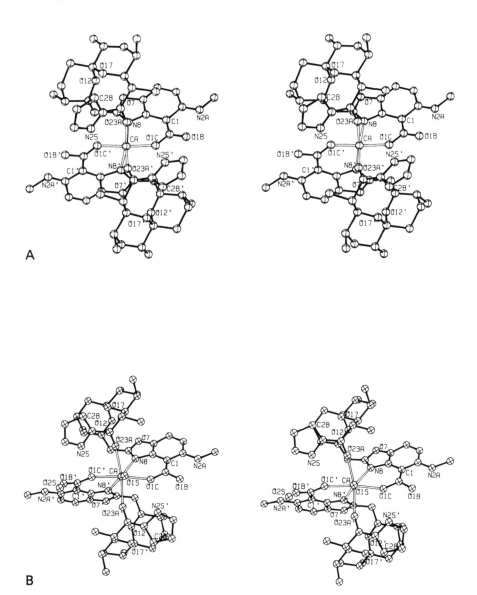

A

B

Figure 11 Stereoscopic views of the two calcium salts of A 23187.
(a) The diethanolate. (b) The dihydrate. In each case the pseudo
twofold axis is virtually normal to the plane of the paper.

Table 6 Distances (Å) and Angles (°) Defining the Octahedron in the Two Calcium Salts of A23187

Diethanolate

Ca^{2+}—O(1C)	2.00(2)		Ca^{2+}—O(1C')	1.93(2)
Ca^{2+}—N(8)	2.22(3)		Ca^{2+}—N(8')	2.21(2)
Ca^{2+}—O(23A)	2.10(2)		Ca^{2+}—O(23A')	2.03(3)
O(1C)—Ca^{2+}—N(8)	83.5(8)		O(1C')—Ca^{2+}—N(8')	84.1(9)
O(1C)—Ca^{2+}—O(23A)	89.1(8)		O(1C')—Ca^{2+}—O(23A')	90.4(9)
N(8)—Ca^{2+}—O(23A)	85.1(8)		N(8')—Ca^{2+}—O(23A')	87.0(9)
O(1C)—Ca^{2+}—O(23A)	99.7(8)		O(1C')—Ca^{2+}—N(8)	96.3(8)
O(1C)—Ca^{2+}—O(23A')	89.7(8)		O(1C')—Ca^{2+}—O(23A)	87.1(8)
N(8)—Ca^{2+}—N(8')	95.5(9)		O(23A)—Ca^{2+}—O(23A')	93.5(8)
N(8)—Ca^{2+}—O(23A')	173.1(9)		N(8')—Ca^{2+}—O(23A)	171.2(9)
O(1C)—Ca^{2+}—O(1C')	176.2(9)			

Dihydrate

Ca^{2+}—O(1C)	2.27(1)		Ca^{2+}—O(1C')	2.28(1)
Ca^{2+}—N(8)	2.69(1)		Ca^{2+}—N(8')	2.58(1)
Ca^{2+}—O(23A)	2.37(1)		Ca^{2+}—O(23A')	2.38(1)
Ca^{2+}—O(1S)	2.38(1)			

O(1C)—Ca^{2+}—N(8)	68.4(4)	O(1C)—Ca^{2+}—N(8')	70.6(4)
O(1C)—Ca^{2+}—O(23A)	106.7(5)	O(1C')—Ca^{2+}—O(23A')	89.8(4)
N(8)—Ca^{2+}—O(23A)	75.9(4)	N(8')—Ca^{2+}—O(23A')	76.0(4)
O(1C)—Ca^{2+}—N(8')	109.8(4)	O(1C')—Ca^{2+}—N(8)	118.9(4)
O(1C)—Ca^{2+}—O(23A')	87.7(4)	O(1C')—Ca^{2+}—O(23A)	79.0(5)
N(8)—Ca^{2+}—N(8')	77.0(4)	O(23A)—Ca^{2+}—O(23A')	153.4(4)
N(8)—Ca^{2+}—O(23A')	130.2(4)	N(8')—Ca^{2+}—O(23A)	121.4(4)
O(1C)—Ca^{2+}—O(1C')	172.0(5)	O(1C')—Ca^{2+}—O(1S)	90.5(5)
O(1C)—Ca^{2+}—O(1S)	85.5(5)	N(8')—Ca^{2+}—O(1S)	148.5(5)
N(8)—Ca^{2+}—O(1S)	134.5(5)	N(23A')—Ca^{2+}—O(1S)	79.1(5)
O(23A)—Ca^{2+}—O(1S)	76.9(5)		

distances; the four Ca^{2+}——O (anion) distances are in the range 2.27 to 2.38(1) Å, the two Ca^{2+}——N distances are 2.58(1) and 2.69(1) Å, while the Ca^{2+}——O (water) distance is 2.38(1) Å. The angles that would be 90° in a regular octahedron vary by as much as from 68.4(4) to 153.4(4)°, while the angles that would be 180° vary from 121.4(6) to 172.0(6)°. The position and orientation of the O(1C)——Ca^2——O(1C') vector are relatively unaffected by the addition of the water molecule.

Torsion angles that define the conformation of the ionophore are given in Table 7. There is a very significant difference between the conformation of the ionophore in the uncomplexed free acid form and that found in the complexed ionic forms. This difference is accomplished mainly by changes in the torsion angles around C(9)-C(10) and C(10)-C(11), and also by changes around C(22)-C(23); the alteration in shape of the ionophore by rotation about these bonds is shown in Figure 12, which looks down on the plane of the fused ring system in the free acid and in one of the anions in the diethanolate. The torsion angles in all four cyrstallographically independent anions are quite similar. Differences between the torsion angles in the anions in the two distinct salts are comparable to the differences between the angles in the two anions in a single salt. In all forms of A23187 investigated, the N(H)——C$\equiv$O group is in the cis configuration. There are some interesting changes in the hydrogen-bonding patterns in going from the free acid to the salts. The N(2A)---O(1B) hydrogen bond is present in all the structures, although it is significantly shorter (2.55 to 2.64 Å) in the salts as compared to 2.72 Å in the free acid. The ionization of the carboxylic acid group in the salts prevents the formation of the O(1C)---N(8) hydrogen bond found in the acid, although the distances remain quite short, 2.78 to 2.82 Å. The conformational changes that occur upon metal complex formation do not permit formation of the N(25)---O(1C) hydrogen bond within a single A23187 anion as was found in the acid. However, this hydrogen bond is replaced by N(25)---O(1C') and N(25')---O(1C) hydrogen bonds between the two anions in the complex. The dimensions of the hydrogen bonds in the salts are found in Table 8.

The packing of the free acid A23187 molecules is shown in Figure 13. The molecule crystallizes without incorporation of solvent and the packing is largely dominated by nonpolar contacts. There is a relatively short contact between the carboxylic acid group in the reference molecule and the ring oxygen atom O(7) in the molecule at $\bar{x}$, $-\frac{1}{2} + y$, $1 - z$; the O(1C)---O(7) distance is 3.19(1) Å. However, the geometry is inappropriate for hydrogen bonding, as O(7) lies above the plane of the carboxyl group with a C(1)——O(1C)---O(7) angle of 71.9(2)°.

The structure of the Ca^{2+} salt of A23187 in the dihydrate form has a relatively open region where one of the water molecules, O(1S), is complexed to Ca^{2+} (see Figure 11b). In the crystal two salts related

Table 7 Torsion Angles in A23187 Derivatives

Torsion angle	Free acid	Ca^{2+} salt diethanolate		Ca^{2+} salt dihydrate	
		Unprimed	Primed	Unprimed	Primed
O(1C)-C(1A)-C(1)-C(6)	0.3	11.6	25.1	2.2	12.4
N(8)-C(9)-C(10)-C(11)	-46.3	73.8	78.3	90.3	80.5
C(9)-C(10)-C(11)-O(12)	174.4	64.4	56.0	50.7	55.7
C(10)-C(11)-O(12)-C(13)	-173.9	-174.9	-172.7	-173.3	-173.4
C(11)-O(12)-C(13)-O(17)	59.6	61.3	57.5	62.1	58.1
O(12)-C(13)-O(17)-C(18)	60.1	55.4	60.0	58.0	62.3
C(13)-O(17)-C(18)-C(22)	-173.4	-169.2	-171.7	-169.3	-170.2
O(17)-C(18)-C(22)-C(23)	65.7	61.9	72.9	62.5	57.3
C(18)-C(22)-C(23)-O(12A)	30.9	79.1	65.9	67.0	79.1
C(18)-C(22)-C(23)-C(24)	-158.0	-102.1	-110.2	-115.7	-96.0
C(22)-C(23)-C(24)-N(25)	-170.5	164.8	165.1	-173.1	171.9

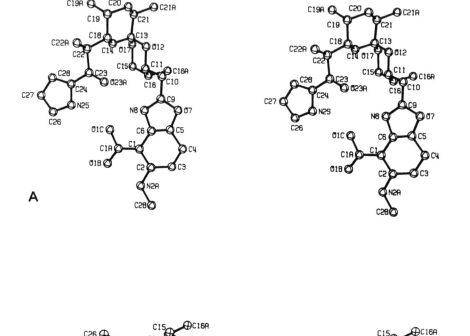

Figure 12 (a) Stereoscopic view of a single molecule of the A23187 free aicd. (b) Stereoscopic view of one of the A23187 anions in the Ca^{2+} salt ethanolate.

Table 8 Hydrogen-Bonding Distances (Å) in the Ca^{2+} Salts of A23187

	Dihydrate	Diethanolate
N(2A)---O(1B)	2.56(3)	2.55(3)
N(2A')---O(1B')	2.64(2)	2.58(4)
N(25)---O(1C')	2.82(2)	2.77(3)
N(25')---O(1C)	2.85(2)	2.91(3)

by the twofold crystallographic axis come together, with these regions adjacent to each other (Figure 14). The two crystallographically related noncomplexed water molecules O(2S) and O(2S)[I] (I designates the atoms related by x̄, y, 1 − z to the reference ones) are involved in hydrogen bonds that serve to link the two salts and thus hold the "dimer" together. The noncomplexed water molecule O(2S)[I] accepts a hydrogen bond from the complexed water molecule O(1S) and in turn acts as a donor in a hydrogen bond to O(1B')[I]. The O(1S)---O(2S)[I] and O(2S)[I]---O(1B')[I] distances are 2.84(4) and 2.51(3) Å, respectively. A schematic view of the hydrogen-bonding arrangement is shown

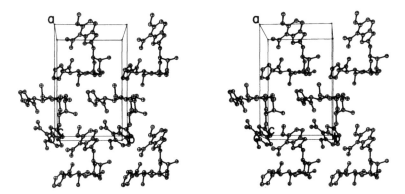

Figure 13 A stereoscopic view of the packing of the free acid A23187 molecules in the crystal. The reference molecule is inside the cell to the lower right of the cell. Its bonds have been blackened.

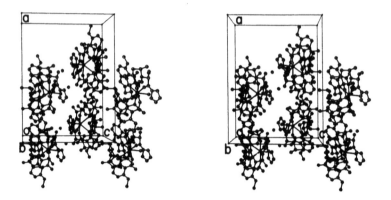

Figure 14   Stereoscopic view of the packing in the Ca²⁺ salt of A23187 dihydrate. The reference molecule is the one at the lower left of the picture.

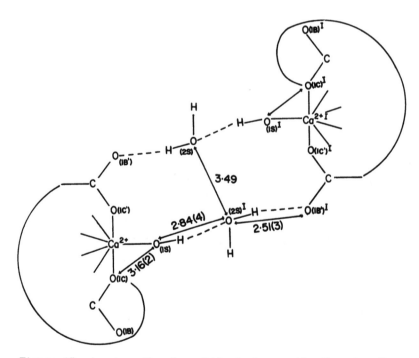

Figure 15   A schematic view of the hydrogen bonding that links the two Ca²⁺ salts of A23187 in the dihydrate crystal. The superscripts I refer to the molecule at x̄, y, 1 − z.

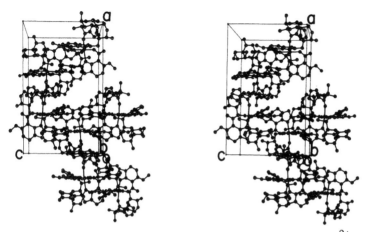

Figure 16 Stereoscopic view of the packing of the Ca^{2+} salt of A23187 diethanolate. The reference molecules are to the near lower right-hand corner of the cell. The volume occupied by the two disordered ethanol molecules can be seen to the near center and toward the lower right of the cell.

in Figure 15. There is no strong evidence for additional hydrogen bonds involving these water molecules. The O(2S)---O(2S)^I distance is 3.49(4) Å and would involve a disordered arrangement for the hydrogen atoms as it passes across the two-fold axis. O(1S) may be involved in a very weak intracomplex hydrogen bond to O(1C); the O(1S)---O(1C) distance is 3.16 Å and the O(1C)---O(1S)---O(2S)^I angle is 173(1)°; if this contact did correspond to a hydrogen bond, it would be along the edge of the Ca^{2+} ion coordination sphere.

The packing of the Ca^{2+} salt in the diethanolate form is shown in Figure 16. In this crystal the two ethanol molecules were disordered. While it appears that at least the oxygen atoms were located, atomic coordinates for the atoms of the solvent molecules were not published (Chaney et al., 1976). There is no evidence in this structure for the hydrogen-bonded dimers present in the dihydrate crystal. One of the ethanol molecules is hydrogen bonded to O(1B)' of the complex, while the second ethanol is hydrogen bonded to the first (Chaney et al., 1976). The space in the crystal occupied by the solvent molecules can be seen in Figure 16 at the center of the cell and toward the lower-right-hand corner.

4. Acanthifolicin

The structure of an antibiotic, acanthifolicin, obtained from marine sources having many of the features of a polyether ionophore has been

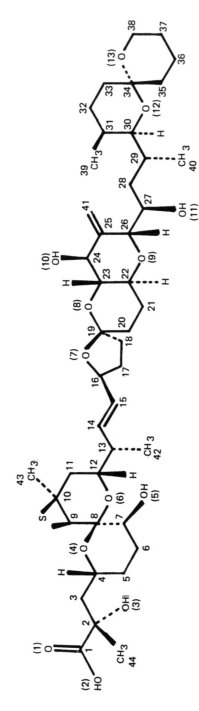

Figure 17 A drawing of the structure of acanthifolicin showing the atom numbering. (Source: van der-Helm, 1981.)

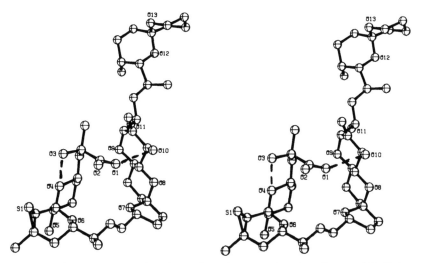

Figure 18 Stereoscopic view of a single molecule of acanthifolicin. Intramolecular hydrogen bonds are shown by distoncinuous lines and oxygen atoms are blackened. (Source: van der Helm, 1981.)

reported recently (Schmitz et al., 1981). The structure of the $C_{44}H_{68}O_{13}S$ molecule is shown in Figure 17. Acanthifolicin has a terminal carboxylic acid group, seven ether rings, and three hydroxyl groups. The molecule has a 38-carbon chain and two unusual features, an episulfide ring and two fused six-membered ether rings. It is thus the first potential polyether ionophore to contain sulfur. The molecule also contains fewer alkyl side groups than is the case for almost all the other compounds described in this chapter.

The x-ray structure analysis was carried out on a crystal of the free acid obtained from a chloroform:benzene mixture and which contained two disordered benzene molecules of crystallization. A stereoscopic view of the structure is shown in Figure 18. In the free acid form part of the molecule adopts a circular conformation stabilized by a hydrogen bond of 2.93 Å between the $O(10)$——H hydroxyl group and the carboxylic acid group. The circular cavity so produced is lined with a number of oxygen molecules and is of the appropriate size to complex metal ions. As of yet, however, there is no information on the metal-complexing ability of acanthifolicin. The rest of the molecule (C-26 to C-38) is pointed away from the polar cavity. There appears to be intermolecular hydrogen bonding involving $O(2)$ and $O(5)$.

5. Alborixin

As the coordinates for the potassium salt have not been publihsed and were not available to us, a detailed discussion of the structure of alborixin is not possible. The structure of the potassium salt (mp 209-

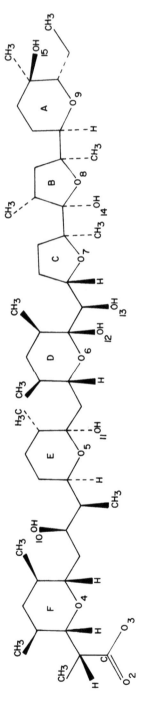

Figure 19   The structure of alborixin with the atom numbering used in the discussion.

Table 9 K^+——O Distances (Å) in the K^+ Salt of Alborixin[a]

K^+——O(2)	2.89	K^+——O(10)	2.71
K^+——O(7)	3.07	K^+——O(11)	2.98
K^+——O(8)	2.81	K^+——O(12)	2.69
K^+——O(9)	2.76	K^+——O(15)	2.76

[a]Standard deviations were not published.
Source: Data are taken from Alléaume et al. (1975).

210°C) has been determined by Alleaume et al. (1975); the free acid is
an amorphous solid (mp 100-115°C). No picture of the structure of
the salt was published. Alborixin (Figure 19) is closely related to
X-206 and the conformation of the backbone in these two ionophores
is very similar.* The backbone "describes a path similar to that of
the seam of a tennis ball" (Alléaume et al., 1975). The hydrogen
bonding and coordination of the cations are slightly different between
alborixin and X-206. The conformation of alborixin is stabilized by
intramolecular hydroben bonding; head to tail between the hydroxyl
group on the terminal ring A [O(15)] and a carboxylate oxygen [O(2)]
of length 2.64 Å, a hydrogen bond between the hydroxyl group [O(12)]
attached to ring D and the other carboxylate oxygen atom [O(3)] of
length 2.58 Å, and one between the hydroxyl groups O(11) and O(14)
of length 2.78 Å. The potassium ion complexes with eight oxygen atoms
in a distorted cubic arrangement; distances ranging from 2.69 to 3.07
Å are listed in Table 9. It is of interest to note that in the case of this
salt the potassium ion is coordinated to one of the carboxylate oxygen
atoms [O(2)] as well as to three ether oxygen atoms and four hydroxyl
oxygen atoms. It has been stated (Clark, 1963) that metal coordination
to two oxygen atoms hydrogen bonded to each other is unusual; however, in this salt such a coordination occurs involving O(2) and O(15).

6. Antibiotic 6016

Antibiotic 6016 is isolated as a crystalline sodium salt (mp 192-195°C
decomp.) and the structure was determined by a x-ray analysis of
the thallium salt (Otake et al., 1978). The absolute configuration was
determined also. The molecular structure is shown in Figure 20.

---

*As this review was being completed a note was published (Seto et al.,
1979) giving a revised structure for alborixin. This corrected structure is shown in Figure 19.

Antibiotic 6016 is unusual in having a hydroxyl group at C(2), i.e., at the α-carbon to the carboxyl group, and also a sugar group at ring D. The structure of the thallium salt (Figure 21) has the familiar head-to-tail hydrogen bond between a hydroxyl [O(14)] on ring F and one of the carboxylate oxygen atoms O(2); the O(14)---O(2) length is 2.75 Å. The Tl$^+$ ion is complexed with six oxygen atoms, both carboxylate oxygens and four ether oxygens; the Tl$^+$—O distances are given in Table 10. The other two hydroxyl groups [i.e., O(3) and O(5)] appear to be involved in hydrogen bonding to the carboxylate group to the other side from the Tl$^+$ ion. The O(5)---O(2) distance is 2.61 Å and the C(3)—O(5)---O(2) angle is 85.7°, while the O(3)---O(1) distance is 2.60 Å, and the C(2)—O(3)---O(1) angle is 65.9°. Both of these hydrogen bonds must be significantly non-linear. Possibly these hydrogen bonds are important in holding the carboxylate group in an orientation whereby both oxygen atoms can enter the coordination sphere of the metal ion. Ring G appears to play no role in the metal complex formation and points away from the generally circular shape of the complex. Also, ring A is in a short loop and does not participate in coordination to Tl$^+$, although the ring ether oxygen atom [O(4)] is directed toward the center of the complex. However, the ether oxygen, O(6), and the three ether oxygen groups in or attached to ring G [O(11), O(1'), and O(2')] are all to the exterior of the salt.

There is a spiro ring junction at C(13); the limits of the bond angles are C(14)-C(13)-O(9) at 104.4° and C(12)-C(13)-C(14) at 115.1°.

The packing of the Tl$^+$ salt of antibiotic 6016 is shown in Figure 22. Ring G can be seen to point into a cavity surrounded by several other ionophore moieties, but none of its oxygen atoms are involved in short contacts. Thus the packing of the salt contains no obvious clues as to the role of ring G in the biological activity.

7. Carriomycin

The structure of carriomycin was determined by the x-ray analysis of the Tl$^+$ salt (Otake et al., 1977). The free acid was obtained as crystalline needles (mp 120-122°C) and the sodium salt melts at 180-182°C. The absolute configuration was obtained by anomalous dispersion. The molecular structure of carriomycin is shown in Figure 23.

The molecule is wrapped around the Tl$^+$ ion in the usual way (Figure 24). There are eight Tl$^+$—O distances of less than 3.25 Å (Table 11), and six, which might be considered to be coordinated, are less than 3.02 Å. The Tl$^+$ coordinates with both carboxylate oxygen atoms, and with four ether oxygen atoms [O(7), O(8), O(10), and O(11)]. The Tl$^+$—O(12) and Tl$^+$—O(13) distances of 3.17(1) and 3.23(1) Å, respectively, are considered too long to represent genuine coordinations, although they are the only oxygen atoms close to the Tl$^+$ ion in

Table 10 Tl⁺—O Distances (Å) in the Tl⁺ Salt of Antibiotic 6016[a]

Tl⁺—O(1)	2.88	Tl⁺—O(9)	2.86
Tl⁺—O(2)	2.94	Tl⁺—O(10)	2.92
Tl⁺—O(8)	2.84	Tl⁺—O(12)	2.81

[a] Standard deviations for the atomic coordinates were not available.

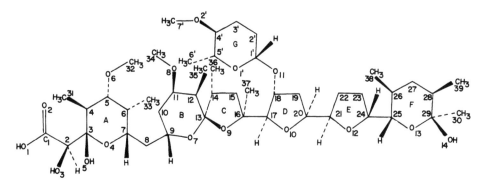

Figure 20 The structure of antibiotic 6016 showing the atom number-ing used in the discussion.

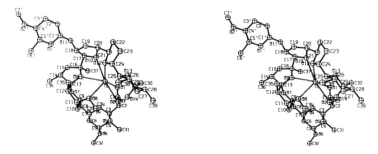

Figure 21 A stereoscopic view of the Tl⁺ salt of antibiotic 6016. The Tl⁺—O coordination is shown by open lines. Ring G is to the upper left of the figure and the ring A "loop" is to the bottom.

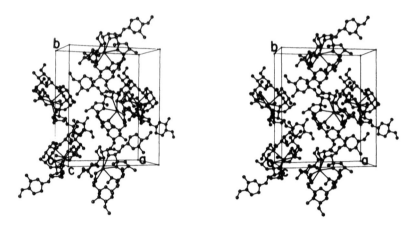

Figure 22 A stereoscopic view of the packing of the Tl$^+$ salt of antibiotic 6016. The reference molecule is to the lower left of the cell.

that area of the molecule. There is a head-to-tail hydrogen bond between the hydroxyl on ring F, O(13), and the carboxylate oxygen
O(2); the O(13)---O(2) distance is 2.76(2) Å. There is probably also
a hydrogen bond between the β-hydroxyl, O(4), and O(2); the
O(4)---O(2) distance is 2.60(2) Å. This latter hydrogen bond is possibly responsible for holding the carboxylate group in an orientation
whereby both oxygens are complexed to Tl$^+$, as the C(31)-C(2)-C(1)-
O(2) torsion angle is 171°.* Ring G is in a position well to the outside
of the complex. The oxygen atoms of ring G, O(5), O(1'), and O(2'),
and the ether oxygen atoms O(3) and O(9) appear to play no role in
metal coordination and tend to lie on the surface of the complex. The
bond angles at the spiro ring junction, C(13), lie in the range 106 to
115(1)° and are more uniform than is often the case at such junctions.

8. Dianemycin

The crystallography of four salts (Na$^+$, K$^+$, Rb$^+$, and Tl$^+$) of dianemycin has been studied by Czerwinski and Steinrauf (1971). Unfortunately, atomic coordinates have not been published and are not available to us; therefore our discussion has to be based entirely on the

---

*This is the value given by Ōtake et al. (1977). Using the coordin-
ates deposited with this paper, we have been unable to reproduce this
value. The problem appears to be with the coordinates of C(31), most
probably the y coordinate. We have arbitrarily repositioned C(31) in
the drawings such that the dimensions are reasonable.

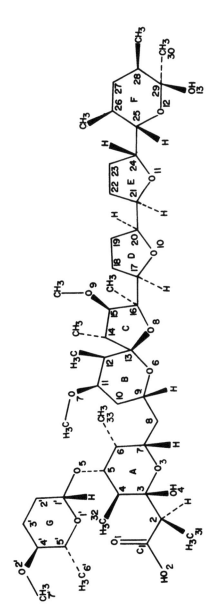

Figure 23 The structure of carriomycin showing the atom numbering used in this discussion.

Table 11 The Tl⁺——O Distances (Å) in the Tl⁺ Salt of Carriomycin

Tl⁺——O(1)	2.73(1)	Tl⁺——O(10)	3.01(1)
Tl⁺——O(2)	3.00(1)	Tl⁺——O(11)	2.85(1)
Tl⁺——O(7)	2.82(1)	Tl⁺——O(12)[a]	3.17(1)
Tl⁺——O(8)	2.87(1)	Tl⁺——O(13)[a]	3.23(1)

[a]These contacts probably do not correspond to coordinations.

single preliminary published account in 1971. The structural formula
of dianemycin is shown in Figure 25. All four salts examined are said
to be isomorphous in the space group $P2_12_12_1$, and cell data were given
for the potassium salt (Table 1). The potassium salt and, presumably,
the other three salts crystallize as monohydrates. Structure analyses
were carried out on the sodium, potassium, and thallium complexes,
and at the stage of the publication R factors in the range 0.13 to 0.15
were obtained. A view of the "dianemycin complex" (Czerwinski and
Steinrauf, 1971) is shown in Figure 26. The antibiotic has the familiar
circular shape stabilized by head-to-tail hydrogen bonding involving
the ——CH₂OH group attached to the terminal six-membered ring (A)
and one of the carboxylate oxygen atoms. There is also a hydrogen
bond from the secondary hydroxyl group of the same ring to a water
molecule, which in turn forms a hydrogen bond with the other carboxylate oxygen atom. There also appears to be a hydrogen bond between the hydroxyl group attached to ring E and the second carboxylate oxygen atom, which has a further stabilizing influence on the

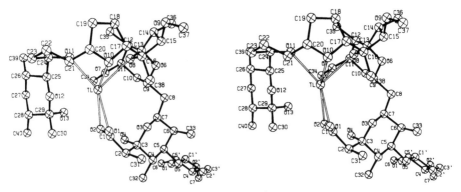

Figure 24 A stereoscopic view of the Tl⁺ salt of carriomycin. The
Tl⁺——O coordinations are shown as open lines.

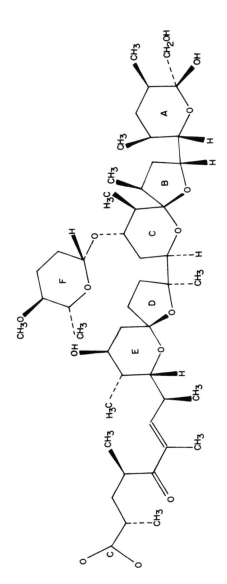

Figure 25 The structure of dianemycin. No atom numbering was given in the original paper.

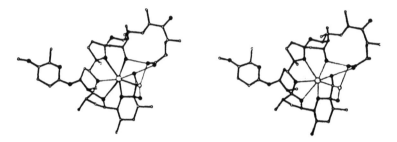

Figure 26 Stereoscopic drawing of the dianemycin complex. (Source: Czerwinski and Steinrauf, 1971.)

conformation of the ionized ionophore. The cation is seven-coordinated to four ether oxygen atoms, two hydroxyl oxygen atoms, and the water molecule; significantly, the carboxylate group is not involved in the coordination. No hydrogen-bonding distance nor metal—oxygen distances were given in the publication. Ring F, which is joined to the main backbone by an ether linkage, is not involved in the metal coordination or intramolecular hydrogen bonding and would seem to have a very minor role to play in the action of metal coordination.

9. Grisorixin

While the coordinates for x-ray structures on this antibiotic have not been published and were not available to us, short descriptions of the free acid monohydrate (Alléaume, 1974), a silver salt (Alléaume and Hickel, 1970), and a monohydrated thallium salt (Alléaume and Hickel, 1972) have

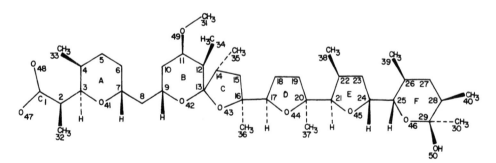

Figure 27 The structure of grisorixin showing the atom numbering used in the discussion.

been published. The structure of grisorixin is shown in Figure 27, which indicates the atom numbering used in this discussion. The absolute configuration was determined. The conformations of grisorixin in the free acid form and as the Ag^+ and Tl^+ salts are effectively the same. Views of the Tl^+ salt structure and the free acid are shown in Figures 28 and 29. The structures have the by-now familar features. The molecule is held together in the salts by O(50)——H---O(48) (carboxylate) hydrogen bonding (2.64 Å for the Ag^+ salt and 2.73 Å for the Tl^+ salt); in the free acid the same donor-acceptor arrangement appears to exist, although the distance was not given. Grisorixin has only one hydroxyl group; hence there are no opportunities for further stabilization of the conformation by additional hydrogen bonds.

In the Ag^+ salt the cation is enclosed in a hydrophilic cavity with a five-coordinated arrangement. The Ag^+——O(47) (carboxylate) distance is 2.20 Å, while the four Ag^+——O(ether) distances lie between 2.4 and 2.7 Å. In the case of the nonisomorphous Tl^+ salt monohydrate the Tl^+ ion is coordinated to the same five oxygen atoms [O(43), O(44), O(45), O(47), and O(49)], but the Tl^+——O distances are longer (2.6 to 3.0 Å). The enlargement of the oxygen-lined pocket is accomplished by rotations of approximately 10° about the C(16)-C(17), C(20)-C(21), and C(24)-C(25) bonds; these three bonds link ether-containing rings.

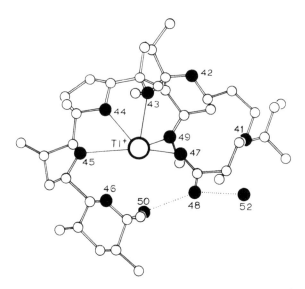

Figure 28 A view of the structure of the Tl^+-grisorixin salt. The oxygen atoms are blackened. Tl^+——O coordinations are indicated by thin lines, while hydrogen bonds are shown by dashed lines. O(52) is a water of crystallization.

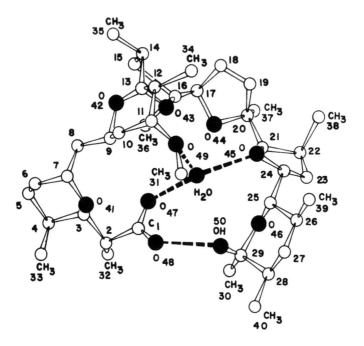

Figure 29   A drawing of the structure of the free acid of grisorixin monohydrate. The oxygen atoms are blackened. Hydrogen bonds are shown by discontinuous lines.

The slightly larger pocket "forces out" the outermost of the two carboxylate oxygen atoms [O(48)] such that it is in a position to form a hydrogen bond to the water molecule O(52) (see Figure 28); the O(48)---O(52) distance is 2.87 Å. In the free acid structure the cavity or pocket is of the same shape and size as in the Ag⁺ complex and is filled with a water molecule. The water molecule donates a hydrogen to form hydrogen bonds to the ether oxygen atoms, O(45) and O(49), and accepts a hydrogen bond from the un-ionized carboxyl group, O(47). The O---O distances lie in the range 2.5 to 2.8 Å. The O(50)——H---O(48) hydrogen bond found in the salts persists in the free acid (Alléaume and Hickel, 1970).

It is of interest that the structure of the *free acid monohydrate* of *grixorixin* was solved by virtue of its isomorphism with the structure of the Ag⁺ salt of *nigericin*; nigericin and grisorixin differ only in nigericin having a CH_2OH group at C(29) instead of a CH_3 group.

10. Ionomycin

Ionomycin is a particularly interesting ionophore, with several distinctive features. The structural formula is shown in Figure 30. The

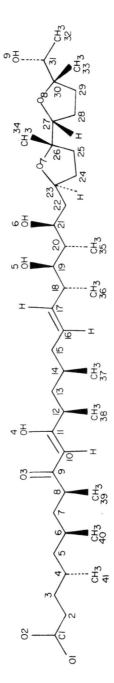

Figure 30 The structure of ionomycin showing the atom numbering used in the present discussion.

molecule has only two rings but has an ethylenic double bond as part of the main chain and an enolzied βdiketone group also in the main chain. This latter feature permits the ionophore to act as a dibasic acid in complexing Ca^{2+} and Cd^{2+} ions. Unlike other ionophores, such as A23187 and lasalocid, which coordinate divalent cations, ionomycin does so as a 1:1 complex. The unsaturation in the main chain also undoubtedly adds to the rigidity of the backbone and contributes to the conformational integrity which is such a major feature of metal ion-ionophore complexes. The crystallography of the metal salts of ionomycin is quite complex and has been carefully studied and fully described by Toeplitz et al. (1979). These authors have carried out structure analyses on a Ca^{2+} salt and on two distinct modifications of a Cd^{2+} salt. The Ca^{2+} salt and one of the forms of the Cd^{2+} salt are isomorphous, crystallizing in the orthorhombic space group $P2_12_12_1$. In this form two of the ionomycin-M^{2+} complexes are related by an exact crystallographic twofold rotation axis and indeed form a dimer by virtue of intermolecular hydrogen bonding. The other form of the Cd^{2+} salt crystallizes in the monoclinic space group $P2_1$, but with two crystallographically independent ionomycin-Cd^{2+} complexes. These two complexes are related by a pseudo (*but* noncrystallographic) twofold rotation axis and are once again joined by intermolecular hydrogen bonding. By carrying out x-ray analyses on both forms of the Cd^{2+} salt and the orthorhombic Ca^{2+} salt, Toeplitz et al. (1979) obtained results on four crystallographically distinct examples of an ionomycin-metal ion complex, although two are isomorphous and the other two are in the same crystal. The structures of all four complexes so obtained are very similar, as are the modes of dimer formation.

The three-dimensional structure of the orthorhombic Cd^{2+} salt is shown in Figure 31. The absolute configuration was determined by x-ray methods. As the metal coordination and internal hydrogen bonding are virtually identical in all "four" complexes, our discussion will describe the orthorhombic Cd^{2+} salt with the relevant dimensions for the other complexes given in Tables 12 and 13. The Cd^{2+} ion is complexed to seven oxygen atoms: one of the carboxylate oxygens, O(2); the two oxygen atoms of the enolized β-diketone, O(3) and O(4); two hydroxyl groups, O(6) and O(9); and two ether groups, O(7) and O(8) (Table 12). A strong case may be made for the Cd^{2+} to be only six-coordinated, as six of the Cd^{2+}——O distances lie in the range 2.25 to 2.39 Å and the seventh, O(8), is 3.05 Å from the Cd^{2+}. The arrangement of oxygen atoms around Cd^{2+} is close to octahedral, with O(7) and O(8) appearing to "share" one coordination site (Figure 31). The ionophore wraps around the metal ion, providing full three-dimensional protection. There is a head-to-tail hydrogen bond between the hydroxyl group O(9)——H and O(1) of the carboxylate group (Table 13). There is also an intramolecular hydrogen bond between the hydroxyl groups O(6)——H and O(5)——H, with O(6) acting as donor. O(5)——H acts as a donor in an intermolecular hydrogen bond (see below). All

Table 12 Metal Ion——O Distances (Å) in the Ca^{2+} and Cd^{2+} Salts of Ionomycin

	Orthorhombic		Monoclinic[a,b]	
	Ca^{2+}	Cd^{2+}	Cd^{2+}	Cd^{2+}
M^{2+}——O(2)	2.28(3)	2.29(1)	2.28(3)	2.38(3)
M^{2+}——O(3)	2.28(4)	2.24(2)	2.15(4)	2.17(14)
M^{2+}——O(4)	2.26(4)	2.25(2)	2.34(11)	2.40(11)
M^{2+}——O(6)	2.43(4)	2.38(2)	2.48(13)	2.15(14)
M^{2+}——O(7)	2.44(4)	2.38(2)	2.71(14)	2.34(12)
M^{2+}——O(8)	2.83(4)	3.05(2)	3.05(11)	3.24(10)
M^{2+}——O(9)	2.44(4)	2.39(2)	2.28(6)	2.47(1)

[a] There are two crystallographically independent sets of Cd^{2+}——O distances in this crystal.
[b] Coordinates and standard deviations for the monoclinic form were generously provided by Professor J. Z. Gougoutas.
Source: Reprinted with permission from Toeplitz et al., 1979, *J. Am. Chem. Soc. 101*:3344-3353. Copyright 1979, American Chemical Society.

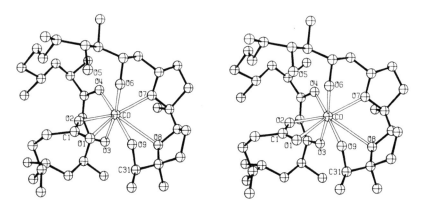

Figure 31 Stereoscopic view of the orthorhombic Cd^{2+}-ionomycin salt. The "polar" face is toward the viewer.

Table 13 Hydrogen-Bonding Distances (Å) in the Ca^{2+} and Cd^{2+} Complexes of Ionomycin

	Orthorhombic		Monoclinic[a,b]	
	Ca^{2+}	Cd^{2+}	Cd^{2+}	Cd^{2+}
O(9)——H---O(1)	2.66(5)	2.69(3)	2.29(14)	2.45(14)
O(6)——H---O(5)	2.70(4)	2.59(3)	2.3(2)	2.83(14)
O(5)——H---O(1)[c]	2.57(4)[d]	2.60(3)[d]	2.57(18)	2.66(14)

[a] There are two crystallographically independent sets of O——O distances in this crystal.
[b] Coordinates and standard deviations for the monoclinic form were generously provided by Professor J. Z. Gougoutas.
[c] This is an intermolecular hydrogen bond responsible for dimer formation.
[d] These values calculated by us are slightly different from those published by Toeplitz et al. (1979).
Source: Reprinted with permission from Toeplitz et al., 1979, *J. Am. Chem. Soc.*, *101*:3344-3353. Copyright 1979, American Chemical Society.

the oxygen atoms are directed toward the "inside" of the complex, excepting those at the "face" shown nearest the viewer in Figure 31. At that face O(5), O(6), O(1), and O(9) are quite exposed, a fact that assists dimer formation. Despite the relative lack of rings, the ionophore adopts rather similar conformations in all four forms. The greatest differences in backbone torsion angles between the orthorhombic Ca^{2+} and Cd^{2+} salts are of 35° for O(8)-C(30)-C(31)-O(9) and 34° for C(23)-O(7)-C(26)-C(27); the greatest difference in torsion angles between the two independent molecules for the monoclinic Cd^{2+} salt is of 54° for the C(26)-C(27)-O(8)-C(30) angle. When all four ionophore molecules are considered, the greatest difference in torsion angle is of 55° for the C(14)-C(15)-C(16)-C(17) torsion angle, between the value of −66° for the orthorhombic Ca^{2+} salt and that of −121° for one of the molecules of the monoclinic Cd^{2+} salt. The overall similarity in conformation is clearly enhanced by the ethylenic group and the enolized β-diketone group; in the latter group the seven atoms C(8)-C(12), O(3), and O(4) are planar within the accuracy of the analysis.

Dimer formation is observed in all three crystalline salts, with the polar face, referred to above, being the region of contact. In the orthorhombic salts the dimer is held together by two O(5)——H---O(1) hydrogen bonds, related by the two-fold crystallographic axis and of

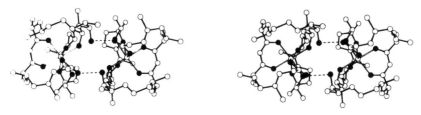

Figure 32 A stereoscopic drawing of the dimer of the Cd^{2+}-ionomycin structure in the orthorhombic form. The oxygen atoms are blackened and the hydrogen bonds that link the two ionomycin anions are shown by discontinuous lines.

length 2.63 Å. The same two hydrogen bonds, although in this case unrelated by symmetry, hold the dimer together in the monoclinic Cd^{2+} salt. A drawing of the dimer of the orthorhombic Cd^{2+} salt is shown in Figure 32. The dimer, by joining the polar faces of the two ionophore-

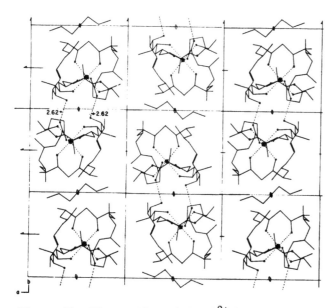

Figure 33 The packing of the M^{2+}-ionomycin complex in the orthorhombic form. (Source: reprinted with permission from Toeplitz et al., 1979, *J. Am. Chem. Soc. 101*:3349. Copyright 1979, American Chemical Society.)

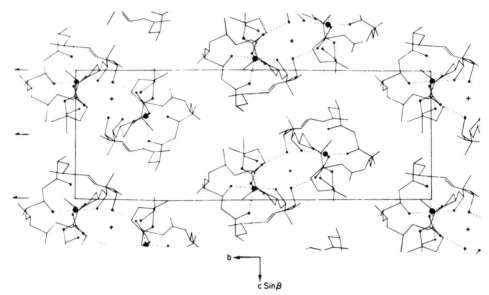

b ←
        ↓
    c Sinβ

Figure 34   The molecular arrangement of the complexed ionophore as
the Cd salt hexane solvate in the monoclinic crystal, viewed down the
a axis. The two molecules of the asymmetric unit are joined through
two hydrogen bonds about a pseudo twofold axis normal to the drawing
and passing through the cross (+).   Virtually the same "dimeric" lipophilic structure is evident about the space group twofold axis in the
orthorhombic structure. (Source: reprinted with permission from
Toeplitz et al., 1979, *J. Am. Chem. Soc. 101*:3352. Copyright 1979,
American Chemical Society.)

M^{2+} salts, presents an entirely nonpolar surface. No data have been
presented to indicate whether these dimers of ionomycin salts persist
in nonpolar solutions as is the case with certain dimers of lasalocid
(see later). The orthorhombic crystals are obtained with half a molecule of n-heptane per asymmetric unit, thus requiring the n-heptane
molecules to lie across a two-fold axis, while the monoclinic crystals
contained one molecule of n-hexane per asymmetric unit and thus one-
half molecule per Cd^{2+}-ionomycin species. While the positions of the
atoms of the solvent molecules could be obtained, they were not included in the refinement process. In both types of crystal structure
(i.e., monoclinic and orthorhombic) the nonpolar solvent molecules
lie outside the dimer structure and have contacts with its nonpolar
surface. Views of the packing of both forms are shown in Figures 33
and 34.

It should be emphasized that the quality of the crystals of these salts was rather poor and loss of solvent complicated the x-ray analyses. Only by virtue of the tenacity of Gougoutas and colleagues are we fortunate to have such well-defined structures for these salts.

11. K-41

The structure and absolute configuration of K-41 (Figure 35) were determined by x-ray analysis of the p-iodo- and p-bromobenzoates at the α-hydroxyl group of the sodium salt (Shiro et al., 1978).* Thus, as the ionophore has been derivatized, one should be more careful than usual when trying to draw conclusions regarding the biological action of the ionophore from the structure in the crystal. The p-iodo and p-bromo derivatives belong to different orthorhombic space groups ($P2_12_12$ in the case of the p-iodo derivative and $P2_12_12_1$ for the p-bromo), hence the crystal structures are not isomorphous. Each form crystallized with one molecule of water and one molecule of n-hexane in the crystal asymmetric unit, but these solvent molecules were not located in the x-ray analyses. The antibiotic K-41 has been shown to be identical to one A32887 isolated by the group at Eli Lilly (Occolowitz et al., 1978).

The molecular structures of the two complexes are very similar (see Figures 36 and 37). We shall discuss the molecular structure of the p-bromo derivative with the dimensions from the p-iodo one included in Tables 14 and 15. The usual circular conformation is stabilized by an O(54)——H---O(63) carboxylate-hydrogen bond. The β-hydroxyl group, O(66)——H, is also involved in a hydrogen bond to the carboxylate oxygen, O(63) (Table 14). The sodium ion is complexed to six oxygen atoms, both carboxylate oxygens and four ether oxygens, O(46), O(47), O(48), and O(57); the Na^+——O distances are given in Table 15. There appears to be a rather large "loop" of the antibiotic chain that does not interact closely with Na^+ in the region C(3)-C(13), including both rings A and B. Ring G and the derivative p-bromobenzoate ring both point toward the exterior of the complex. Several oxygen atoms, O(50), O(51), O(52), O(45), O(55), O(59), O(61), and O(68), lie near the surface of the molecule, making it more polar than many ionophores. In some other ionophores the presence of an α-hydroxy group often serves to hold the carboxylate group in an eclipsed position, possibly so that both oxygen atoms can interact with the metal ion. Derivatization of this hydroxy group has not had a great effect on the conformation in this region, possibly on account of the presence of a β-hydroxy group, which can also form a hydrogen

---

*The available coordinates for the p-iodo derivative correspond to the absolute configuration given in Figure 37. However, those for the p-bromo derivative correspond to the mirror image. The dimensions given in the following discussion were obtained from the transformed coordinates.

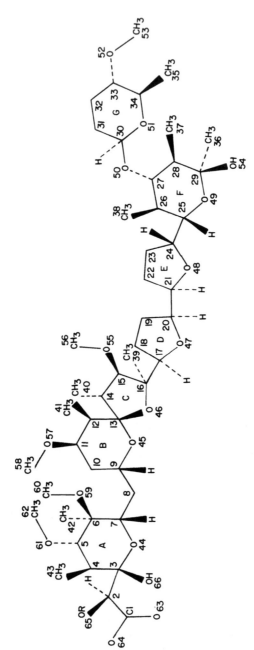

Figure 35   The structure of K-41 showing the atom numbering.

Table 14 O---O Distances (Å) Involved in Hydrogen Bonding in the p-Bromo- and p-Iodobenzoates of the Na⁺ Salt of K-41[a]

	p-Bromo	p-Iodo
O(54)---O(63)	2.74	2.71
O(66)---O(63)	2.60	2.64

[a]Standard deviations in the atomic parameters were not available.

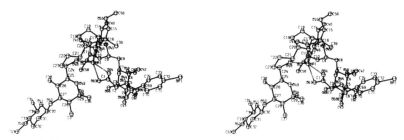

Figure 36 A stereoscopic view of the structure of the p-bromobenzoate of the Na⁺ salt of K-41. The Na⁺—O coordinations are shown by open lines. The coordinates associated with the paper by Shiro et al. (1978) corresponded to the enantiomer of the natural configuration.

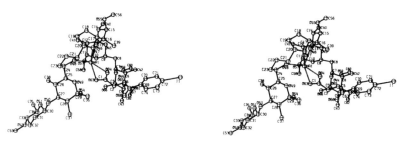

Figure 37 A stereoscopic view of the structure of the p-iodobenzoate of the Na⁺ salt of K-41. The Na⁺—O coordinations are shown by open lines.

Table 15 Na$^+$——O Distances (Å) in the p-Bromo- and p-Iodobenzoates of the Na$^+$ Salt of K-41[a]

	p-Bromo	p-Iodo
Na$^+$——O(63)	2.55	2.50
Na$^+$——O(64)	2.52	2.56
Na$^+$——O(46)	2.48	2.51
Na$^+$——O(47)	2.48	2.51
Na$^+$——O(48)	2.42	2.41
Na$^+$——O(57)	2.45	2.40

[a]Standard deviations in the atomic parameters were not available.

bond to the carboxylate group; the O(64)-C(1)-C(2)-O(65) torsion
angle is 18.7° in the p-bromo derivative and −3.0° in the p-iodo. The
spiro ring junction at C(13) results in wide variations of the bond
angle, 101-119° in the p-bromo and 98-117° in the p-iodo. The smallest angle is C(12)-C(13)-O(46) in the p-bromo and C(14)-C(13)-O(46)
in the p-iodo; the largest angle is O(45)-C(13)-O(46) in both derivatives.

12. Lasalocid (X-537A)

Lasalocid, originally called X-537A, was one of the three antibiotics
isolated as crystalline salts by Berger et al. at Roche Laboratories in
1951. It is also the ionophore which has been most extensively studied
by x-ray diffraction techniques. The structure of lasalocid showing
the atom numbering used in the present discussion is given in Figure
38, as well as the atom numbering proposed by Westley (1976) based on
biogenetic arguments. As most of the x-ray structural data is based
on the earlier numbering system, it will be used in the present discussion. X-ray analyses have been carried out on a Ba^{2+}L$_2^-$·H$_2$O
(L = lasalocid) salt (Johnson et al., 1970b), and Ag$_2^+$L$_2^-$·2CH$_3$·CO·CH$_3$
salt (Maier and Paul, 1971), an Ag$_2^+$(5-NO$_2$L)$_2^-$·CH$_3$OH salt (C. I.
Hejna, E. N. Duesler, and I. C. Paul, unpublished data, 1972), two
forms of a Na$_2^+$(5-BrL)$_2^-$ salt (Schmidt et al., 1974), a Na$_2^+$·L$_2^-$·2H$_2$O
(Smith et al., 1978a), a Na$^+$L$^-$·CH$_3$OH salt (Chiang and Paul, 1977), a
Cs$^+$L$^-$ salt (W. F. Paton and I. C. Paul, unpublished data, 1978), and
on a 1:1 salt of (R)-1-amino-1-(4-bromophenyl)ethane (Westley et al.,
1977). In addition, x-ray analyses have been carried out on four acid
crystals. These are (5-BrL)$_2$·H$_2$O (Bissell and Paul, 1972), 5-BrL·
C$_2$H$_5$OH (C. C. Chiang and I. C. Paul, unpublished data, 1976), and

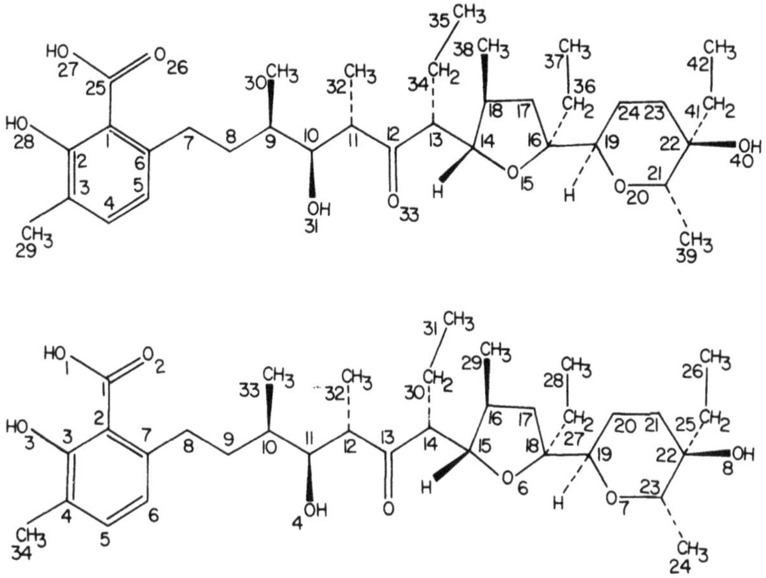

Figure 38 A drawing of the structure of lasalocid showing (top) the atom numbering used in the present discussion and (below) that proposed by Westley (1976).

two forms of L·CH$_3$OH (Friedman et al., 1979). Studies have also been carried out on the 5-bromo derivative of isolasalocid (Westley et al., 1974). The structure of lasalocid was established by the x-ray analysis of the Ba^{2+} salt (Johnson et al., 1970a) and the absolute configuration was determined by chemical degradation (Westley et al., 1970).

Lasalocid has several unusual features. It is a relatively small molecule for an ionophore, C$_{34}$H$_{54}$O$_8$, with a molecular weight of 590.6, and has an aromatic ring to which the carboxyl group is attached; there is a phenolic hydroxyl in an ortho position to the carboxyl group. With the exception of the isolasalocid structure, which will be discussed separately, the ionophore adopts virtually the same conformation in all its forms. This conformation is almost invariably stabilized by head-to-tail hydrogen bonding between the tertiary hydroxyl, O(40)——H, and the carboxyl group and reinforced by a hydrogen bond between the secondary hydroxyl, O(31)——H, and the carboxyl group and a "salicylic acid-type" hydrogen bond between O(28)——H and the carboxyl group. A schematic view of the conformation and the usual hydrogen-bonding assignments are shown in Figure 39. Hydrogen-bonding distances for the various salts are given in Table 16, and those for the acids in Table 17. Lasalocid also has a very strong tendency

Table 16 The O---O Distances (Å) in Hydrogen Bonds in Lasalocid Anions

	Ba^{2+} salt		Ag^+ salt		$Ag^+ 5\text{-}NO_2L$ salt		Form
	Unprimed	Primed	Unprimed	Primed	Unprimed	Primed	Unprimed
O(40)——H---O(26)	2.82(2)	3.26(2)	2.63(2)	2.71(1)	3.08(2)	2.62(2)	3.29(4)
O(40)——H---O(27)	2.71(1)	2.76(3)	3.75(2)	3.62(2)	2.75(2)	3.31(2)	2.87(4)
O(31)——H---O(26)	2.63(2)	2.86(2)	2.81(2)	2.94(2)	2.79(2)	2.65(2)	2.94(4)
O(28)——H---O(27)	2.44(2)	2.42(2)	2.38(2)	2.40(2)	2.51(2)	2.48(2)	2.38(4)
O(W)——H---O(20)	5.59(2)	2.80(2)	—	—	—	—	—
O(W)——H---O(33)	2.84(3)	3.13(2)	—	—	—	—	—
O(40)——H---W_2	—a	—	—	—	—	—	—
W_1——H---O(26)	—	—	—	—	—	—	—
W_2——H---O(26')	—	—	—	—	—	—	—
W(2)——H---O(27)	—	—	—	—	—	—	—
O(methanol)——H---O(26)	—	—	—	—	—	—	—

aA dash means that type of hydrogen bonding is not applicable to that particular compound.

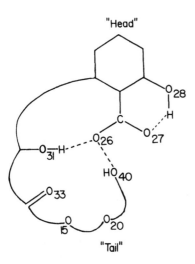

"Head"

028

C

O27

H

O$\overline{3|}$ H

O26

HO40

O33

O

15

O20

"Tail"

Figure 39 Schematic view of the general arrangement and hydrogen bonding usually found in lasalocid. When the ionophore is ionized, O(40) is the donor and either O(26) or O(27), or both, the acceptor in the head-to-tail hydrogen bond. In the neutral form O(26) can be the donor and O(40) the acceptor.

| Na$^+$5-Br L salt | | | Na$^+$·L$^-$·H$_2$O salt | | | | |
| I | Form II | | | | | | Lasalocid:amine salt |
Primed	Unprimed	Primed	Unprimed	Primed	Na$^+$L$^-$·CH$_3$OH	Cs$^+$ salt	salt
2.96(4)	2.63(3)	2.77(2)	3.55(1)	2.92(1)	3.021(4)	3.20(2)	3.48(1)
2.84(4)	3.33(3)	2.73(2)	4.32(1)	3.11(2)	2.811(4)	2.81(2)	2.75(1)
2.94(4)	2.63(3)	2.70(2)	3.23(1)	3.00(1)	2.709(4)	2.65(2)	2.69(1)
2.47(4)	2.40(3)	2.37(3)	2.42(1)	2.42(2)	2.477(5)	2.48(2)	2.45(1)
—	—	—	—	—	—	—	—
—	—	—	—	—	—	—	—
—	—	—	2.72(1)	—	—	—	—
—	—	—	2.61(1)	—	—	—	—
—	—	—	2.73(1)	—	—	—	—
—	—	—	2.73(1)	—	—	—	—
—	—	—	—	—	2.73(4)	—	—

to form dimers; this is true not only when it complexes divalent ions such as Ba^{2+}, but also when it complexes monovalent ions, often forming 2:2 rather than 1:1 salts. In addition, one form of the free acid of the 5-bromolasalocid also crystallizes as a dimer. We believe that the tendency to dimerize is a consequence of the conformational integrity shown by the ionophore in most of its salts, and also of its relatively small size. This latter feature prevents a single molecule from adopting a conformation that can surround its polar groups with a hydrophobic exterior. A single molecule can provide effectively *one* hydrophobic "side" or "face" for an ionic complex, but not *two*. Thus, even in the monomeric structures that have been reported, the other face is occupied by a molecule such as methanol, ethanol, or an organic amine that can help provide nonpolar protection. The Cs$^+$ salt is unusual in having a polymeric structure. Of the seven dimeric structures reported, none exhibits crystallographic two-fold symmetry, although in several cases the overall symmetry of the complex is very close to having a twofold axis. This lack of exact twofold symmetry is something of a contrast to the behavior of A23187 and X-14547A, two ionophores which also form dimers. Another feature of lasalocid structural chemistry that is especially interesting is the propensity to form different entities, monomer versus dimer or dimer I versus dimer II, depending somewhat on the solvent conditions used for crystallization. In some cases solution NMR studies in parallel with crystallographic work have shown that approximately the same entities found in the

Duesler and Paul

Table 17 O——O Distances (Å) in Hydrogen Bonds in Lasalocid Free Acids

| | $(5Br-L)_2 \cdot H_2O$ | | $5Br-L \cdot C_2H_5OH$ | $L \cdot CH_3OH$ | |
	Unprimed	Primed		Form I	Form II
O(26)——H--O(40)	2.51(2)	2.57(2)	2.601(14)	2.618(3)	2.698(7)
O(31)——H--O(26)	3.14(2)	3.06(2)	3.209(5)	3.208(4)	3.356(7)
O(28)——H--O(27)	2.43(2)	2.48(2)	2.505(6)	2.499(4)	2.527(8)
O(40)——H--O(33')	3.04(1)	3.52(2)	—	—	—
O(40')——H--O(W)	—	2.95(2)	—	—	—
O(W)——H--O(40)	3.09(1)	—	—	—	—
O(W)——H--O(33)	3.01(2)	2.99(1)	—	—	—
O(31)——H--O(alc)	—	—	2.847(4)	2.929(4)	2.927(7)
O(40)——H--O(alc)	—	—	2.727(4)	2.739(4)	2.716(7)
O(alc)——H--O(15)	—	—	2.774(4)	2.818(4)	2.895(7)

crystal are also present in solution. We shall describe in turn the dimer salts, the monomer salts, the polymer salt, the dimer acid, and the monomer acids. Finally, the rather different structure found for iso-lasalocid will be discussed.

The only crystal structure reported for a divalent ion is that of the Ba^{2+} salt, which crystallizes as a dimer monohydrate (Johnson et al., 1970b). A view of this structure is shown in Figure 40, with a schematic drawing in Figure 41. The Ba^{2+} ion is ninefold coordinated; however, it lies somewhat closer to one lasalocid anion, which provides six coordinating oxygen atoms, than to the other, which provides only two, with the water molecule completing the coordination. The Ba^{2+} ion is complexed with both carboxylate groups. The Ba^{2+}——O distances range from 2.63 to 3.07 Å (Table 18). The water molecule forms two hydrogen bonds to the less-complexed lasalocid anion (Figure 40). There are no hydrogen bonds between the two ionophore anions in the dimer. If one refers to the aromatic ring as the "head" of the molecule and the oxacyclohexane ring as the "tail," the dimer can be described as head to tail. There was no evidence for any further association of the dimers in the crystal.

The Ag^+ salt of lasalocid also crystallizes as a dimer which encloses the two Ag^+ ions shown in Figure 42 (Maier and Paul, 1971). A schematic view of the complex is shown in Figure 43. The salt very closely approaches twofold symmetry, with the dimer being organized in a head-to-tail fashion, i.e., the phenyl ring of one ion is opposite the ether ring of the other ion. The coordination of each Ag^+ ion is virtually identical. The Ag^+ sits in a "basket" provided by five oxygen

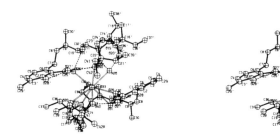

Figure 40 A stereoscopic view of the Ba^{2+} lasalocid dimer monohydrate. The Ba^{2+}——O coordination bonds are shown by open lines and hydrogen bonds are shown by discontinuous lines. The water molecule is hydrogen bonded to the primed molecule and complexed to the Ba^{2+} ion.

Table 18 Ba^{2+}——O Distances (Å) in the Ba^{2+}·L$_2^-$·H$_2$O Salt

Ba^{2+}——O(26)	2.81(2)	Ba^{2+}——O(40)	2.72(2)
Ba^{2+}——O(31)	3.07(2)	Ba^{2+}——O(26')	2.63(2)
Ba^{2+}——O(33)	2.81(2)	Ba^{2+}——O(40')	2.84(2)
Ba^{2+}——O(15)	2.99(2)	Ba^{2+}——O(W)	2.75(2)
Ba^{2+}——O(20)	2.85(2)		

Source: Reprinted with permission from Johnson et al., 1970b, *J. Am. Chem. Soc.* 92:4428-4435. Copyright 1979, American Chemical Society.

atoms, O(15), O(20), O(31), O(33), and O(40) (i.e., excluding the carboxylate oxygens) from one ionophore; the other side of the Ag$^+$ ion is involved in a π complex to a bond, C(5)-C(6), in the aromatic ring; Ag$^+$——O and Ag$^+$——C distances are in Table 19. The Ag$^+$---Ag$^+$ distance within the dimer is quite long, 7.108(2) Å. There is no intra-complex hydrogen bonding. The acetone of crystallization is to the outside of the dimer (see below) and there are no dimer-dimer specific interactions in the crystal. In order to remove the possibility of a

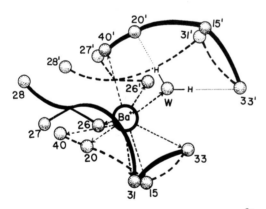

Figure 41 A schematic view of the Ba^{2+} lasalocid salt monohydrate. The covalent backbone is represented by curved lines, continuous nearer to the viewer and discontinuous farther away, The Ba^{2+}——O coordination is shown by discontinuous arrow-headed lines and the hydrogen bonds by dotted lines. (Source: reprinted with permission from Johnson et al., 1970b, *J. Am. Chem. Soc* 92:4428-4435. Copyright 1970, American Chemical Society.)

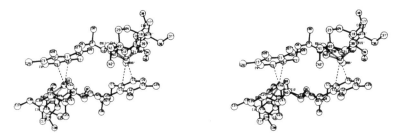

Figure 42 Stereoscopic view of the dimer of the Ag$^+$ salt of lasalocid. The Ag$^+$——O coordinations are shown by open bonds, while the Ag$^+$——C≡C interaction is shown by dashed lines.

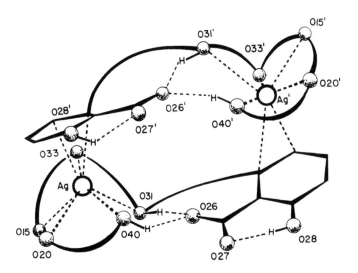

Figure 43 Schematic drawing of the coordination of the Ag$^+$ salt of X-537A. The covalent backbone of the molecule is shown by thick solid lines, the coordination bonds by discontinuous lines. The hydrogen-bonding assignments are also shown. (Source: Maier and Paul, 1971.)

Table 19 Ag$^+$——O and Ag$^+$——C Distances (Å) in the Ag$^+$·Lasalocid· Acetonate Complex and the Ag$^+$·5-Nitrolasalocid·Methanolate Complex

	$Ag_2^+ \cdot L_2^- \cdot CH_3 \cdot CO \cdot CH_3$		$Ag_2^+(5\text{-}NO_2L)_2^- \cdot CH_3OH$	
	Unprimed	Primed	Unprimed	Primed
Ag$^+$——O(15)	2.48(1)	2.47(1)	2.61(1)	2.50(1)
Ag$^+$——O(20)	2.56(1)	2.55(1)	2.54(1)	2.62(1)
Ag$^+$——O(31)	2.87(1)	2.78(1)	3.50(1)	3.27(2)
Ag$^+$——O(33)	2.85(1)	3.03(1)	2.70(1)	2.50(1)
Ag$^+$——O(40)	2.34(1)	2.36(1)	2.43(1)	2.43(1)
Ag$^+$——O(26')[a]	4.77(1)	4.80(2)	3.48(1)	2.36(1)
Ag$^+$——O(27')[a]	5.34(1)	5.32(2)	2.42(2)	4.13(2)
Ag$^+$——O(40')[a]	6.60(1)	6.50(1)	2.69(1)	4.35(1)
Ag$^+$——C(5')	2.40(2)	2.46(2)		
Ag$^+$——C(6')	2.76(2)	2.64(2)		

[a]In the case of the primed molecules these distances refer to the corresponding Ag'——O contacts.

Ag$^+$——C$\equiv$C interaction of the type found in this crystal, a study of the Ag$^+$ salt of 5-nitrolasalocid was undertaken (C. I. Heija, E. N. Duesler, and I. C. Paul, unpublished data, 1972). A view of the structure is shown in Figure 44 and a schematic drawing is given in Figure 45. Once again the structure is dimeric. One can think of obtaining the structure of the Ag$^+$ · 5-NO$_2$ lasalocid from the Ag$^+$·lasalocid structure by "breaking" the Ag$^+$——C$\equiv$C bonds and translating the resulting Ag$^+$·L$^-$ monomer, the Ag$^+$ still attached to most of the oxygen atoms that comprised the basket, by approximately 3.5 Å, such that the Ag$^+$---Ag$^+$ distance is now 3.565(2) Å. The complexing of the two Ag$^+$ ions in the 5-nitro dimer is slightly different. One Ag$^+$ ion, Ag$^+$, is six-coordinated, being complexed with O(15), O(20), O(33), and O(40) in the unprimed anion but not to O(31). This Ag$^+$ ion is also complexed with O(27') and O(40') in the primed molecule. The other Ag$^+$ ion, Ag'$^+$, is only five-coordinated, being complexed with O(15'), O(20'), O(33'), and O(40') in the primed lasalocid anion and with O(26) in the unprimed ion. The nitro groups lie to the outside of the dimer, thus presenting a more polar surface to the exterior than other lasalocid dimers; they are also twisted out of the planes of the respective phenyl rings by 47.6 and 37.3° in the two lasalocid anions.

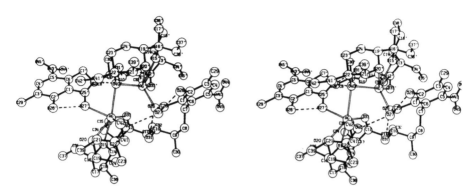

Figure 44 Stereoscopic view of the Ag$^+$-5-nitrolasalocid dimer. The Ag$^+$——O coordinations are shown by open bonds, the hydrogen bonds by discontinuous lines.

twisted out of the planes of the respective phenyl rings by 47.6 and 37.3° in the two lasalocid anions.

The Na$^+$ salt of 5-bromolasalocid was obtained in two crystallographically distinct modifications (Form I and Form II) by Schmidt et al. (1974). Form I tended to crystallize more readily from nonpolar solvents such as carbon tetrachloride, while Form II was more readily obtained from acetone. However, frequently crystals of both were found. In both crystals the salt exists as a dimer, but in Form I the dimer is head to tail, while in Form II it is head to head (Figures 46

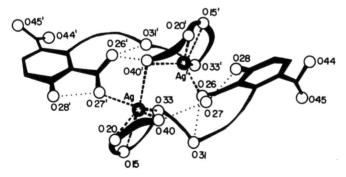

Figure 45 A schematic view of the Ag$^+$-5- nitrolasalocid dimer. The Ag$^+$——O coordination bonds are shown by dashed lines; the hydrogen bonds are shown by dotted lines.

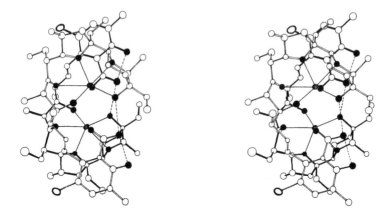

Figure 46 Stereoscopic drawing of the Form I (head-to-tail) structure of the dimer of the Na$^+$ salt of 5-bromolasalocid. The Na$^+$ ions are open circles and the oxygen atoms are solid circles. The Na$^+$—O coordinations are shown on thin lines, and the hydrogen bonds by discontinuous lines. (Source: reprinted with permission from Schmidt et al., 1974, *J. Am. Chem. Soc. 96*:6189. Copyright 1974, American Chemical Society.)

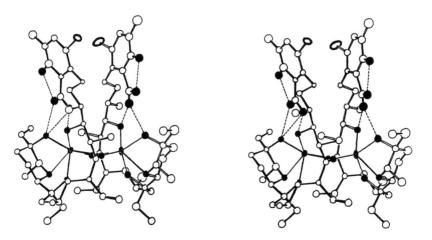

Figure 47 Stereoscopic drawing of the Form II (head-to-head) structure of the dimer of the Na$^+$ salt of 5-bromolasalocid. The Na$^+$ ions are open circles and the oxygen atoms are solid circles. The Na$^+$—O coordinations are shown on thin lines, and the hydrogen bonds by discontinuous lines. (Source: reprinted with permission from Schnidt et al., 1974, *J. Am. Chem. Soc. 96*:6189. Copyright 1974, American Chemical Society.)

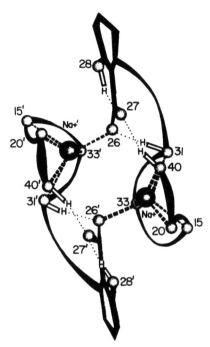

Figure 48 Schematic view of Form I (head-to-tail) structure of the
dimer of the Na⁺ salt of 5-bromolasalocid. Only the Na⁺ and oxygen
atoms are shown, with the covalent backbone represented by curved
lines. The Na⁺——O coordinations are shown by discontinuous lines,
and the hydrogen bonds by dotted lines.

and 47). Schematic drawings of the two structures are shown in Figures 48 and 49. In each form the Na⁺ ion sits in the basket provided
by the five oxygen atoms O(15), O(20), O(31), O(33), and O(40);
Na⁺——O distances are given in Table 20. In Form I (i.e., head to
tail) the other side of the Na⁺ ion is complexed with a carboxylate
oxygen, O(26), with the Na⁺——O(26) vector almost normal to the
"plane" of the basket. The Na⁺---Na⁺ distance is 3.83(2) Å. In Form
II (i.e., head to head) the ketone oxygen, O(33), acts as a bridge
between the two Na⁺ ions and provides a sixth coordination; the
Na⁺---Na⁺ distance in this dimer is 3.78(1) Å. There is no intracomplex interionophore hydrogen bonding. Both dimers closely approach
twofold symmetry.

NMR studies (Schmidt et al., 1974) provided evidence that a structure similar to the head-to-tail dimer exists in nonpolar solvents. This
preliminary NMR work was greatly extended by Patel and Shen (1976)
and by Shen and Patel (1976).

Table 20 Na$^+$—O Distances (Å) in the two Na$_2$·(5Br-Lasalocid)$_2$ Dimers, the Na$_2$·L$_2$·2H$_2$O Dimer, and the Na·L·CH$_3$OH Monomer

| | Na$_2$·(5BrL)$_2$ | | | | Na$_2$·L$_2$·2H$_2$O | | Na·L·CH$_3$OH |
| | Form I | | Form II | | | | |
	Unprimed	Primed	Unprimed	Primed	Unprimed	Primed	
Na$^+$—O(15)	2.44(3)	2.53(3)	2.34(2)	2.42(2)	2.42(1)	2.40(1)	2.399(3)
Na$^+$—O(20)	2.49(3)	2.54(3)	2.52(2)	2.58(2)	2.47(1)	2.44(1)	2.589(3)
Na$^+$—O(31)	2.57(3)	2.58(3)	2.43(2)	2.57(2)	2.67(1)	2.47(1)	2.653(3)
Na$^+$—O(33)	2.75(3)	2.51(3)	2.68(2)	2.77(2)	2.67(1)	2.93(1)	2.620(3)
Na$^+$—O(40)	2.46(3)	2.51(3)	2.29(2)	2.29(2)	2.56(1)	2.72(1)	2.358(3)
Na$^+$—O(26')	2.30(3)	2.29(2)	4.88(2)	5.74(2)	5.48(1)	4.08(1)	
Na$^+$—O(33')	4.52(3)	4.28(2)	2.29(2)	2.33(2)	2.42(1)	5.11(1)	
Na$^+$—O(W$_1$)					2.45(1)	2.37(1)	
Na$^+$—O(W$_2$)					3.79(1)	2.40(1)	
Na$^+$—O(methanol)							2.317(3)

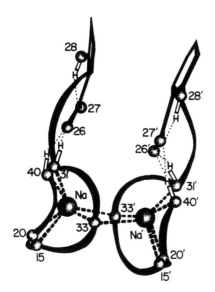

Figure 49 Schematic view of Form II (head-to-head) structure of the dimer of the Na⁺ salt of 5-bromolasalocid. Only the Na⁺ and oxygen atoms are shown, with the covalent backbone represented by curved lines. The Na⁺——O coordinations are shown by discontinuous lines, and the hydrogen bonds by dotted lines.

The crystal structure of a hydrated Na⁺ salt of lasalocid dimer has been reported by Smith et al. (1978a). The crystals were obtained from 95% ethanol. A view of the structure is shown in Figure 50 and a schematic drawing is given in Figure 51. This dimer is unusual in several respects. The two water molecules are an integral part of the dimer structure. The dimer is less symmetrical than those of the other 2:2 salts, particularly as regards the coordination to Na⁺. Also, the head-to-tail hydrogen bonding that is such a feature of lasalocid geometry is modified in this structure. One of the Na⁺ ions, Na-1⁺ is seven-coordinated, sitting in the usual basket provided by O(15), O(20), O(31), O(33), and O(40), with the other side complexed with a water molecule (W-1) and with the ketone oxygen, O(33'), of the second ionophore. The other Na⁺ ion, Na-2⁺, is only six-coordinated, complexing with O(15'), O(20'), O(31'), and O(40') [but not O(33')], with the other side complexed with both water molecules. In the unprimed ionophore anion there is no direct O(40)——H---O(carboxylate) hydrogen bond, as a water molecule (W-2) is interposed between O(40) and the carboxylate group; there is O(40)——H---(W-2)---O(27) hydrogen bonding. There is also an O(31)——H---O(26) carboxylate hydrogen bond. In the primed ionophore ion there is probably a direct O(40')——H---O(26') carboxylate hydrogen bond and also an O(31')——H---O(26') carboxylate hydrogen bond.* One of the water molecules (W-1) forms a hydrogen bond to the carboxylate group, O(26), of the unprimed ionophore, while the other water molecule (W-2) in addition to accepting a hydrogen bond from O(40)——H, donates hydrogen bonds to the other oxygen of the carboxylate group, O(27), and to the carboxylate group O(26') in the primed molecule. The dimer is thus held together by a combination of Na——O coordination bonds and hydrogen bonds from the water molecules; one water (W-1) is coordinated with both Na^+ ions, O(33') is coordinated with the Na-1$^+$ ion that is mainly associated with the unprimed ion, and W-2 is hydrogen bonded to both carboxyl groups. The Na^+---Na^+ distance in the dimer is 3.745(6) Å. There are no direct intracomplex interionophore hydrogen bonds. There are no specific interactions between different dimers in the crystal.

Crystallization of sodium lasalocid from methanol gave a monomeric 1:1 methanolate salt (Chiang and Paul, 1977). The quality of the crystals was excellent and all the hydroxylic hydrogen atoms could be positioned with confidence, thus allowing a *definite* assignment of the hydrogen-bonding patterns as shown in Figure 52 (Chiang and Paul, 1977; Friedman et al., 1977). The Na^+ ion is coordinated with five oxygen atoms from the lasalocid anion, O(15), O(20), O(31), O(33), and O(40), and to the oxygen atom of the methanol molecule. The Na^+——O distances are very similar to those found in the two Na_2^+(5-BrL)$_2^-$ dimers (see Table 20). The conformation of the lasalocid anion

---

* In this analysis, as with most others of lasalocid dimers, the positions of the hydroxyl hydrogen atoms were not determined and hence an unambiguous assignment of the hydrogen bonding cannot be made. In the paper by Smith et al. (1978a) it was noted that the three oxygen atoms O(40'), O(31'), and O(26') "form a nearly equilateral triangle" and hence "the exact nature of the hydrogen bonding scheme within the ion is unknown." However, a hydrogen bond O(40')——H---O(31') or O(31')——H---O(40') would place the proton along the edge of the Na^+ coordination sphere, a situation which is unlikely (Clark, 1963). Also, the C(10')-O(31')---O(26') and C(22')-O(40')---O(27') angles, 96.7(6) and 116.9(7)°, are both reasonable for hydrogen bonding, while the C(10')-O(31')---O(40') and C(22')-O(40')---O(31') angles are not favorable, 153.2(7) and 138.2(8)°. The C(22')-O(40')---O(27') angle would suggest that the O(40') hydrogen is pointed at both oxygens of the carboxyl group rather than solely to the closer O(26'), as the C(22')-O(40')---O(26') angle is 158.8(6)°. Both on these arguments and from the results on other structures, it seems highly probable that O(40')——H and O(31')-H are *both* hydrogen bonded to the carboxylate group.

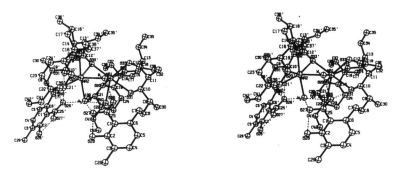

Figure 50 A stereoscopic view of the Na⁺-lasalocid-hydrate dimer. The Na⁺——O coordinations are shown by open bonds; hydrogen bonds are indicated by discontinuous lines.

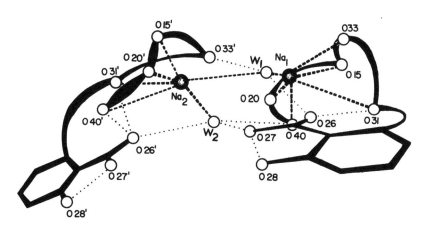

Figure 51 Schematic view of the hydrated sodium lasalocid dimer. The Na⁺——O coordination bonds are shown by dashed lines; the hydrogen bonds are shown by dotted lines.

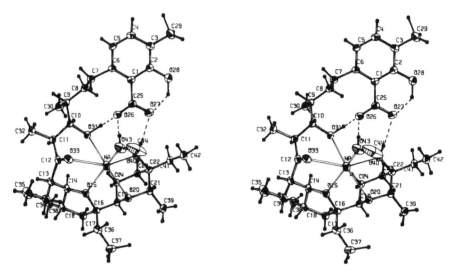

Figure 52 A stereoscopic view of the Na⁺-lasalocid:methanolate complex. The Na⁺——O coordinations are shown by open bonds; hydrogen
bonds are indicated by discontinuous lines. (Source: Chiang and
Paul, 1977. Copyright 1977, American Association for the Advancement
of Science.)

is virtually identical to those found in most of the structures discussed
previously. In addition to the O(40)——H---O(27) and O(28)——H---
O(27) hydrogen bonds within the anion, there are hydrogen bonds between O(31)——H and the methanol oxygen and a hydrogen bond between the hydroxyl group of the methanol to the carboxylate O(26).
The methanol molecule sits above the Na⁺ ion and, in addition to complexing with the Na⁺ ion, its methyl group provides a partial protec-
tive nonpolar surface for the polar region of the ionophore.

In summary, in all the examples studied of Na⁺ and Ag⁺ ion coordination the metal ion is complexed mainly by the ether and hydroxyl
oxygen atoms of a single lasalocid ion. There are no examples of
M⁺——carboxyl coordination with the *same* anion; however, the M⁺ ion
is sometimes coordinated with a carboxyl group of the other lasalocid
ion making up the dimer and *always* coordinated with at least one other
atom from either a second lasalocid anion or a solvent molecule.

Crystals of a cesium lasalocid salt were obtained by crystallization
from a dichloromethane:hexane mixture (W. F. Paton and I. C. Paul,
unpublished data, 1978). A view of the structure is shown in Figure
53. This salt is unusual in being polymeric. The lasalocid anion adopts

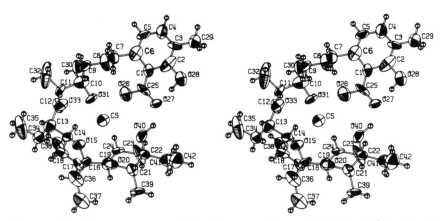

Figure 53 The structure of the "monomeric part" of the Cs⁺ lasalocid salt. The Cs⁺ ion is coordinated with O(26), O(33), O(15), O(20), and O(40).

the usual circular conformation and the Cs⁺ ion sits above the center of the circle. It is coordinated with five oxygen atoms from this anion, O(15), O(20), O(33), O(40), and O(26), with Cs⁺——O distances ranging from 2.94(1) to 3.14(1) Å; the Cs⁺——O(31) distance of 3.36(1) Å is probably too long to represent a genuine coordination. Thus the greater radius of the Cs⁺ ion can involve both the hydroxyl and ether oxygen atoms of the "tail" *and* the carboxylate oxygen in the same molecule. The other side of the Cs⁺ ion is coordinated to the phenolic oxygen, O(28), in another molecule; the Cs⁺——O(28) distance is 3.10(1) Å. It is this additional coordination that gives rise to the polymeric structure.

Crystals (mp 205-207°C) of the 1:1 lasalocid:(R)-1-amino-1-(4-bromophenyl) ethane salt were obtained from a solution of the racemic amine and lasalocid in methylene dichloride and n-hexane (Westley et al., 1977). It was found that the preferential crystallization of the R-salt provided a method for resolution of the racemic amine that could be extended to other primary amines. A view of the structure is shown in Figure 54. Lasalocid adopts the usual circular conformation, with O(40)——H---O(27), O(31)——H---O(26), and O(28)——H---O(27) hydrogen bonding. The ammonium slat* is hydrogen bonded by

---

*The hydrogen atoms were located in the analysis and there appears no doubt that proton transfer from the carboxyl group to the amino group has occurred, resulting in salt formation.

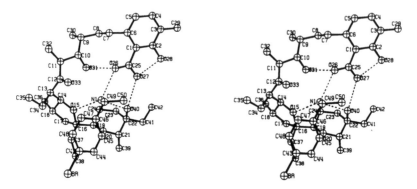

Figure 54 Stereoscopic view of the 1:1 lasalocid:(R)-1-amino-1-(4-bromophenyl)ethane salt. The hydrogen bonds are shown by discontinuous lines.

three N^+---O distances of 2.90(1), 2.81(1), and 2.80(1) Å, respectively. It appears that the enantiomeric selectivity of the lasalocid for the R-amine results from placing the small volume occupied by C——H bond of the asymmetric α-carbon of the amine in the direction of the ketone group, C(10)——O(33), which points up to the side complexed by the amine, while the largest group attached to the asymmetric carbon, the p-bromophenyl substituent, lies in the depression created in the region of the five- and six-membered rings. The third substituent, the methyl group, is directed over the O(40)——H---O(27) hydrogen bond.

While four different crystal structures of free acids have been carried out, the structures of the acid in three of these are very similar. These three are the 5-bromolasalocid·ethanol complex and the two forms of the lasalocid·methanol complex; the fourth structure is the dimer of 5-bromolasalocid·hemihydrate.

Crystals of the (5-BrL)$_2$·H$_2$O dimer were obtained from a hexane:methylene dichloride mixture (Bissell and Paul, 1972). Although water was not specifically added to the solvent, no rigorous attempt was made to exclude it and the crystals proved to correspond to a hemihydrate. The crystals deteriorated fairly rapidly in the x-ray beam, so the resulting analysis, while clearly providing the gross structure, failed to provide the hydroxyl hydrogen atom positions and hence failed to give an unambiguous assignment of the hydrogen bonding. The structure (Figure 55) is a head-to-head dimer, with the two bromolasalocid molecules enclosing the water molecule. The most reasonable

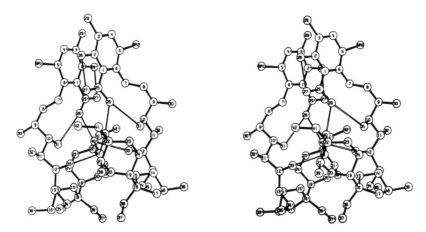

Figure 55   A stereoscopic view of the structure of the 5-bromolasa-
locid hemihydrate structure.   Hydrogen bonds are shown by open
lines.   (Source: Bissel and Paul, 1972.)

hydrogen-bonding assignment does indicate some intradimer hydrogen
bonding. The conformations of the two 5-bromolasalocid molecules are
almost identical and are stabilized by head-to-tail O(26)——H---O(40)
and also by O(31)——H---O(26) hydrogen bonds. As the carboxyl
group acts as the donor in the head-to-tail hydrogen bond, the
O(40)——H hydrogen is free to participate in other hydrogen bonds.
In one molecule (unprimed) there is an O(40)——H---O(W) hydrogen
bond, while in the other there is an intermolecular O(40')——H---O(33)
linkage. The water molecule acts as a donor in the O(W)——H---O(33')
and O(W)——H---O(40') hydrogen bonds. The O——O distances are
given in Table 17. The O(33')——O(W)---O(40') angle is 113.8(5)°.

Crystals of a monomeric 5-bromolasalocid:ethanolate were obtained
from ethanol solution, and two forms of a monomeric lasalocid:methano-
late were obtained from methanol. The structures of the 5-BrL·C_2H_5OH
complex and the two forms of the lasalocid·CH_3OH complex are all
monomeric (see Figure 56). To a very high degree the conformations
of the lasalocid molecules and the mode of association of the complexes
are very similar. In these crystals hydroxyl hydrogen atoms could be
located and hence the hydrogen-bonding assignments are definite. The
usual circular conformation of the lasalocid entities is stabilized by
head-to-tail O(26)——H---O(40) hydrogen bonding. The secondary
hydroxyl group O(31)——H and the tertiary O(40)——H are both involved in hydrogen bonds to the methanol or ethanol oxygen atom; the

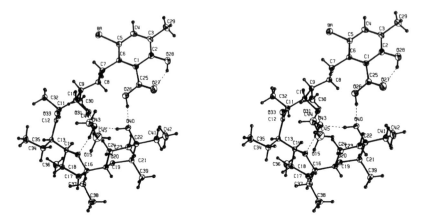

Figure 56 A stereoscopic drawing of the 5-bromolasalocid·ethanolate structure. Hydrogen atoms were located and hydrogen bonds are shown by discontinuous lines.

alcohol hydroxyl hydrogen, in turn, forms a hydrogen bond to O(15). The methyl or ethyl group of the complexed alcohol provides a partial nonpolar protection for the polar regions of the lasalocid molecule. It is of interest to note that in the 5-bromolasalocid:ethanol complex the terminal methyl group of the ethanol molecule lies over the region of the lasalocid molecule with the five- and six-membered ether rings, a region very similar to that occupied by the phenyl group in the 4-bromophenyl amine complex.

The existence of two forms of the lasalocid:methanol complex was first detected by infrared and Raman spectra (Friedman et al., 1979). The Raman spectra showed a very clear distinction in the ketone [C(10)—O(30)] stretching frequencies, 1724 cm^{-1} in form A and 1713 cm^{1-} in form B. However, when the crystal structures were determined, there was no clear intramolecular structural difference in this region to account for the spectral shift.* A possible explanation of the spectral shift may lie in the different intermolecular environments of the ketone group. While the space groups of the two forms are the same ($P2_12_12_1$), the crystal structures are clearly different. In form

---

*Crystal structures of the deuterium-labeled molecules in both forms revealed that they were essentially identical with the H forms (C. C. Chiang, E. N. Duesler, and I. C. Paul, unpublished data, 1979).

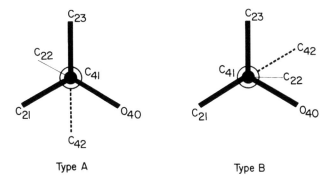

Type A   Type B

Figure 57 Views of the two arrangements for the C(41)——C(42)
ethyl group. The torsion angles are viewed along the C(22)——C(41)
bond.

A there is a contact of 3.42 Å between O(33) in the reference molecule
and C(30) in a molecule at $\frac{1}{2} - x$, $1 - y$, $\frac{1}{2} + z$; while this contact is
equal to the sum of the appropriate van der Waals radii, it is 0.2 Å
shorter than any contact involving O(33) in form B. The C(30) atom
in form A is positioned such that any steric compression from this contact would tend to shorten the C====O bond and thus raise the stretching frequency. The most significant difference noted between the molecular structures in the two forms was in the orientation of the ethyl
group, C(41)——C(42), attached to C(22). In form A the C(42) atom
is in a conformation that bisects the C(21) and O(40) bonds to C(20),
while in form B the C(42) atom bisects the C(23) and O(40) bonds to
C(20); this corresponds to a difference in the torsion angles of 120°
(see Figure 57).

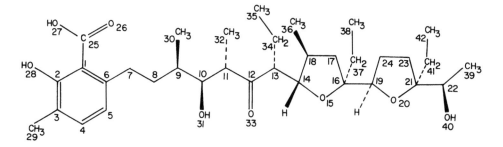

Figure 58 The structure of isolasalocid showing the atom numbering
used in the present discussion.

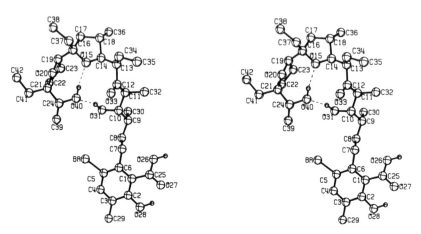

Figure 59   Stereoscopic view of the 5-bromoisolasalocid molecule. Only
the hydroxyl hydrogen atoms are shown. Hydrogen bonds are shown
by discontinuous lines. The carboxylic acid group is involved in
intermolecular hydrogen bonding.

   Isolasalocid is a natural structural isomer and differs from lasalocid
in that the terminal ring is five membered rather than six membered
and the hydroxyl group at that end of the molecule is secondary rather
than tertiary (see Figure 58). A x-ray analysis was carried out on
the 5-bromo derivative (mp 185 to 186°) obtained from acetone:hexane
(Westley et al., 1974). A view of the structure is shown in Figure 59.
The structure is monomeric. The molecular conformation is quite different from that usually adopted by lasalocid. The carboxylic acid
hydrogen is not involved in intramolecular hydrogen bonding and the
group points toward the outside of the molecule. Thus the familiar
circular conformation is not present. The O(40)——H hydroxyl forms
a hydrogen bond to the O(15) ether oxygen and the O(31)——H hydroxyl forms a hydrogen bond to O(40); the O(40)---O(15) and
O(31)---O(40) distances are 2.85 and 2.76 Å, respectively. The
O(28)——H---O(27) hydrogen bond is also present, with an O(28)---
O(27) distance of 2.52 Å. The most dramatic change in the conformation is in the orientation of the phenyl group, which in 5-bromoiso-
lasalocid has the bromine atom pointing toward the tail of the molecule.
This conformation results in the carboxylic acid group being involved
in an intermolecular hydrogen bond to O(31) (see below).
   If one excludes the isolasalocid structure, the conformations of the
lasalocid ions in all the salts are very similar. The most notable exception is that of the primed anion in the $Ag^+(5-NO_2L)^-$ dimer. There

are significant differences in the angles of twist in the region where the main chain leaves the phenyl ring (Figure 44). In the unprimed anion the C(1)——C(6)——C(7)——C(8) torsion angle is $-76°$ (a value which is typical of all the other lasalocid anions); however, in the primed anion this angle is $70°$, indicating that the main chain bends at C(7) to the opposite side of the phenyl ring from the usual situation. Similarly, the C(7)——C(8)——C(9)——C(10) torsion angle is $94°$ in the primed anion, whereas a more typical value of $-63°$ is found in the unprimed anion. Apart from these two large differences, the greatest variation in the torsion angles of the bonds in the molecular backbone among all 15 different lasalocid anions is $26°$. In any single dimer, again with the exception of the $Ag^+(5-NO_2L)^-$ dimer noted above, the greatest difference in torsion angle between the two anions is $24°$ for the C(12)——C(13)——C(14)——O(15) torsion angle in the Ba^{2+} salt.

The six-membered oxygen-containing ring is always in the chair conformation in the lasalocid salts. The five-membered ring is in an envelope conformation, with C(18) lying out of the plane of the other four atoms. The greatest difference from the ideal envelope conformation is found in the primed molecule of the hydrated dimeric sodium salt, where the C(14)——O(15)——C(16)——C(17) torsion angle is $-10°$ instead of the ideal value of $0°$; this latter distortion is toward a halfchair conformation.

Another significant difference in conformation among lasalocid anions is found in the orientation of the C(41)——C(42) ethyl group. In some of the anions the C(41)——C(42) bond lies in a position which bisects the angle between the C(21)——C(22) and C(22)——O(40) bonds when viewed down the C(22)——C(41) bond (position A), while in others the C(41)——C(42) bond bisects the angle between the C(22)—— O(40) and C(22)——C(23) bonds (position B) Figure 57). Position A is found in both molecules in the $Ba^{2+}L_2^- \cdot H_2O$, $Ag_2^+L_2^- \cdot 2CH_3 \cdot CO \cdot CH_3$, and Form II of the $Na_2^+(5-BrL)_2^-$ dimers, and also in the $Na^+ \cdot L^- \cdot CH_3OH$ monomer and in the Cs^+ salt polymer. Position B is found in both molecules in Form I of the $Na_2^+(5-BrL)_2^-$ dimer, in the $Na_2^+L_2^- \cdot 2H_2O$ dimer, and in the amine salt. The $Ag^+5-NO_2 \cdot L^-$ salt is the only dimer which has the C(41)——C(42) group in position A in one molecule and position B in the second molecule.

In general, the carboxylate group is coplanar with the plane of the phenyl ring; the greatest exceptions are found in the dimeric Ba^{2+} salt and in the $Ag^+(5 \cdot NO_2L)^-$ dimer, where dihedral angles of 25 to $32°$ are obtained. In the latter example the angles of twist are in opposite directions ($30°$ in the unprimed molecule and $31°$ in the other), once again showing that the Ag^+ nitrolasalocid derivative is among the least symmetrical of the dimers.

The conformations of the lasalocid molecules in the un-ionized form are quite similar to those found in the salts; however, there is greater uniformity among the acids and virtually no unusual features. The greatest variation in torsion angle in the backbone is 15°. The five-membered ring is in the same envelope conformation, with C(18) lying out of the plane. However, the five-membered ring in the unprimed molecule in the 5-bromolasalocid hemihydrate dimer is distorted some-what toward the halfchair conformation. All the acids have the C(41)——C(42) ethyl group in position A, with the exception of form B of the lasalocid:methanolate monomer.

It is noteworthy that the only other example found of two crystal-line modifications of the same chemical structure being obtained from the same solvent systems, namely, the $(5\text{-BrL}^- \cdot \text{Na}^+)_2$ dimers, has *both* ions with one conformation for C(41)——C(42) in one form and *both* ions with the other conformation for C(41)——C(42) in the other form. One may speculate that the crystalline form is dictated by the confor-mation of the molecules in that region in solution.

The carboxylic acid group is within 12° of coplanarity with the phenyl ring in all the free acid molecules.

The packing in the crystal of some of the lasalocid derivatives merits discussion. When the x-ray structure determination of the di-meric Ag^+-lasalocid salt was undertaken, it was realized that it was an acetonate with one acetone molecule per lasalocid moeity (Maier and Paul, 1971). When the analysis was complete, no significant electron density could be recognized that corresponded to acetone molecules. However, when the arrangement of the dimers in the cell was examined, it was apparent that there were infinite "empty" channels running along the crystal in the a-direction (Figure 60). These channels, ap-

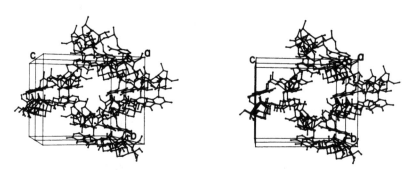

Figure 60   A stereoscopic view of the packing of the Ag^+-lasalocid acetonate. The acetone molecules were not located in the analysis and must be disordered. They must occupy the apparently open channels running along the a-direction between stacks of Ag^+-lasalocid dimer.

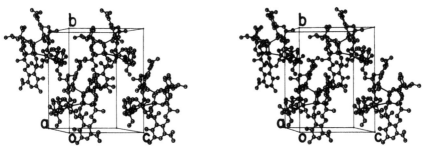

Figure 61   A stereoscopic view of the packing in the Ag⁺-5-nitro-lasalocid methanolate structure. The reference molecule is to the lower left-hand corner of the unit cell. The molecules of methanol are disordered and were not located by the analysis. They must occupy pockets between the dimers such as are seen to the right central part of the cell.

proximately 8 $\overset{\circ}{A}$ in diameter, must contain the acetone molecules in an almost totally disordered structure. The continued presence of the acetone in virtually the full stoichiometric amount was established by NMR spectroscopy. In a similar but less spectacular fashion, the methanol of crystallization in the dimer of the Ag⁺ salt of 5-nitro-lasalocid must be locked in the crystal in a disordered structure (C. I.

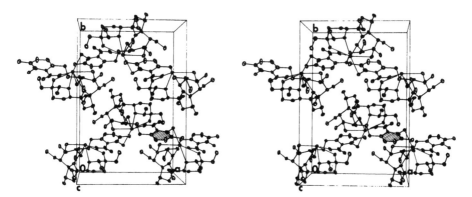

Figure 62   A stereoscopic view of the packing in the Cs⁺-lasalocid structure. The phenyl ring of the reference molecule has been shaded. The polymeric structure runs along the a direction.

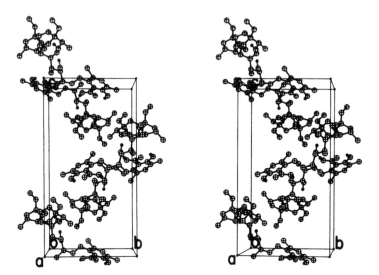

Figure 63 The packing of 5-bromoisolasalocid molecules in the unit
cell. The reference molecule is to the rear of the cell (from the viewer) and about halfway along the c axis. The intermolecular hydrogen
bond between the carboxylic acid group of the reference molecule and
the hydroxyl group of the molecule at $\frac{1}{2}$ + x, $1\frac{1}{2}$ − y, 1 − z is shown
by a thin line. These intermolecular hydrogen bonds result in chains
of molecules running in the a direction.

Hejna, E. N. Duesler, and I. C. Paul, unpublished data, 1972). However, in this case the solvent must occupy discrete pockets. A view of
the packing of this structure is shown in Figure 61.

The polymeric structure for the Cs^{+} salt is generated by the coordination of the Cs^{+} principally associated with one lasalocid anion
to the phenolic hydroxyl, O(28), of the adjacent lasalocid anion along
the a-direction (W. F. Paton and I. C. Paul, unpublished data, 1978).
A view of part of this polymer structure is shown in Figure 62. The
Cs^{+}——O(28) contact is between the reference molecule and that related by $-\frac{1}{2}$ + x, $\frac{1}{2}$ − y, −z.

The carboxylic acid group in 5-bromoisolasalocid is involved in
intermolecular hydrogen bonding. The conformation adopted by the 5-
bromoisolasalocid places the carboxylic group to the outside of the molecule and it forms a hydrogen bond to the O(31)——H hydroxyl group
in an adjacent molecule in the a-direction (Figure 63). The O(26)——
H---O(31) ($\frac{1}{2}$ + x, $1\frac{1}{2}$ − y, 1 − z) distance is 2.61 Å. While O(31)——H
is a donor in intramolecular hydrogen bonding, the O(26)——H---O(31)
hydrogen bonds form a polymeric chain along the a-axis.

13. *Lonomycin*

The history of this ionophore is rather involved. Riche and Pascard-Billy (1975) published the structure and named the ionophore emericid. Coordinates were not published. The structure is shown in Figure 64. Sodium and silver salts were examined by x-ray methods and were reported to be "nearly isomorphous"; cell data are given in Table 1. The absolute configuration was determined by anomalous dispersion methods on the Ag^+ salt, but the better refinement appears to have been achieved on the Na^+ salt. Shortly after, Yamazaki et al. (1976) determined the structure by x-ray analysis of an Ag^+ salt apparently as a methanolate; they named the ionophore DE-3936. Coordinates were not published. At about the same time, Ōtake et al. (1975b) determined the structure and absolute configuration of the Tl^+ salt, crystallized apparently without solvent. These workers named the ionophore lonomycin and published the atomic coordinates. In the present discussion we will follow the name and numbering system used by Ōtake et al. (1975b).

The space group of the Ag^+ salt methanolate (Yamazaki et al., 1976) and the Tl^+ salt (Ōtake et al., 1975b) is $P2_12_12_1$ and the cell data are quite similar. The available evidence suggests that the two salts are isostructural. Reference is made in both papers to crystal decomposition, yet only in the case of the Ag^+ salt is the presence of solvent of crystallization acknowledged. The space group of the unsolvated Ag^+ and Na^+ salts studied by Riche and Pascard-Billy (1975) is $P2_1$, and while the a and c axes are about the same length as those studied in Japan, the b axis length is about half of that for the Ag^+-methanolate and the Tl^+ salt.

A view of the structure of the Tl^+ salt is shown in Figure 65. The Tl^+ ion is complexed to six oxygen atoms, with distances in the 2.6 to 3.0 Å range (Table 21); they are the two carboxylate oxygen atoms and four ether oxygen atoms. The Tl^+—O(12) and Tl^+—O(14) dis-

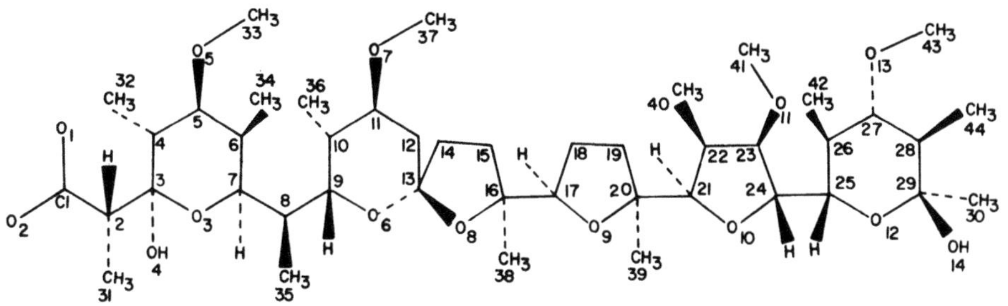

Figure 64 The structure of lonomycin showing the atom numbering used in the present discussion.

Table 21 Metal Ion——O Distances (Å) in the Salts of Lonomycin

	Tl^+	Ag^+ (unsolvated)	Na^+ (unsolvated)
M^+——O(1)	2.71(2)	2.41[a]	2.38[a]
M^+——O(2)	3.03(3)	2.65	2.45
M^+——O(7)	2.83(2)	2.70	2.50
M^+——O(8)	2.79(2)	2.55	2.40
M^+——O(9)	2.95(2)	2.77	2.51
M^+——O(10)	2.88(2)	2.50	2.45
M^+——O(12)	3.21(2)		
M^+——O(14)	3.45(2)		

[a]Standard deviations were not given in the paper by Riche and Pascard-Billy (1975).

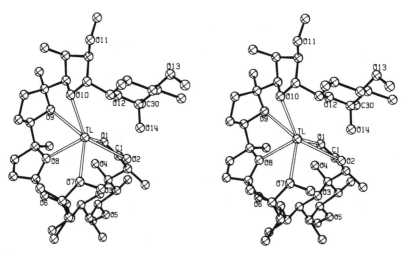

Figure 65 A view of the Tl^+ salt of lonomycin. The Tl^+——O coordinations are drawn as open lines.

tances of 3.21 and 3.45 Å are probably too long to be considered as coordination.

In the unsolvated Na^+ and Ag^+ salts studied by Riche and Pascard-Billy (1975) the Na^+ and Ag^+ ions are coordinated with the same six oxygen atoms; distances are given in Table 21. In every case the Na^+——O distance is shorter than the Ag^+——O distance, which is in turn shorter than the Tl^+——O distance. From the brief description, it appears that the metal coordination in the Ag^+-methanolate salt is identical to those of the others. In the Tl^+ salt the ionophore is held in the head-to-tail conformation by O(14)——H---O(2) hydrogen bonding; the O(14)---O(2) distance is 2.75(3) Å. There is also a hydrogen bond between the β-hydroxyl group, O(4), and the carboxylate oxygen, O(1); the O(4)---O(1) distance is 2.60(3) Å. As is the case of several ionophores with α- or β-hydroxy groups, this hydrogen bond may help to fix the orientation of the carboxylate group; the C(31)——C(2)——C(1)——O(2) torsion angle is 1.3°. The same patterns of hydrogen bonding are found in the other salts. Several of the methoxyl ether oxygen atoms, O(5), O(11), and O(13), lie to the outside of the complex. The arrangement of bond angles at the C(13) spiro ring junction shows a smaller spread than is often the case, 106 to 115°.

From the brief report on the structure of the Ag^+-methanolate salt (Yamazaki et al., 1976) no differences between it and the Tl^+ salt are apparent.

14. Lysocellin

Lysocellin is among the smaller acid ionophore molecules. It has a formula of $C_{34}H_{60}O_{10}$ and a molecular weight of 628.9. The free acid is an amorphous powder, while the sodium and silver salts were obtained as crystalline hemihydrates with melting points of 158-160°C

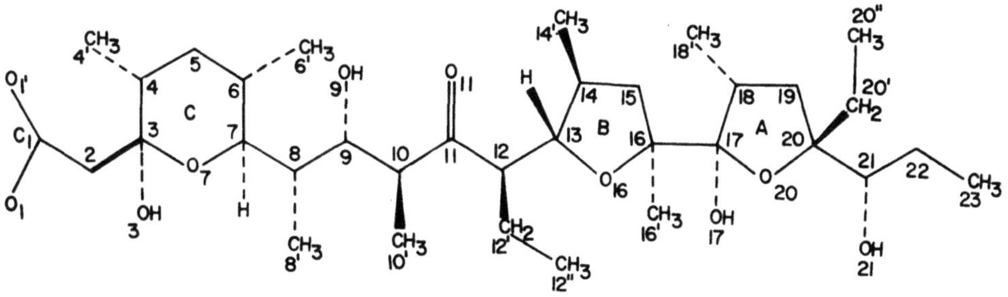

Figure 66 The structure of lysocellin showing the atom numbering used in the discussion.

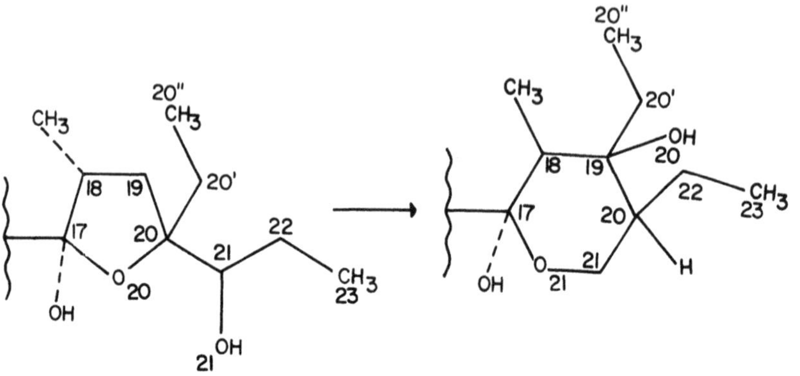

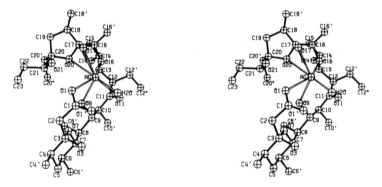

Figure 67 A drawing of the rearrangement that takes place in lysocellin.

and 123°C (decomposed) by O̅take et al. (1975a). The structure of
lysocellin is shown in Figure 66. When the free acid is dissolved in
methanol, isomerization of the five-membered ring A into a six-membered ring gradually takes place, with bond formation between O(21)
and C(17) instead of O(20) and C(17) (Figure 67); at the same time
decarboxylation and methylation at O(3) also take place (Koenuma

Figure 68 A stereoscopic view of the structure of the Ag⁺ salt of lysocellin. The Ag⁺——O coordination bonds are shown by open lines.

Table 22 Ag^+—O Distances (Å) in the Ag^+ Salt of Lysocellin

Ag^+—O(1)	2.55(1)	Ag^+—O(17)	2.45(1)
Ag^+—O(9)	2.55(1)	Ag^+—O(20)	3.05(1)
Ag^+—O(11)	3.00(1)	Ag^+—O(W)	2.39(1)
Ag^+—O(16)	2.46(1)		

et al., 1976). There appears to be a discrepancy regarding the water of crystallization. In both publications on this structure (Otake et al., 1975a; Koenuma et al., 1976) the salt is referred to as a hemihydrate, yet it appears that the water molecule is complexed (with Ag^+) with an individual lysocellin molecule. The space group of the crystal, $P2_12_12_1$, has no special sites for a water molecule. It is possible that the complex should ideally be a 1:1 hydrate but that ~ 50% of the water was lost prior to elemental analysis. A view of the Ag^+ salt of lyocellin is shown in Figure 68.

The ionophore is wrapped around the Ag^+ ion in typical fashion. The Ag^+ ion is complexed with six oxygen atoms in the ionophore and with the water molecule of crystallization.* The Ag^+ ion complexes with the carboxyl group, O(1), with three hydroxyl groups, O(9), O(11), and O(17), and with two ether oxygens, O(16) and O(20); Ag^+—O distances are given in Table 22. The circular conformation of the lysocellin anion is stabilized by a head-to-tail hydrogen bond between O(21)—H---O(1); the O(21)---O(1) distance is 2.62(3) Å. There are probably also intramolecular hydrogen bonds between O(3)—H---O(1'), O(9)—H---O(7), and O(17)—H---O(21); the O(3)---O(1'), O(9)---O(7), and O(17)---O(21) distances are 2.64(2), 2.68(1), and 2.78(3) Å, respectively, and the C(3)—O(3)---O(1'), C(9)—O(9)---O(7), and the C(17)—O(17)---O(21) angles are 88(1), 80(1), and 98(1)°. The water molecule, in addition to being coordinated with Ag^+, is probably involved in two hydrogen bonds, with O(1') and O(11). The O(W)---O(1') and O(W)---O(11) distances are 2.65(3) and 2.94(2) Å, respectively, and the O(1')—(W)---O(11) angle is 122.3(8)°. In many ways the structure of lysocellin is reminiscent of those for lasalocid or isolasalocid; the molecular weights are roughly comparable and there are similarities in the substituent pattern. However, lysocellin does not have an aromatic group.

---

*In the publication by Koenuma et al. (1976) it was stated that Ag^+ was surrounded by six oxygen atoms, with distances from 2.39 to 2.99 Å; however, as the Ag^+—O(20) distance is 3.05 Å, we believe it to be more appropriate to consider the Ag^+ ion to be seven-coordinated.

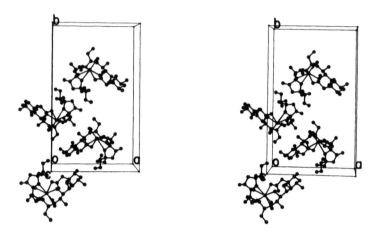

Figure 69 A stereoscopic view of the packing in the Ag^+-lysocellin salt. The water molecule is complexed to the Ag^+ ion and does not participate in intermolecular hydrogen bonding. The reference molecule is the upper one in the unit cell.

A view of the packing of the Ag^+ salt is shown in Figure 69. There are no unusually short contacts and the water molecule interacts with only one salt entity.

15. Monensin

The elucidation of the structure of monensin by x-ray analysis of its silver salt (Agtarap et al., 1967) opened the door to the structures of the organic acid ionophores. Since then the crystallography of monensin and its derivatives has been examined by several groups. Pinkerton and Steinrauf (1970) reported two types of crystals for monovalent metal salts and designated them type Na and type K. Dihydrates of sodium and silver salts were obtained as type Na in the monoclinic space group $P2_1$, while dihydrates of potassium, silver, and thallium salts were obtained as type K in the orthorhombic space group $P2_12_12_1$. The a and c axes of the two types had effectively the same length, but the b axis virtually doubled in going from the monoclinic to the orthorhombic form. A full x-ray analysis was carried out on the silver salt to establish the molecular structure. Poor crystals of a Rb^+ salt were reported as possibly belonging to a third form. A very recent preliminary report by Smith and Duax (1979) announces the determination of the structure of the sodium salt as a dihydrate in, apparently, Steinrauf's type K form. Smith and Duax (1979) also re-

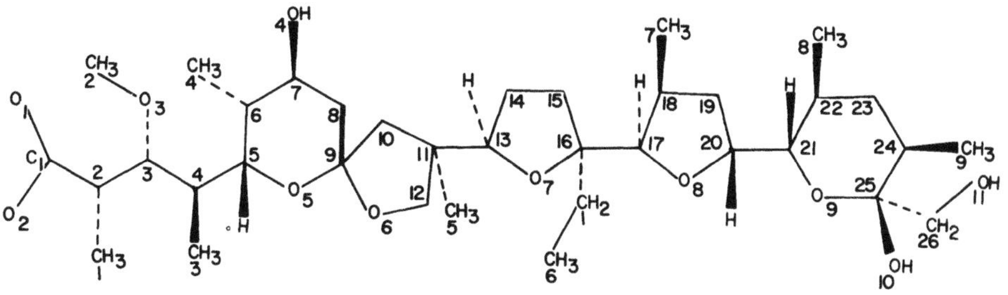

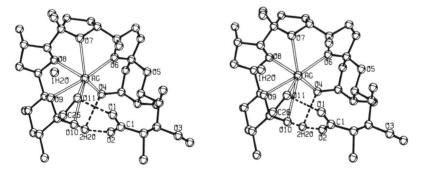

Figure 70 The structure of monensin showing the atom numbering.

port the determination of the structure of an anhydrous sodium salt with cell dimensions and space group in agreement with type Na. Lutz et al. (1971) determined the structure of the free acid as a mono-hydrate, while Ward et al. (1978) have described the structure of a NaBr complex of the free acid. The cell dimensions of this latter complex are similar to those of Steinrauf's type K and the space group is the same. On the basis of a statistical comparison of the structural parameters of the dihydrated Ag^+ salt with those of the anhydrous Na^+Br^- complex, Ward et al. (1978) concluded that the "crystal structures are very similar."

Figure 71 Stereoscopic view of a single molecule of Ag^+-monensin dihydrate. The Ag^+——O coordinations are shown by open bonds; the hydrogen bonds are shown by dashed lines.

Table 23 Ag^+—O, Na^+—O, and H_2O—O Distances (Å) in the
Ag^+ Salt, the NaBr Complex, the Sodium Salt Dihydrate, the Anhydrous Na^+ Salt, and the Free Acid of Monensin

	Ag^+ salt·$2H_2O$	NaBr complex	Na^+ salt·$2H_2O$	Na^+ anhydrous	Free acid[a]
X—O(4)[b]	2.427(10)	2.350(7)	2.336(7)	2.346(2)	3.48
X—O(6)	2.407(9)	2.366(7)	2.358(6)	2.411(2)	3.40
X—O(7)	2.692(9)	2.503(7)	2.543(7)	2.529(2)	2.85
X—O(8)	2.583(9)	2.472(8)	2.443(7)	2.408(2)	3.77
X—O(9)	2.560(10)	2.438(7)	2.447(7)	2.513(2)	3.73
X—O(11)	2.455(10)	2.418(8)	2.449(7)	2.381(2)	2.64
X—O(1)	3.864(12)	4.163(9)			2.90
X—O(2)	3.842(11)	4.308(8)			3.84

[a]No standard deviations were given in the paper by Lutz et al.
(1971).
[b]In the Ag^+ salt X = Ag^+; in the NaBr complex and in the Na^+ salts
X = Na^+; in free acid X = H_2O.

The molecular structure of monensin is shown in Figure 70, which
also gives the atom numbering used in the discussion. Monensin represents a unique situation in that all the research groups used the
same numbering system. The structure of the Ag^+ salt (Pinkerton and
Steinrauf, 1970) is illustrated in Figure 71. The anion of the ionophore
is wrapped around the Ag^+ ion in typical fashion. The Ag^+ ion is coordinated to six oxygen atoms; they are two hydroxyl, O(4) and O(10),
and four ether oxygens, O(6), O(7), O(8), and O(9) (Table 23). It
is not coordinated with the carboxyl group; the shortest Ag^+—O
(carboxyl) distance is 3.84(1) Å. The circular conformation of the
ionophore is stabilized by *two* head-to-tail hydrogen bonds, one between O(10)—H---O(2) and the other O(11)—H---O(1); the O(10)---
O(2) and O(11)---O(1) distances are 2.65(2) and 2.51(2) Å, respectively. The hydroxyl oxygen atom, O(4), is probably involved in a
hydrogen bond to one of the water molecules of crystallization (H_2O-2);
the O(4)—O-2 distance is 2.84(2) Å and the C(7)—O(4)---O—2 angle
is 106.6(1)°. This water molecule probably also acts as a donor in a hydrogen bond to O(10), with a O—2---O(10) distance of 2.89(2) Å. The
other water molecule, H_2O-1, acts as a donor in hydrogen bonds to
O(11) in the reference molecule and O(3) in the molecule at $-\frac{1}{2} + x$,
$1\frac{1}{2} - y$, $-z$; the O—1---O(11) and O—1---O(3) distances are 2.82 and

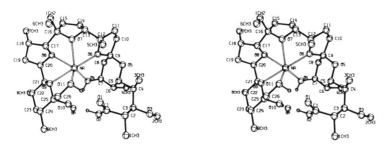

Figure 72 The structure of the NaBr·monensin complex. The Na⁺——O coordination is shown by open lines. The Br⁻ anion lies to the lower rear portion of the figure.

2.93(1) Å, respectively, and the O(11)——O-1——O(3) angle is 95.0(1)°. In addition, the two water molecules are hydrogen bonded to each other, with H_2O-2 acting as donor to H_2O-1 associated with the molecule at $\frac{1}{2}$ + x, $1\frac{1}{2}$ − y, 1 − z; the O-2---O-1 distance is 2.78(2) Å, and the O(10)——O-2---O-1 angle is 133.7(1)°. This arrangement of hydrogen bonds does provide the crystal with some relatively unusual polar intermolecular contacts. Only the oxygen atoms involved in hydrogen bonding to the water molecules lie to the outside of the circular shape.

The crystal structure of the NaBr complex of monensin (Figure 72) is virtually identical to that of the Ag⁺ salt. A halfnormal probability comparison of the positional parameters for the two structures gave a linear plot which indicates a great similarity in the structures (Ward et al., 1978). The only significant deviations were in two of the coordinates for the Na⁺ and Ag⁺ ions. However, there are interesting *chemical* differences. In the NaBr complex the carboxylic group is not ionized and the two water molecules of the Ag⁺ salt are replaced by the Br⁻ ion. The Na⁺——O coordination is very similar to that of Ag⁺——O in the Ag⁺ salt, although the distances are slightly shorter (Table 23). While the O(11)—H---O(1) hydrogen bond is retained in the NaBr complex, O(2) acts as the donor in a hydrogen bond to O(10); the O(11)---O(1) and O(2)---O(10) distances are 2.731(10) and 2.757(9) Å, respectively. These distances are significantly longer than the ones found in the Ag⁺ salt. The hydroxyl groups O(10) (now acting as a *donor*) and O(4) form O——H---Br⁻ hydrogen bonds. The O(10)---Br⁻ and O(4)---Br⁻ distances are 3.192(6) and 3.216(7) Å, respectively. Thus the Br⁻ ion occupies the position of the (H_2O)-2 water molecule in the Ag⁺ salt; there is no atom corresponding to the position of (H_2O)-1. The intermolecular interactions between mole-

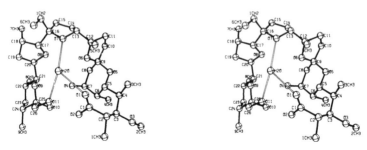

Figure 73   A stereoscopic view of the monensin:water complex. The
hydrogen bonds involving the water molecule are shown by open lines.

cules through hydrogen bonds found in the Ag^+ salt are not present
in the NaBr complex.

At the spiro ring junction, C(9), there is considerable deviation
from tetrahedral angles; the smallest angle is O(6)——C(9)——C(10),
103.3(6)°, and the greatest is C(8)——C(9)——C(10), 115.8(8)°.

The crystal structure of the free acid of monensin monohydrate
(Lutz et al., 1971) is different from those of the salt and the complex, although the space groups are the same. A view of the free
acid monohydrate is shown in Figure 73. The neutral molecule has a
rather similar conformational arrangement to those found in the salt
and has the water molecule enclosed in the center rather than the Ag^+
and Na^+ cations. However, there is only *one* head-to-tail hydrogen
bond, between O(2)——H and O(11); the O(2)---O(11) distance is
2.65 Å. There are additional intramolecular hydrogen bonds between
O(10)——H---O(4) and O(4)——H---O(6); the O(10)---O(4) and
O(4)---O(6) distances are 2.77 and 2.80 Å, respectively, and the
C(25)——O(10)---O(4) and C(7)——O(4)---O(6) angles are 109.1 and
82.9°, respectively. The enclosed water molecule is also involved in
acting as a hydrogen bond donor to O(1) and O(7) and as an acceptor
from O(11). The H_2O---O(1), H_2O---O(7), and O(11)---H_2O distances
are 2.90, 2.85, and 2.64 Å, respectively, and the O(1)——H_2O---O(7)
angle is 126°. The distances between the water molecule and many of
the oxygen atoms in the molecule are given in Table 23. Comparison of
these distances with the Ag^+——O and Na^+——O distances in the other
two compounds reveals a very significant difference in the relative
position of the water molecule with respect to the ionophore when compared to positions of the Ag^+ and Na^+ ions. A schematic view of this
difference is shown in Figure 74 (Lutz et al., 1971).

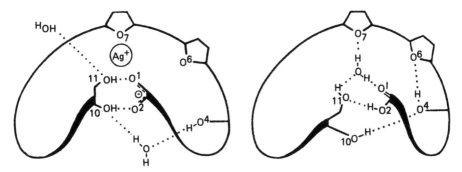

Figure 74 Schematic representation of hydrogen-bonding patterns in monensin silver salt and free acid. Not all of the hydrogen positions indicated have been confirmed from difference syntheses, which tend to show electron-density accumulation close to both oxygen atoms in each hydrogen bond, possibly as the result of disorder in the hydrogen atom arrangement. (Source: Lutz et al., 1971.)

The differences in the conformations of the monensin entities in the three crystals are quite small. The torsion angles that show differences of 10° or greater are given in Table 24. In all cases these differences involve the free acid. The greatest difference is 18° in the O(8)—C(20)-C(21)—O(9) angle. However, the changes in conformation are made by relatively small changes in a large number of torsions, rather than by a major change in a few.

There are no unusual intermolecular contacts in the NaBr complex or the free acid of monensin. However, in the Ag^+ monensin dihydrate structure as mentioned above there are intermolecular hydrogen bonds involving the water molecules of crystallization. One of the water molecules, H_2O-2, forms two hydrogen bonds to O(4) and O(10) in the reference molecule, while the other water molecule, H_2O-1, is on the other side of the molecule (Figure 71) and forms a hydrogen bond to O(11) in the reference molecule and one to O(3) in the molecule at $-\frac{1}{2} + x$, $1\frac{1}{2} - y$, $-z$. The water molecule, H_2O-2, associated with the reference molecule acts as a donor in a hydrogen bond to H_2O-1 associated with the molecule at $\frac{1}{2} + x$, $1\frac{1}{2} - y$, $1 - z$. This system of hydrogen bonds results in layers of complexes held together by the water molecules of crystallization in the a-c plane. Part of this network and some of the intermolecular hydrogen bonds are illustrated in Figure 75.

After this chapter was submitted we received a manuscript from W. L. Duax describing the structures of the sodium salt dihydrate of monensin and that of the anhydrous sodium salt of monensin (Duax et al., 1980). As mentioned earlier in the chapter, the sodium salt

Table 24 Torsion Angles (°) Where There Are Differences in the Angles in the Ag$^+$ Salt, the NaBr Complex, and the Free Acid of 10° or More[a]

	Ag$^+$ salt 2H$_2$O	NaBr complex	Na$^+$ salt 2H$_2$O	Na$^+$ anhydrous	Free acid
O(1)-C(1)-C(2)-C(3)	-123	-121	-122	-107	-111
C(2)-C(3)-C(4)-C(5)	-86	-83	-82	-77	-76
C(13)-O(7)-C(16)-C(15)	25	30	24	33	17
O(7)-C(16)-C(15)-C(14)	-3	-6	-1	-13	9
C(13)-C(14)-C(15)-C(16)	-19	-17	-20	-10	-29
C(16)-C(17)-O(8)-C(20)	-161	-167	-164	-162	-156
O(8)-C(20)-C(21)-O(9)	53	46	51	51	64
C(21)-O(9)-C(25)-C(24)	-60	-49	-58	-59	-63
O(9)-C(25)-C(24)-C(23)	56	51	58	53	61

[a]The corresponding angles for the sodium salt dihydrate and the anhydrous sodium salt are also given.

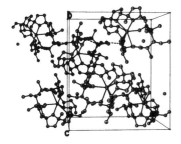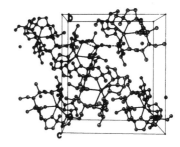

Figure 75   A stereoscopic view of the packing in the Ag⁺-monensin dihydrate structure. The reference molecule is inside the cell to the upper left of the cell. The oxygen atoms involved in hydrogen bonding are blackened and some of the intermolecular hydrogen bonds are shown by discontinuous lines. The two water molecules serve as hydrogen-bonded links among molecules in the a-c plane and form layers in this plane.

dihydrate belongs to Steinrauf's type-K classification (Pinkerton and Steinrauf, 1970), although it was not reported by them, while the anhydrous sodium salt corresponds to the type-Na classification, although Steinrauf and Pinkerton reported only a sodium salt dihydrate in that classification (monoclinic, $P2_1$). As might be expected from the earlier work, the crystal of the sodium salt dihydrate is closely isostructural with that of the silver salt dihydrate (Pinkerton and Steinrauf, 1970). The coordination spheres of the metal in the two

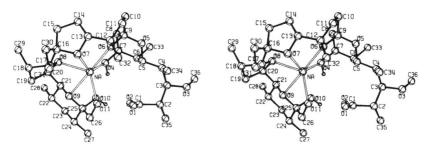

Figure 76   Stereoscopic view of the anhydrous Na⁺-monensin salt. (Source: Duax et al., 1980.)

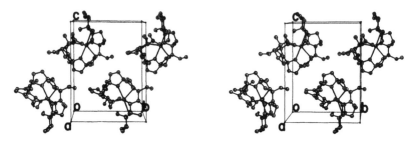

Figure 77 Stereoscopic view of the packing of the anhydrous Na^+-monensin salt (Source: Duax et al., 1980).

new sodium salts are the same as those in the silver salt dihydrate and the NaBr complex. The Na^+——O distances in the anhydrous and dihydrate salts are very similar to those in the NaBr complex, but in all three Na^+ salts the M^+——O distances are, on the average, significantly shorter than those in the Ag^+ salt (see Table 23).

Views of a single molecule and of the packing of the anhydrous sodium salt are shown in Figure 76 and 77.

16. Nigericin

Nigericin was one of the first of the family of acid ionophores to be studied by x-ray diffraction. The structure of Ag^+ salt was carried out and published by two different groups at almost the same time (Kubota et al., 1968; Steinrauf et al., 1968). Steinfauf et al. (1968) reported that the silver and sodium salts of nigericin were isomorphous and determined the structure of the Ag^+ salt. Kubota et al. (1968) also described the Ag+ salt and named the molecule polyetherin A. Shiro and Koyama (1970) subsequently published a full description of the crystal structure, including atomic coordinates, of the Ag^+ salt, and it is from this paper that most of this discussion is based. While the name nigericin will be used in this discussion, we will use the atom numbering described by Shiro and Koyama (1970) (Figure 78). It is also of interest that one of the three ionophore antibiotics (X-464) isolated by Berger et al. at Roche in 1951 turned out to be nigericin (Stempel et al., 1969).

The structure of the Ag^+ salt of nigericin is shown in Figure 79. The conformation of the salt has the usual features: a nonpolar exterior and a polar interior, and the circular conformation held together by head-to-tail hydrogen bonding. The Ag^+ ion is complexed to five oxygen atoms, four of them are ether oxygens and the fifth is one of the carboxyl oxygen atoms; the Ag^+——O distances are given in Table 25. The major hydrogen bond is between the hydroxyl oxygen atom

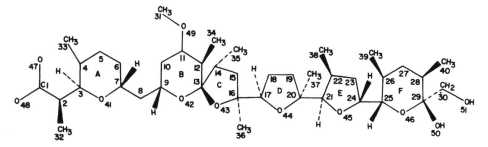

Figure 78 The structure of nigericin showing the atom numbering.

O(50) and the other carboxyl oxygen atom, O(48); the O(50)---O(48) length is 2.58(2) Å.

Although not mentioned in the paper by Shiro and Koyama (1970), O(51)——H is probably involved in intramolecular hydrogen bonding to either O(48) or O(50). The O(51)---O(48) and O(51)---O(50) distances are 2.79(2) and 2.77(2) Å, respectively, while the C(30)-O(51)---O(48) and C(30)-O(51)---O(50) angles are 92(1) and 62(1)°, respectively. On the basis of the geometry, the more probably hydrogen-bonding assignment is O(51)——H---O(48), which would correspond to a second head-to-tail hydrogen bond.

Rings B and C have a spiro ring junction; the largest bond angle is C(12)——C(13)——C(14) at 114(1)°, while the smallest is the endocyclic angle in the five-membered ring, C(14)——C(13)——O(43), at 103(1)°. The three six-membered ether rings have the expected chair conformation, two of the five-membered rings (D and E) are in the envelope conformation, while ring C is a half chair.

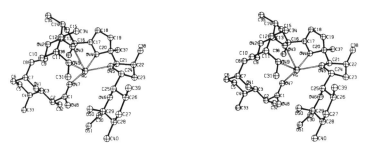

Figure 79 A stereoscopic view of the Ag$^+$ salt of nigericin. The Ag$^+$——O coordination bonds are shown by open lines.

Table 25 Ag$^+$——O Distances (Å) Less Than 2.7 Å in the Ag$^+$-Nigericin Salt

Ag$^+$——O(47)	2.26(1)	Ag$^+$——O(49)	2.62(1)
Ag$^+$——O(45)	2.47(1)	Ag$^+$——O(44)	2.66(1)
Ag$^+$——O(43)	2.60(1)		

There do not appear to be any unusual features in the molecular packing. The shortest intermolecular contact is of 3.31(1) Å between the methyl carbon of C(37) and the ether oxygen O(41) in the molecule at $1 - x$, $-\frac{1}{2} + y$, $1\frac{1}{2} - z$.

17. Salinomycin

Salinomycin is a crystalline compound (mp 112.5-113.5°C), but no crystalline salts could be prepared (Kinashi et al., 1973, 1975). Consequently, the structure analysis was carried out on a p-iodophenacyl derivative at the carboxyl position. While this is a very effective procedure for determination of structure and absolute configuration, the resulting crystal structure will probably have little relevance for biological activity. The molecular structure of salinomycin is shown in Figure 80. The structure is novel in having three rings, B, C, and D in spiro linkages and in having a double bond in ring C. Ring A and its substituents and the β-ketol position of the backbone [C(18)——C(22)] are similar to those found in lasalocid (Kinashi et al., 1975).

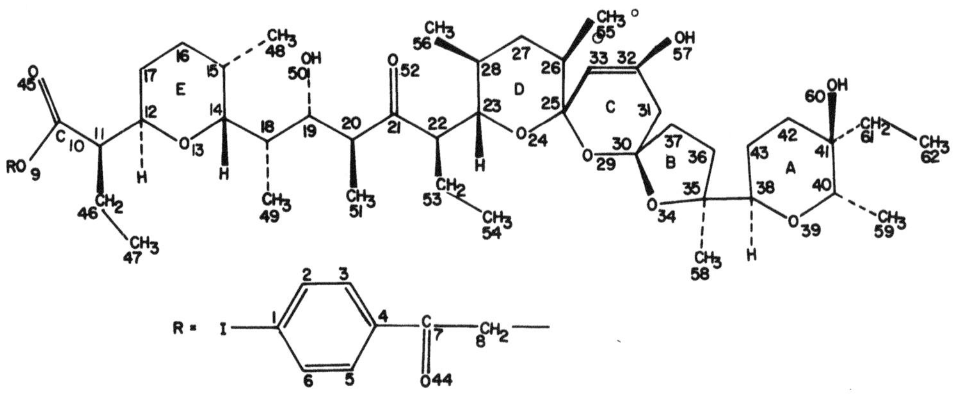

Figure 80 A drawing of the molecular structure of salinomycin showing the atom numbering, including that of the p-iodophenylacyl group.

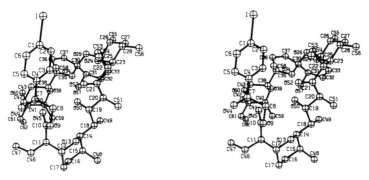

Figure 81   A stereoscopic view of the p-iodophenacyl ester of salino-mycin.

A view of the structure of the p-iodophenacyl derivative of salino-mycin is shown in Figure 81. As the carboxyl group is substituted, there is no head-to-tail hydrogen bonding between O(60)——H and the carboxyl group. The molecule adopts a "helical" arrangement (Kinashi et al., 1975) rather than the usual circular one. This arrangement is stabilized by probable hydrogen bonds between O(50)——H and O(34) and between O(57)——H and O(39); the O(50)---O(34) and O(57)---O(39) distances are 2.81 and 2.91 Å, respectively, and the C(19)——O(50)---O(34) and C(31)——O(57)---O(39) angles are 144.1 and 114.3°. The O(50)——H---O(34) hydrogen bond appears somewhat more prob-able than one within the β-ketol group, i.e., O(50)——H---O(52). The O(50)---O(52) distance is 2.93(2) Å and the C(19)——O(50)---O(52) angle is 66.1(6)°. Most of the oxygen atoms in the structure are di-rected toward the interior, making one suspect that the molecule should be capable of complexing metal ions.

The molecular packing appears to be dominated by contacts between nonpolar groups. There is no evidence for specific intermolecular as-sociations.

18. *Septamycin*

Although isolated as the Na$^+$ salt, septamycin was characterized as the p-bromophenacyl derivative at the carboxyl position (Pletcher and Weber, 1974). Hence, while the chemical structure and absolute stereo-chemistry were determined, the carboxyl group that normally plays a major role in the determination of conformation has been altered. The structure of septamycin is shown in Figure 82.

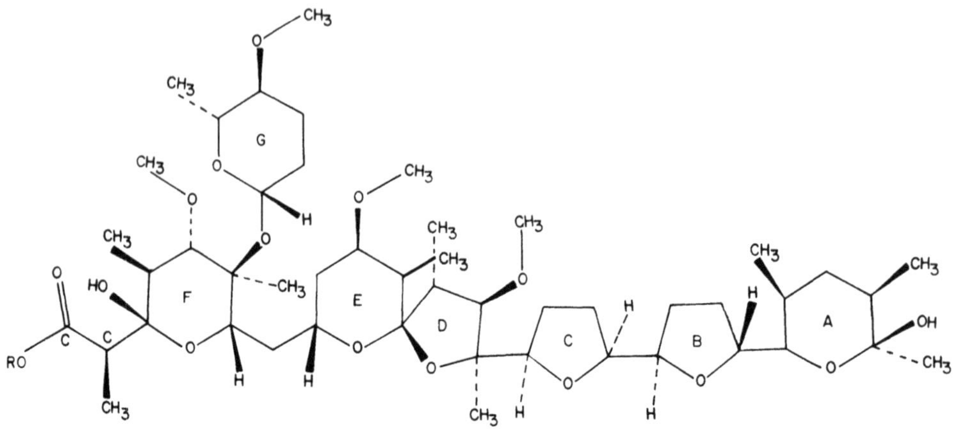

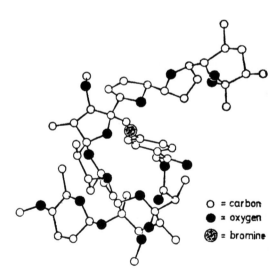

Figure 82   The structure of septamycin. No atom numbering was given in the paper.

Coordinates were not published and there is very little discussion of the conformation in the paper by Pletcher and Weber (1974). A drawing of the structure of the p-bromophenacyl derivative is shown in Figure 83. The molecule in this picture appears to adopt a relatively

O = carbon
● = oxygen
◉ = bromine

Figure 83   Projection of p-bromophenacylseptamycin down the crystallographic a axis. (Source: Pletcher and Weber, 1974.)

open arrangement. The chemical structure is very similar to that of
A204A (Jones et al., 1973); septamycin lacks a methoxyl on ring A,
and ring G has a different configuration and point of attachment. On
the basis of a space-filling model of the unsubstituted molecule,
Pletcher and Weber (1974) reason that the folding is similar to those
of nigericin and A204A; they assume that ring G would not be involved
in metal coordination and would hang out as a tail.

19. X-206

X-206 was one of the three ionophores originally isolated by Berger
et al. in 1951. It forms sodium, potassium, silver, and barium salts.
The structure of X-206 was first reported from x-ray analysis of the
Ag^+ salt (Blount and Westley, 1971). The space group, $P6_3$, was
rather unusual for an acid ionophore and the amount of data was very
small for a reliable determination. A subsequent analysis (Blount and
Westley, 1975) of the hydrate of the free acid of X-206 showed that the
analysis of the Ag^+ salt had failed to detect three methyl groups and
that a hydroxyl group had been previously mistaken as a methyl group.
The correct structure, including absolute configuration, for X-206 is
shown in Figure 84. The three methyl groups omitted from the previous formulation (Blount and Westley, 1971) were those at C(20),
C(28), and C(30), while there is a secondary hydroxyl at C(22)
rather than a methyl group.

Atomic coordinates have not been published for either the Ag^+ salt
or the free acid, and they are not available to us. A stereoscopic
picture of the slightly incorrect Ag^+ salt structure is shown in Figure 85 (Blount and Westley, 1971). The molecule provides effective
three-dimensional protection for the Ag^+ ion, with the backbone describing "a path similar to that of the seam of a tennis ball" (Blount
and Westley, 1971). There is a head-to-tail hydrogen bond of length
2.69 Å from the O(14)——H to one of the carboxyl oxygen atoms, O(2).
The Ag^+ ion is coordinated to six oxygen atoms, one of the carboxyl
oxygens, O(1), three hydroxyl oxygens, O(4), O(6), and O(8), and
two ether oxygens, O(12) and O(13); the Ag^+——O distances range from
2.5 to 2.8 Å. On the basis of Figure 85 there are probably hydrogen
bonds between O(8) and O(1) and between O(11) and O(6); in addition,
there may be hydrogen bonds between O(6) and O(7) and between
O(4) and O(3). The misidentified hydroxyl group, O(9), points away
from the center of the moleculr and does not appear to be involved in
intramolecular hydrogen bonding. No details or figures of the conformation of the free acid were published (Blount and Westley, 1975).

A report has recently been published that shows the very close
similarity of alborixin and X-206 (Seto et al., 1979). Apparently, in
the report on the structure of alborixin (Alléaume et al., 1975) the
stereochemistry of the O(13)H hydroxyl (alborixin numbering) was
incorrectly shown in the structural drawing; it was this same hydroxyl

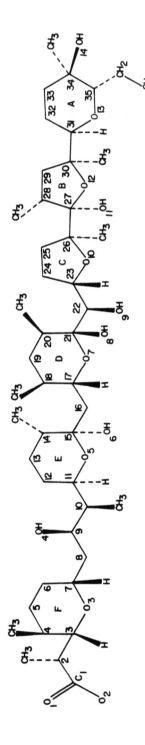

Figure 84 The structure of X-206 showing the atom numbering used in the discussion.

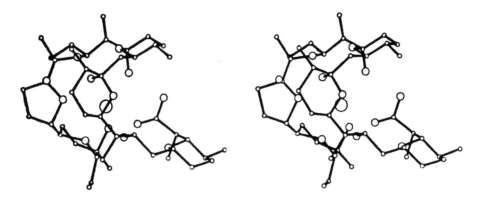

Figure 85 A stereoscopic drawing of the Ag⁺ salt of X-206. The structure is slightly incorrect in that three methyl groups are missing and an ——OH group is misidentified as a methyl (see text). (Source: Blount and Westley, 1971.)

that was originally identified as a methyl group for X-206. The hydrogen-bonding assignments in the Ag^+ salt of X-206 and in the K^+ salt of alborixin are the same and the metal coordination in the two salts are quite similar. However, in the K^+ salt of alborixin the metal ion is complexed with the hydroxyl attached to ring A and to the ether

Figure 86 The structure of X-14547A showing the atom numbering used in the discussion. The structure of the p-bromophenylamine is also shown.

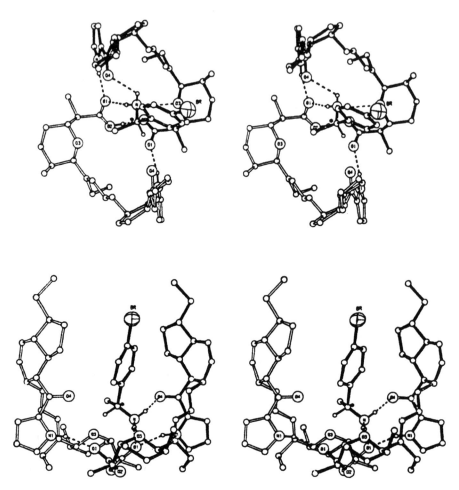

Figure 87 Two stereoscopic views of the structure of the 2:1
X-14547A:bromophenylethylamine salt. Hydrogen bonds are shown by
discontinuous lines. For clarity, the bonds of one of the X-14547A
molecules and of the amine have been blackened. (Source: Westley
et al., 1979; *J. Antibiot.*)

oxygen of ring C in addition to the other six oxygen atoms with which
Ag^+ is coordinated; it should be noted that the K^+——O distance to
that ether oxygen is the longest in the eight coordination sphere described for alborixin.

20. *X-14547A*

X-14547A has a number of very unusual features for an acid ionophore. The structure is shown in Figure 86 (Westley et al., 1979). X-14547A (free acid mp 138-141°C) is a relatively small molecule, $C_{31}H_{43}NO_4$, with a molecule weight of only 493.7. It has only four oxygen atoms and has the nitrogen-containing five-membered ring found previously in A23187. It has, in addition, two novel features, a 1,3-diene system in the main chain and a trans-fused tetrahydroindane ring. As a result of several of these features, there will be less conformational flexibility in this molecule than in many other ionophores.

While a Ca^{2+} salt has been reported, the structure analysis was carried out on a 1:2 amine salt (mp 128-131°C) of X-14557A; the amine used was the chiral R(+)-1-amino-1-(4-bromophenyl)ethane (see Figure 86) (Westley et al., 1979). The absolute configuration was established. Coordinates were not published, but the paper contained considerable structural detail. The 1:2 complex crystallizes in the space group $P4_34_12$, with the two ionophore entities being related by a crystallographic twofold axis. Thus, while in any individual complex or dimer one ionophore is ionized and the other is not, there is a statistical disorder throughout the crystal. The amine lies across the twofold axis and is statistically disordered throughout the crystal. Despite the problems associated with this disorder, it was possible

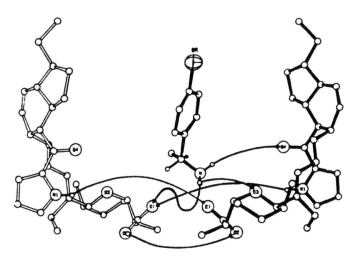

Figure 88 Schematic drawing of the 2:1 X-14547A:amino complex. Hydrogen bonds are shown by the thin curved lines. (Source: Westley et al., 1979, *J. Antibiot.*)

to delineate the details of the complex from the x-ray analysis. Two
stereoscopic views of the complex are shown in Figure 87, while Figure 88 is a more schematic view of the structure. The dimer is relatively open, with the two tetrahydroindane rings facing each other
and providing a "jawlike" protection of the $\overset{+}{\text{p}}$-bromophenyl group of
the amine. The amine nitrogen forms three $\overset{+}{\text{N}}$— H---O hydrogen
bonds; two to the ionized ionophore (designated without primes) and
one to the non-ionized one (designated with primes). The hydrogen
bonds are $\overset{+}{\text{N}}$—H---O(3) (ether), and $\overset{+}{\text{N}}$—H---O(4) (ketone), and
$\overset{+}{\text{N}}$—H---O(1') (carboxylic). In addition, the dimer is stabilized by
the two crystallographically related N(pyrrole)—H---O(1') and
N'—H---O(1) hydrogen bonds and one between the two related carboxylic acid groups O(2')—H---O(2). As was the case with A23187
the N(H)—C$\cong$O group is in the cis arrangement. Because of the
lack of conformational flexibility, the realtively few opportunities for
hydrogen bonds, and the small size of the molecule, one may speculate
that X-14547A, like lasalocid, will have a strong tendency to form dimeric structures. Further structural data on this ionophore are awaited
with interest.

III. CONCLUSION

There are a great many structural similarities among the polyether
antibiotics. In all the salts examined the exterior of the salt or salt
complex is quite nonpolar and the majority of the oxygen atoms are
directed toward the interior. In virtually every case studied, the only
exceptions being where a covalently bound derivative has been prepared, such as in salinomycin and septamycin, the conformation of the
ionophore in the salt is held in a circular or sometimes near-spherical
arrangement by hydrogen bonding between the carboxylate group at
the "head" and a hydroxyl group at the "tail" of the molecule. With
most of the Ag^+, Na^+, K^+, Tl^+, Ba^{2+}, and Cs^+ salts examined the coordination is quite irregular in geometry and it appears that the molecule wraps itself around the metal ion in such a way as to provide the
maximum metal ion-oxygen interaction.

The metal-oxygen distances shown considerable variation. The
shortest Na^+—O distance is 2.29 Å (lasalocid), the shortest Ag^+—O
distance is 2.2 Å (grisorixin), the shortest Tl^+—O distance is 2.6 Å
(grixorixin), the shortest K^+—O distance is 2.69 Å (alborixin), and
the shortest Ca^{2+}—O distance is 1.93 Å (A23817). While it is safe
to say that Tl^+—O distances are generally greater than Ag^+—O
or Na^+—O distances, it is more difficult to make generalizations
among the Na^+—O and Ag^+—O distances. For example, in the Na^+
salt of A204A the six Na^+—O distances lie in the range 2.71 to 2.97 Å,
while in several of the Na^+-lasalocid salts the six distances are all
less than 2.77 Å; in the Ag^+ salt of X-206 the six Ag^+—O distances

are in the range 2.5 to 2.8 Å, while in the Ag^+-nigericin structure
the five Ag^+—O distances are in the range 2.26 to 2.66 Å and for
one of the Ag^+ ions in the 5-nitrolasalocid dimer the five Ag^+—O
distances are in the range 2.36 to 2.62 Å. It certainly appears that
considerable variation in metal ion—O distances can be tolerated to
allow the ionophore to fold in an efficient conformation for metal-ion
coordination. The case of A23187 is an example where increasing the
coordination of the Ca^{2+} ion from six to seven leads to a very significant increase in Ca^+—O distances (from a range of 1.93 to 2.10 Å
to one of 2.27 to 2.38 Å).

In several ionophores the formally negatively charged carboxylate
group is not coordinated to the metal. This is especially true for
smaller ionophores such as lasalocid and monensin. In many cases,
metal ion—carboxylate coordination is assisted by an intramolecular
hydrogen bond between a β-hydroxyl group and the carboxylate ion;
this intramolecular hydrogen bond holds the carboxylate group in a
conformation whereby it can coordinate to the metal ion. This feature
is present in A204A, antibiotic 6016 (both an α and a β-hydroxy
group), carriomycin, K-41, lonomycin, and lysocellin. Several of the
longer and more flexible ionophores such as alborixin and X-206
coordinate the carboxylate group without this feature. It is also noteworthy that only in the case of the large Cs^+ ion can the lasalocid
molecule complex the metal ion with both the tail oxygen atoms and the
head carboxylate group, At least in the cases of the metal ions that
have been examined up to now, the conformation of the anion is only
very slightly altered when one ionophore forms a salt with different
metal ions.

The ionophores A-130, A204A, antibiotic 6016, carriomycin, dianemycin, K-41, and septamycin all have six-membered ether rings attached to a ring in the main chain by means of an ether linkage. In
no case is this attached six-membered ring involved in metal coordination and it is usually pointing outward from the quasi-spherical shape
of the metal ion complex. The role of this type of ring in metal complex formation does not appear significant and the presence of these
rings in the ionophores is somewhat puzzling.

For five ionophores x-ray structure determinations have been carried out on both the free acid and at least one salt. In four of these
cases, A204A, lasalocid, monensin, and X-206, virtually no major conformational changes are observed between the acid and the salt. Hydrogen bonding between the same pairs of oxygen atoms is found, most
of the oxygen atoms are located in the interior, and the exterior is
nonpolar. The free acid and the Ag^+ and Na^+ salts of A204A have the
same space group and virtually the same cell dimensions. The behavior
of A23187 is in marked contrast to those of the other four. A23187
forms salts with Ca^{2+} ions in 2:1 stoichiometry, and while the conformations of the anions in the two distinct Ca^{2+} salts studied are very
similar, a very different conformation is found for the free acid in the

crystal. The smaller and more rigid ionophores, such as A23187, lasalocid, and X-14547A, would clearly have difficulty providing three-dimensional nonpolar protection for a metal ion in a 1:1 complex. The structures of their salts indicate the different ways in which they overcome this difficulty. A23187 appears to complex only with divalent metal ions and thus forms a dimer which has three-dimensional protection. Lasalocid usually also forms dimers, even with univalent metal ions, thus forming 2:2 rather than 1:1 complexes. It can also form a polymer or involve solvent to provide additional protection. X-14547A, at least in its complex with an amine, involves a second neutral molecule to form a 2:1 complex, which provides three-dimensional protection.

In general, the ionophores show little tendency to form significant intermolecular interactions unless that is an integral feature of the metal ion complex, as often is the case with lasalocid complexing with metal salts, X-14547A forming the 2:1 amine complex, and A23187 and lasalocid complexing with divalent ions. The Cs^+-lasalocid salt is unique in crystallizing as a polymer. Ionomycin in an interesting example of an ionophore which forms dimers by hydrogen bonding between the M^{2+}-ionomycin moieties in all the crystals examined. An apparently less specific type of intermolecular hydrogen bonding is found in the case of the crystal of Ag^+-monensin dihydrate, where the water molecules of crystallization link the Ag^+-monensin entities in two-dimensional layers. Only in the case of lasalocid has convincing evidence been thus far presented (Schmidt. et al., 1974; Patel and Shen 1976; Shen and Patel, 1976) that the dimeric structures found in the crystal persist in solution.

Several interesting clues as to the biological action of the ionophores are apparent from the crystal structure studies. The types of structures invariably found in the crystal for the metal salts with the highly nonpolar exterior are obviously well suited to carry metal ions through nonpolar media. There is also good evidence from the structural work on lasalocid, monensin, and A204A that these structures with very little change can accomodate water molecules as a replacement for or even in addition to the metal ions. The crystal structure evidence suggests that in many cases the free acid has virtually the same conformation as the salt. Yet it may be dangerous to draw the conclusion that this is always the case in polar solutions, although in some cases NMR evidence is quite compelling that this is so. However, it should be borne in mind that the crystal structure of a free ionophore acid presents the conformation of that acid in a highly nonpolar environment. It would be very informative if a free acid ionophore could be crystallized with a large number of water molecules of crystallization. Unfortunately, this aim has yet to be accomplished.

In summary, the x-ray evidence does not yet present us with a clear picture of the mechanism of metal ion uptake and release that will be generally true for all the ionophores. However, it does present a persuasive outline, with many details clearly evident. In some specific examples it provides more than that, but additional x-ray studies and, more challengingly, new techniques to produce crystals from different environments will be necessary for the entire picture to be revealed.

ACKNOWLEDGMENT

We wish to thank Dr. John Westley for inviting us to write this chapter and also Dr. Westley and his colleagues at Hoffmann-LaRoche for several generous gifts of samples over the past decade and for many stimulating discussions on the structure of ionophores. Valuable discussions with Dr. Dinshaw Patel and Dr. Denis Rousseau of Bell Laboratories have also helped in the preparation of this chapter. We wish also to thank Professor Jack Gougoutas, Dr. Noel Jones, Dr. William Duax, and Professor Dick van der Helm for providing coordinates and other information prior to publication on ionophores that they had investigated. Susan Botts made many of the drawings included in this chapter. Finally, we wish to recognize the contributions of former members of this laboratory whose work contributed to the determination and understanding of lasalocid structure and behavior, Suzanne Johnson, Carol Maier, Carol Hejna, Ed Bissell, Karen Chiang, Andrew Wang, Paul Schmidt, and Bill Paton.

REFERENCES

Agtarap, A., Chamberlin, J. W., Pinkerton, M., Steinrauf, L. (1967). The structure of monensic acid, a new biologically active compound. *J. Am. Chem. Soc. 89:*5737-5739.

Alléaume, M., and Hickel, D. (1970). The crystal structure of grisorixin silver salt. *Chem. Commun. 1970:*1422-1423.

Alléaume, M., and Hickel, D. (1972). The crystal structure of the thallium salt of the antibiotic grisorixin. *Chem. Commun. 1972:*175-176.

Alléaume, M. (1974). Crystal structure of the antibiotic grisorixin in the free acid form. In *Abstracts of Second European Crystallographic Meeting.* European Committee of Crystallography, Keszthely, Hungary, pp. 405-407.

Alléaume, M., Busetta, B., Farges, C., Gachon, P., Kergomard, A., and Staron, T. (1975). X-ray structure of alborixin, a new antibiotic ionophore. *J. Chem. Soc. Chem. Commun. 1975:*411-412.

Berger, J., Rachlin, A. I., Scott, W. E., Sternbach, L. H., and Goldberg, M. W. (1951). The isolation of three new crystalline antibiotics from streptomyces. *J. Am. Chem. Soc. 73:*5295-5298.

Bissell, E. C., and Paul, I. C. (1972). Crystal and molecular structure of a derivative of the free acid of the antibiotic X-537A. *J. Chem. Soc. Chem. Commun. 1972:*967-968.

Blount, J. F., and Westley, J. W. (1971). X-ray crystal and molecular structure of antibiotic X-206. *Chem. Commun. 1971*:926-928.

Blount, J. F., and Westley, J. W. (1975). Crystal and molecular structure of the free acid form of antibiotic X-206 hydrate. *J. Chem. Soc. Chem. Commun. 1975*:533.

Blount, J. F., Evans, R. H., Jr., Liu, C. -M., Hermann, T., and Westley, J. W. (1975). X-ray structure of Ro 21-6150, a polyether antibiotic related to dianemycin. *J. Chem. Soc. Chem. Commun. 1975*:853-855.

Chaney, M. O., Demarco, P. V., Jones, N. D., and Occolowitz, J. L. (1974). The structure of A23187, a divalent cation ionophore. *J. Am. Chem. Soc. 96*:1932-1933.

Chaney, M. O., Jones, N. D., and Debono, M. (1976). The structure of the calcium complex of A23187, a divalent cation ionophore antibiotic. *J. Antibiotic. 29*:424-427.

Chiang, C. C., and Paul, I. C. (1977). Monomeric forms of the acid ionophore lasalocid A (X-537A) from polar solvents. *Science. 196*:1441-1443.

Clark, J. R. (1963). Water molecules in hydrated organic crystals. *Rev. Pure Appl. Chem. 13*:50-90.

Duax, W. L., Smith, D. M., and Strong, P. D. (1980). Complexation of metal ions by monensin, the crystal and molecular structure of hydrated and anhydrous crystal forms of Na^+-monensin. *J. Am. Chem. Soc. 102*:6725-29.

Czerwinski, E. W., and Steinrauf, L. K. (1971). Structure of the antibiotic dianemycin. *Biochem. Biophys. Res. Commun. 45*:1284-1287.

Dietrich, B., Lehn, J. M., and Sauvage, J. P. (1973). Cryptates: Control over bivalent/monovalent cation selectivity. *J. Chem. Soc. Chem. Commun. 1973*:15-16.

Friedman, J. M., Rousseau, D. L., Shen, C., and Paul, I. C. (1977). Infrared evidence for hydrogen bonding in the sodium salts of lasalocid A(X-537A). *J. Chem. Soc. Chem. Commun. 1977*:684-686.

Friedman, J. M., Rousseau, D. L., Shen, C., Chiang, C. C., Duesler, E. N., and Paul, I. C. (1979). Lasalocid crystallized from methanol: Spectroscopic and x-ray structural evidence for two structures. *J. Chem. Soc. Perkin Trans. 2 1979*:835-838.

Johnson, S. M., Herrin, J., Liu, S. J., and Paul, I. C. (1970a). Crystal structure of a barium complex of antibiotic X-537A, $Ba(C_{34}H_{53}O_8)_2 \cdot H_2O$. *Chem. Commun. 1970*:72-73.

Johnson, S. M., Herrin, J., Liu, S. J., and Paul, I. C. (1970b). The crystal and molecular structure of the barium salt of an antibiotic containing a high proportion of oxygen. *J. Am. Chem. Soc. 92*:4428-4435.

Jones, N. D. Chaney, M. O., Chamberlin, J. W., Hamill, R. L., and Chen, S. (1973). Structure of A204A, a new polyether antibiotic. *J. Am. Chem. Soc. 95*:3399-3400.

Kinashi, H., Otake, N., Yonehara, H., Sato, S., and Saito, Y. (1973). The structure of salinomycin, a new member of the polyether antibiotics. *Tetrahedron Lett. 1973*:4955-4958.

Kinashi, H., Otake, N., Yonehara, H., Sato, S., and Saito, Y. (1975). Studies on the ionophorous antibiotics. I. The crystal and molecular structure of salinomycin p-iodophenacyl ester. *Acta Crystallog. B31*:2411-2415.

Koenuma, M., Kinashi, H., Otake, N., Sato, S., and Saito, Y. (1976). Studies on the ionophorous antibiotics. II. Silver salt of lysocellin. *Acta Crystallogr. B32*:1267-1269.

Koyama, H., and Utsumi-Oda, K. (1977). Crystal and molecular structure of a silver salt of antibiotic A-130A. *J. Chem. Soc. Perkin Trans.* 2:1531-1536.

Kubota, T., Matsutani, S., Shiro, M., and Koyama, H. (1968). The structure of polyetherin A. *Chem. Commun. 1968*:1541-1543.

Leiserowitz, L. (1976). Molecular packing modes. Carboxylic acids. *Acta Crystallogr. B32*:775-802.

Lutz, W. K., Winkler, F. K., and Dunitz, J. D. (1971). Crystal structure of the antibiotic monensin. Similarities and differences between free acid and metal complex. *Helv. Chim. Acta* 54:1103-1108.

Maier, C. A., and Paul, I. C. (1971). X-ray crystal structure of a silver complex of antibiotic X-537A; a structure enclosing two metal ions. *Chem. Commun. 1971*:181-182.

Occolowitz, J. L., Dorman, D. E., and Hamill, R. L. (1978). Structure of the polyether antibiotic K-41 by mass and nuclear magnetic resonance spectrometry. *J. Chem. Soc. Chem. Commun. 1978*:683-684.

Otake, N., Koenuma, M., Kinashi, H., Sato, S., and Saito, Y. (1975a). The crystal and molecular structure of the silver salt of lysocellin, a new polyether antibiotic. *J. Chem. Soc. Chem. Commun. 1975*:92-93.

Otake, N., Koenuma, M., Miyamae, H., Sato, S., and Saito, Y. (1975b). Studies on the ionophorous antibiotics. Part III. The structure of lonomycin. a polyether antibiotic. *Tetrahedron Lett. 1975*:4147-4150.

Otake, N., Nakayama, H., Miyamae, H., Sato, S., and Saito, Y. (1977). X-ray crystal structure of the thallium salt of carriomycin, a new polyether antibiotic. *J. Chem. Soc. Chem. Commun. 1975*:590-591.

Otake, N., Ogita, T., Nakayama, H., Miyamae, H., Sato, S., and Saito, Y. (1978). X-ray crystal structure of the thallium salt of antitiotic-6016, a new polyether ionophore. *J. Chem. Soc. Chem. Commun. 1978*:875-876.

Patel, D. J., and Shen, C. (1976). Structural and kinetic studies of lasalocid A(X-537A) and its silver, sodium, and barium salts in non-polar solvents. *Proc. Nat. Acad. Sci. USA,* 73:1786-1790.

Pinkerton, M., and Steinrauf, L. K. (1970). Molecular structure of monovalent metal cation complexes of monensin. *J. Mol. Biol.* 49:533-546.

Pletcher, T. J., and Weber, H. -P. (1974). X-ray crystal structure and absolute configuration of p-bromophenacylseptamycin monohydrate, a polyether antibiotic. *J. Chem. Soc. Chem. Commun.* 1974:697-698.

Riche, C., and Pascard-Billy, C. (1975). Crystal and molecular structure of emericid: A new polyether antibiotic. *J. Chem. Soc. Chem. Commun.* 1975:951-952.

Schmidt, P. G., Wang, A. H. -J., and Paul, I. C. (1974). A structural study on the sodium salt of the ionophore, X-537A (lasalocid), by x-ray and nuclear magnetic resonance analysis. *J. Am. Chem. Soc.* 96:6189-6191.

Schmitz, F. J., Prasad, R. S., Gopichand, Y., Hossain, M. B., and van der Helm, D. (1981). Acanthifolicin, a new episulfide-containing polyether carboxylic acid from extracts of the marine sponge, *Pandaros acanthifolium*. *J. Am. Chem. Soc.* 103:2467-2469.

Seto, H., Mizoue, K., Otake, N., Gachon, P., Kergomard, A., and Westley, J. W. (1979). The revised structure of alborixin. *J. Antitiot.* 32:970-971.

Shen, C., and Patel, D. J. (1976). Free acid, anion, alkali, and alkaline earth complexes of lasalocid A(X-537A) in methanol: Structural and kinetic studies at the monomer level. *Proc. Nat. Acad. Sci. USA* 73:4277-4281.

Shiro, M., and Koyama, H. (1970). Crystal structure of silver polyetherin A. *J. Chem. Soc. B* 1970:243-253.

Shiro, M., Nakai, H., Nagashima, K., and Tsuji, N. (1978). X-ray determination of the structure of the polyether antibiotic K-41. *J. Chem. Soc. Chem. Commun.* 1978:682-683.

Smith, G. D., and Duax, W. L. (1976). Crystal and molecular structure of the calcium ion complex of A23187. *J. Am. Chem. Soc.* 98:1578-1580.

Smith, G. D., and Duax, W. L. (1979). PA 26: Structure of ionophores and the mechanism of ion capture and release. In *Abstracts of the American Crystallographic Association, Summer Meeting*. American Crystallographic Association, Boston, p. 23.

Smith, G. D., Duax, W. L. and Fortier, S. (1978a). Structure of a hydrated sodium-lasalocid A(X-537A) dimer: An intermediate in complex formation. *J. Am. Chem. Soc.* 100:6725-6727.

Smith, G. D., Strong, P. D., and Duax, W. L. (1978b). The structure of the free acid of antibiotic A204A, *Acta Crystallogr.* B34:3436-3438.

Steinrauf, L. K., Pinkerton, M., and Chamberlin, J. W. (1968). The structure of nigericin. *Biochem. Biophys. Res. Commun.* 33:29-31.

Stempel, A., Westley, J. W., and Benz, W. (1969). The identity of the antibiotics nigericin, polyetherin A and X-474. *J. Antibiot.* 22:384-385.

Toeplitz, B. K., Cohen, A. I., Funke, P. T., Parker, W. L., and Gougoutas, J. Z. (1979). Structure of ionomycin—A novel diacidic polyether antibiotic having high affinity for calcium ions. *J. Am. Chem. Soc.* 101:3344-3353.

Truter, M. R. (1976). Chemistry of the calcium ionophores. In *Symposia of the Society for Experimental Biology, No. XXX: Calcium in Biological Systems.* Cambridge University Press, London, New York, pp. 19-40.

Ward, D. L., Wei, K.-T., Hoogerheide, T. G., and Popov, A. I. (1978). The crystal and molecular structure of the sodium bromide complex of monensin, $C_{36}H_{62}O_{11} \cdot Na^{+}Br^{-}$. *Acta Crystallogr.* B34:110-115.

Westley, J. W. (1976). A proposed numbering system for polyether antibiotics. *J. Antibiot.* 29:584-586.

Westley, J. W. (1977). Polyether antibiotics: Versatile carboxylic acid ionophores produced by streptomyces. In *Advances in Applied Microbiology, Vol. 22.* Academic Press, New York, San Francisco, pp. 177-223.

Westley, J. W. (1978). Polyethers. In *Kirk-Othmer: Encyclopedia of Chemical Technology,* 3rd ed., Vol. 3, M. Grayson (ed.). Wiley and Sons, New York, pp. 47-64.

Westley, J. W., Blount, J. F., Evans, R. H., Jr., Stempel, A., and Berger, J. (1974). Biosynthesis of lasalocid. II. X-ray analysis of a naturally occurring isomer of lasalocid A. *J. Antibiot.* 27:597-604.

Westley, J. W., Evans, R. H., Jr., and Blount, J. F. (1977). Optical resolution of asymmetric amines by preferential crystallization as lasalocid salts. *J. Am. Chem. Soc.* 99:6057-6061.

Westley, J. W., Evans, R. H., Jr., Sello, L. H., Troupe, N., Liu, C. -M., and Blount, J. F. (1979). Isolation and characterization of antibiotic X-14547A, a novel monocarboxylic acid ionophore produced by streptomyces antibioticus NRRL 8167. *J. Antitiot.* 32:100-107.

Yamazaki, K., Abe, K., and Sano, J. (1976). Structure of antibiotic DE-3036. *J. Antibiot.* 29:91-92.

chapter **4**

MASS SPECTROMETRY OF POLYETHER ANTIBIOTICS

J. L. Occolowitz and *R. L. Hamill*
Lilly Research Laboratories, Indianapolis, Indiana

I. INTRODUCTION

The first reported instance of the use of mass spectroscopy to elucidate the structures of polyether antibiotics was the work of Chamberlin and Agtarap (1970), which used a study of the mass spectrometry
of monensin to postulate the structures of several minor factors. It
was not until four years later that physical methods other than x-ray
diffraction were used extensively to elucidate the structures of polyether antibiotics. This time lag was probably due to the empirical
nature of the structure-spectrum relationship for this class of compounds. Once a sufficiently broad data base was established, mass
spectrometry and its powerful collaborator NMR spectroscopy were

used effectively in establishing new structures. Also, for the higher-
molecular-weight members of the class the advent of field desorption
(FD) ion sources helped to provide data which was unobtainable by
electron impact (EI) because of sample stability problems.

Generally, mass spectrometry offers a rapid means of structure
elucidation, provided that the new compound can be related to a known
class, e.g., in metabolism studies or by inspection of the mass spectrum. To date, mass spectrometry has not been used to provide stereochemical information about polyether antibiotics; this has been obtained
by NMR. A study of the reactions of metastable ions in the mass spectrometer by the mass-analyzed ion kinetic-energy spectrometry (MIKES)
or collisional activation mass-analyzed ion kinetic-energy spectrometry
(CA/MIKES) techniques may be of use in differentiating stereoisomers.
At present the structure of a new class of polyether antibiotics has not
been deduced by the use of mass spectrometry or NMR spectroscopy.
However, the two methods have been useful in recognizing changes,
which are sometimes fairly extensive, in the substituents on known
skeletons.

Apart from speed, mass spectrometry offers to the investigator the
advantage of being able to successfully examine impure and noncrystalline samples. Mixtures can be separated in the direct probe of the mass
spectrometer by thermal fractionation or resolved mass-spectrometrical-
ly by high-resolution analysis of ions with the same nominal mass.

II. GENERAL CONSIDERATIONS

The sodium salts of most polyether antibiotics with molecular weights
below 800 to 900 give satisfactory EI spectra containing molecular ions.
The spectra of the acid forms may suffer from two main deficiencies:
the absence of discernible molecular ions and a proclivity to show ions
due to the sodium salt of the acid. If the molecular weight of the compound is not known, the formation of the sodium salt from the acid in
the mass spectrometer can lead to an erroneous conclusion. This can
be further compounded if the accurate mass in mass units (MU) of the
molecular ion is determined. The mass doublet $(2.C-H)-Na$ is separated by only 2.4 mMU, so that within a window of ±3 mMU plaus-
ible but incorrect elemental formulas are generated from high-resolution data. The presence of a peak at m/z 23 (Na^+) in the spectrum of
a polyether usually indicates that it is, at least partially, due to the
sodium salt.

Chamberlin and Agtarap (1970) noted that relatively pure samples
of the potassium and rubidium salts of monensin showed disproportion-
ally high peaks due to sodium monensin in their mass spectra. There
was no evidence of a peak due to sodium monensin in the spectrum of
monensin acid. In contrast, Occolowitz et al. (1976) noted relatively
intense peaks due to sodium narasin in the EI spectrum of pure nara-

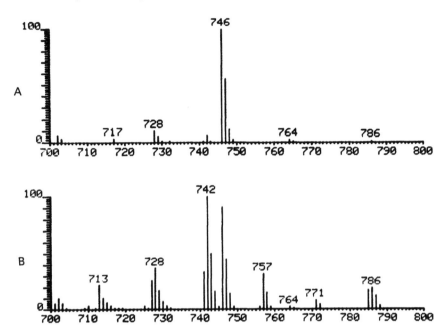

Figure 1 Mass spectrum of narasin acid. (A) Inbeam probe. (B) Regular probe.

sin acid. Evidence that the sodium arises from the ion source is presented in Figures 1A and 1B. The upper figure represents a partial spectrum of narasin obtained by using an in-beam probe which places the sample about 3 mm from the ionizing electron beam of a Varian-MAT 731 mass spectrometer. The lower figure represents a spectrum obtained using the conventional probe, where the sample is just outside the ion-source housing. Use of the in-beam technique results in less ion-source molecule collisions before ionization. The upper spectrum is almost entirely due to narasin acid, $M^{+\cdot}$ = 764, $(M-H_2O)^{+\cdot}$ = 746, while the bottom spectrum contains a substantial contribution from sodium narasin, $M^{+\cdot}$ = 786, $(M-CO_2)^{+\cdot}$ = 742.

The FD spectra of sodium salts of polyether antibiotics contain intense molecular ions, but often little reproducible fragmentation. Structurally significant fragments in FD spectra are obtained from the methyl ester or a derivatized methyl ester. This approach is exemplified in the structure determination of K-41 (Occolowitz et al., 1978). FD spectra of polyether acids show quasimolecular ions as well as cationized molecular ions. Cationization in FD mass spectrometry is often observed in diverse classes of compounds (Beckey, 1977).

The mass spectra of the polyether antibiotics are best described by a rather detailed classification by skeletal type. Generally, the addition or removal of such common substituents as hydroxyl, alkyl, methoxyl, or sugar moieties from the basic skeleton results in no drastic change in the mass spectrum. Not unexpectedly, changes in the basic skeleton can lead to new fragmentations; e.g., the presence of a double bond in the C ring of members of the salinomycin group (Section XI) leads to a prominent fragmentation not observed in the mass spectra of those compounds not having an unsaturated ring system. Common to the EI and FD of many of the compounds, however, are fragmentations resulting in oxonium ion formation (e.g., see below).

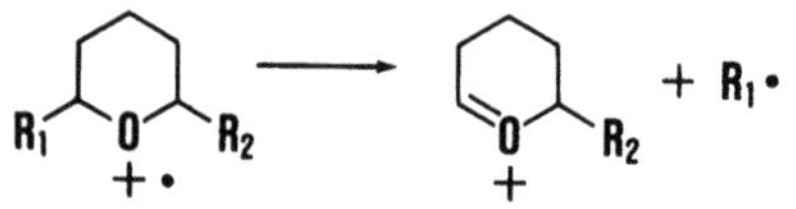

$$R_1 \overbrace{\qquad}^{} O \; R_2 \quad \longrightarrow \quad O \; R_2 \quad + \; R_1\bullet$$

The EI spectra of the sodium salts of the polyethers show ions in which the sodium atom is retained, as well as ions free of sodium. In

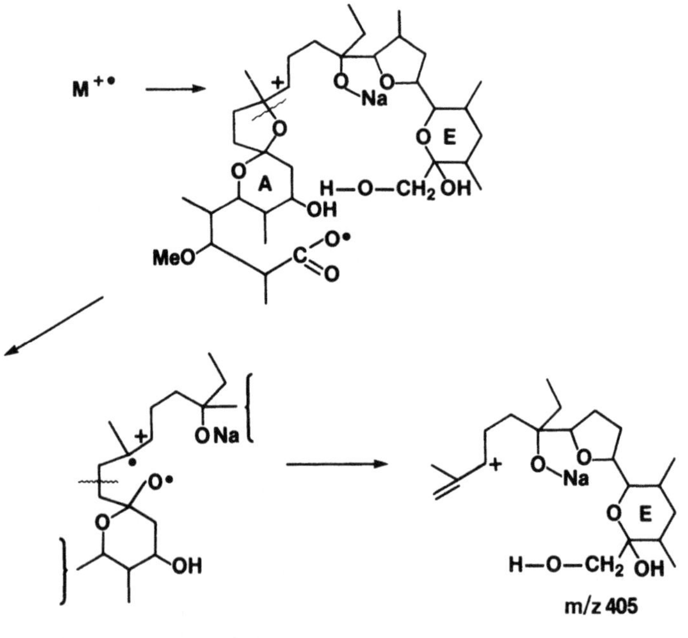

Scheme 1 Formation of m/z 405 in the EI spectrum of sodium monensin. (Source: Chamberlain and Agtarap, 1970.)

effect, the sodium is not localized to any one region of the molecular ion. Chamberlin and Agtarap (1970) have postulated the formation of bonds between the cyclic ether oxygens of sodium monensin and the sodium atom. Formation of the sodium-oxygen bond resulted in fission of a carbon-oxygen bond, and the new charge distribution created by the process resulted in the observed fragmentation. In Scheme 1 this process is depicted for the formation of m/z 405, a prominent peak in the spectrum of sodium monensin.

III. ALBORIXIN GROUP

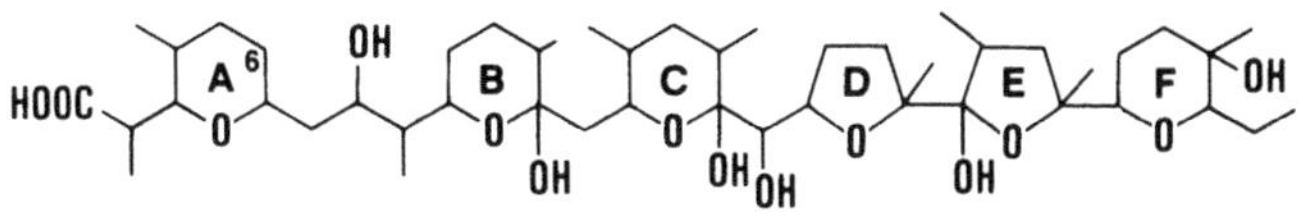

Compound	Substituent 6
Alborixin	Me
X-206	H

The two members of this group differ only by the C-6 substituent and consequently would be expected to have similar mass spectra. Absence of spiro systems and the presence of six secondary or tertiary hydroxyl groups result in spectra showing extensive inter-ring fragmentation and water loss.

Fragmentation of alborixin under electron impact has been discussed by Gachon et al. (1976). Scheme 2 illustrates their summary of the EI spectrum.

Ions containing rings A, E, and F intact were observed in the spectrum of the acid and were consequently useful for structure determination. However, those ions containing rings B, C, and D were observed only after the loss of one or more moles of water, limiting their usefulness for structure determination.

Gachon et al. (1976) also discussed the EI mass spectra of alborixin triacetate, a tetramethylsilyl derivative, two reduction products, and two oxidation products. In the case of the first two compounds the highest mass ion observed was $(M-2H_2O)^{+}\cdot$. No further fragmentation was reported; such fragmentation was apparently of limited structural utility, as the authors were unable to determine the sites of derivatization.

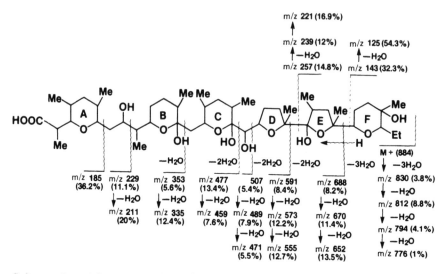

Scheme 2 EI fragmentation of alborixin. (Source: Gachon et al., 1976. With permission from *The Journal of Antibiotics.*)

Reduction resulted in products in which the B and E rings and the B, C, and E rings were opened at the ether oxygens to yield two new hydroxyl groups for each ring opened. Although molecular ions were not seen, the EI spectra of the reduction products proved to be of use in determining their structure.

Oxidation of the reduction product of alborixin (mol wt = 890), in which the B, C, and E rings had been opened, yielded two products, mol wt = 516 and mol wt = 372. The EI spectra of these compounds is summarized in Scheme 3.

Although not reporting the mass spectra of X-206 or its salt, Blount and Westley (1971) used mass spectrometry and NMR to examine two oxidation products. Unfortunately, these data were not sufficiently informative to define the correct structure of the larger product and subsequent structure determination by x-ray diffraction was needed to define the correct structure of X-206 (Blount and Westley, 1975).

The EI mass spectrum of sodium alborixin was reported to show a molecular ion with relative intensity 2.4% (Gachon et al., 1976). Further examination of the EI spectra of the sodium salts of alborixin and X-206 showed that they contained peaks of structural significance (J. L. Occolowitz, unpublished data, 1979). The spectra contained ions in which the B, C, and D rings are intact and thus provide data complementary to that provided by the spectrum of the acids. The spectrum of sodium alborixin and the rationalization of some of the key peaks are shown in Figure 2 and Scheme 4, respectively. Assignments

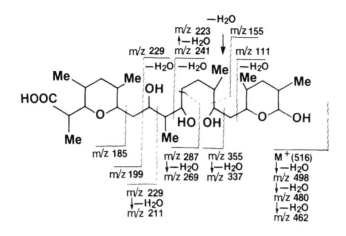

Scheme 3 EI fragmentation of oxidized reduction products of alborix-in. (Source: Gachon et al., 1976. With permission from *The Journal of Antibiotics*.)

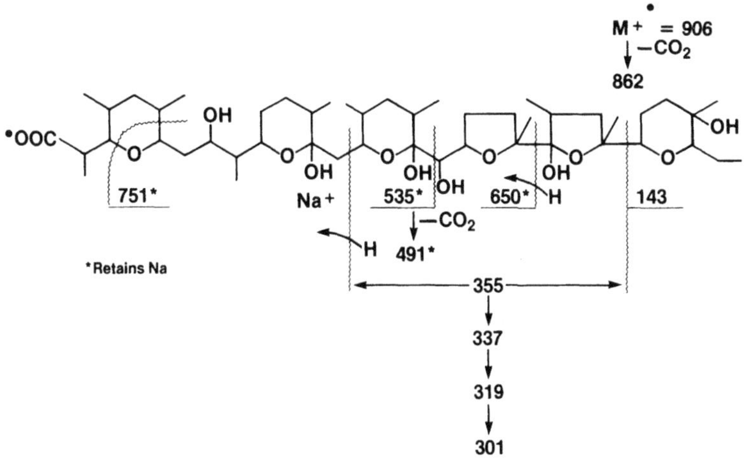

Scheme 4 EI fragmentation of sodium alborixin.

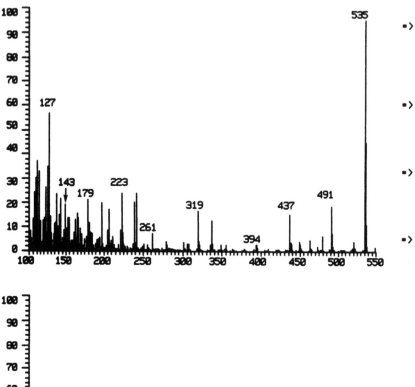

Figure 2   EI spectrum of sodium alborixin.

are supported by observation of appropriate mass shifts in the spectrum of the sodium salts of X-206.

IV. DIANEMYCIN GROUP

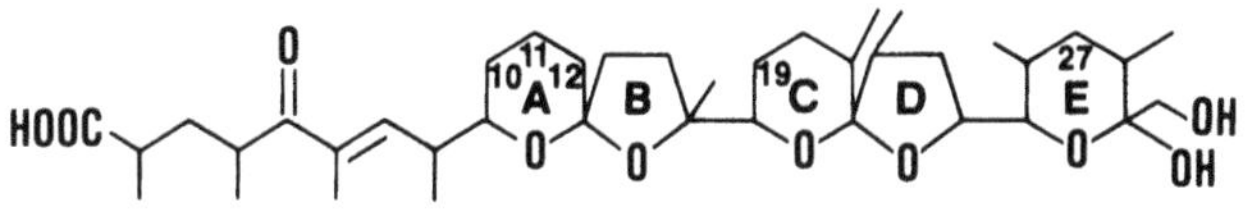

HOOC ... (structure with rings A, B, C, D, E; positions 10, 11, 12, 19, 27; OH, OH)

	Substituent [a]				
Compound	10	11	12	19	27
Dianemycin	Me	OH	H	Sug	H
A-130A (lenoremycin)	H	Sug	Me	H	H
A-130B	H	Sug	Me	H	Sug
A-130C	H	Sug	Me	H	H

[a] Sug denotes the moiety

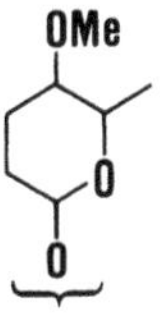

OMe (structure)

as against Sug-H, the molecule

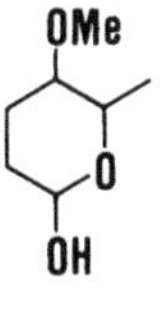

OMe (structure) OH

There is very little published information on the mass spectra of this group. Czerwinski and Steinrauf (1971) reported a mass-spectrometric molecular weight of 888 for dianemycin (sodium salt) and Kubota et al. (1975) reported that A-130A sodium salt gave a molecular ion at m/z 872 and that the highest mass ion in the spectrum of the free acid appeared at m/z 832 $(M-H_2O)$. The following data and interpretation are derived from work performed in the authors' laboratories.

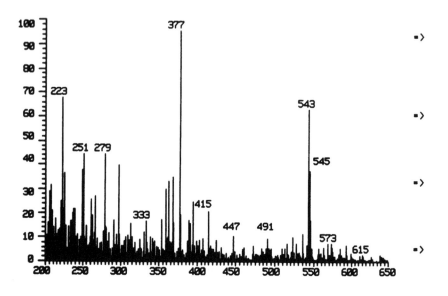

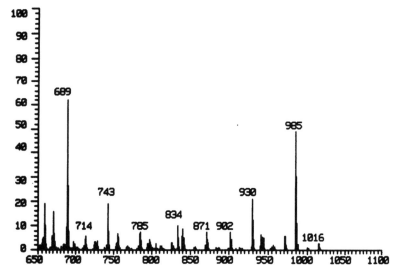

Figure 3   EI spectrum of A-130B.

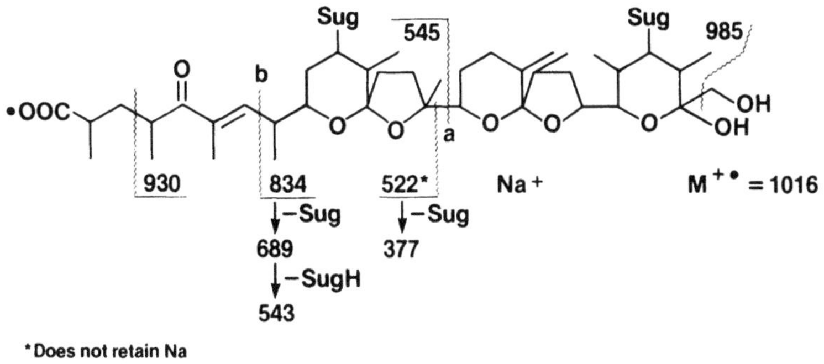

Scheme 5 EI fragmentation of sodium A-130B.

The sodium salts of all four compounds gave EI spectra containing molecular ions. Many of the most intense peaks in the spectra arose from multiple fragmentations of the molecular ions. Figure 3 illustrates the EI spectrum of A-130B sodium salt. The rationalization of the spectrum is shown in Scheme 5.

The peaks at $(M-31)^+$, $(M-86)^{+\cdot}$, $(M-182)^{+\cdot}$, and $(M-182-145)^+$, which occurred at m/z 985, 930, 834, and 689 in the spectrum of A-130B sodium salt, were all prominent in the EI spectra of the sodium salts of the other three compounds. They should be diagnostic in recognizing any new members of this group. In the case of A-130A sodium salt a peak at m/z 545 in its spectrum can arise by two different fragmentations; directly by fragmentation a, or by a two-step process involving fragmentation b followed by loss of the sugar moiety. High-resolution examination of the peak at m/z 545 shows that the two-step path was the predominant one.

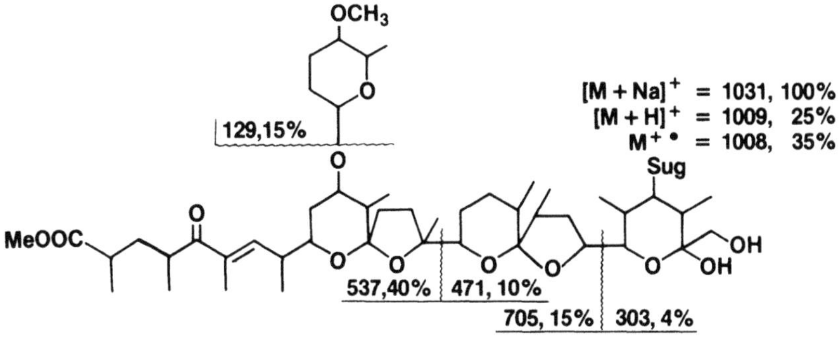

Scheme 6 FD fragmentation of A-130B methyl ester.

The FD spectrum of A-130B methyl ester, taken above the temperature of field desorption emitter (anode) that generates maximum molecular ion currents and minimal fragmentation, best anode temperature (BAT), showed some fragmentation of structural significance. Scheme 6 summarizes the spectrum.

A-130C (Tsuji et al., 1980) differs from A-130A by having an axial methyl at C-28. As might be expected, the EI spectra of the sodium salts of A-130A and A-130C are quite similar (J. L. Occolowitz, unpublished data, 1980).

V. LASALOCID GROUP

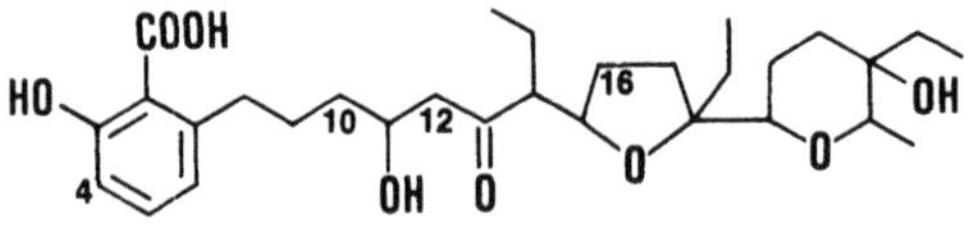

Compound	Substituent			
	4	10	12	16
Lasalocid A	Me	Me	Me	Me
Lasalocid B	Et	Me	Me	Me
Lasalocid C	Me	Et	Me	Me
Lasalocid D	Me	Me	Et	Me
Lasalocid E	Me	Me	Me	Et

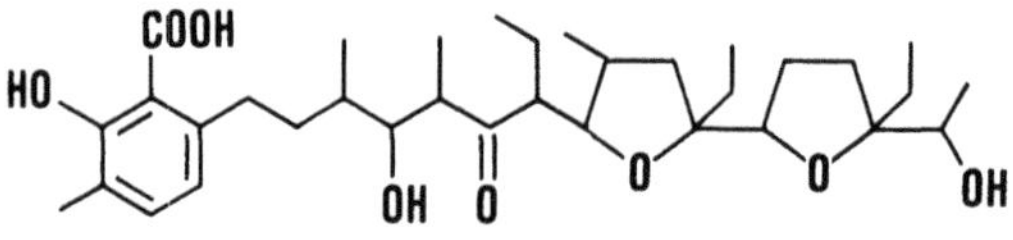

Isolasalocid A

Westley et al. (1974a) have rationalized the EI spectrum of lasalocid A and have used the scheme to deduce the structure of the lasalocids B to E.

Neither the sodium salt of lasalocid A nor the free acid yield a molecular ion under EI conditions. The highest mass peak in the salt spectrum arose from the elimination of Na, CO_2, and H_2O. The highest mass peak in the spectrum of the acid resulted from even more extensive degradation; however, the ions formed were useful for structure elucidation. Fragmentation of lasalocid A has been ration-

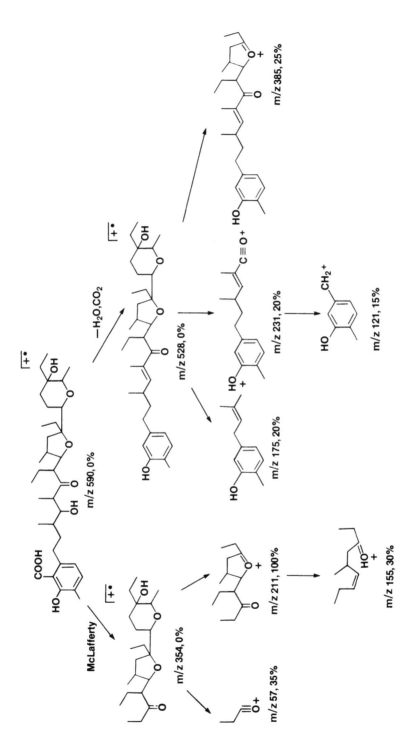

Scheme 7 EI fragmentation of lasalocid A. (From Westley et al., 1974. With permission from *The Journal of Antibiotics*.)

209

alized as proceeding through two major pathways: fragmentation of the bond between C-10 and C-11 by a McLafferty rearrangement to give m/z 354, and decarboxylation and dehydration to give m/z 528 (Scheme 7).

Although neither of these ions were observed, they were assumed to be the progenitors of the most abundant ions in the spectrum. A rearrangement analogous to the McLafferty rearrangement was observed in the pyrolysis of lasalocid A, but molecular ions arising from ultimate products of this reaction, a mixture of isomeric dihydronaphthalens with molecular weight 174, were not reported as present in the mass spectrum. Removal of the hydroxyl group at C-11 suppresses the McLafferty rearrangement. It is not clear whether the decarboxylation-dehydration product, m/z 528, arose by thermal or EI processes or both.

Fragmentation of the other lasalocids occurred in a manner analogous to lasalocid A, and changes in the nature of the substituents were discerned by observing the appropriate mass shift of the ions shown in Scheme 7.

The FD spectrum of sodium lasalocid A was determined by J. L. Occolowitz, (unpublished data, 1979). It showed a molecular ion at m/z 612. At emittter currents beyond the BAT structurally significant fragments were observed in the spectrum, as summarized in Scheme 8.

There is no published mass spectrum of isolasalocid A. However, Westley et al. (1974b) have compared the EI spectra of the retroaldol cleavage products of lasalocid A and isolasalocid A ([1] and [2], respectively, in Scheme 9.).

While the ion at m/z 211 occurred in the spectra of both [1] and [2], the ion at m/z 309 occurred in the spectrum of [2] only. These data suggested structure [2], which was subsequently confirmed by NMR. Similar reasoning was used by Koenuma and Otake (1977) in differentiating two isomeric reaction products of lysocellin (Section VI).

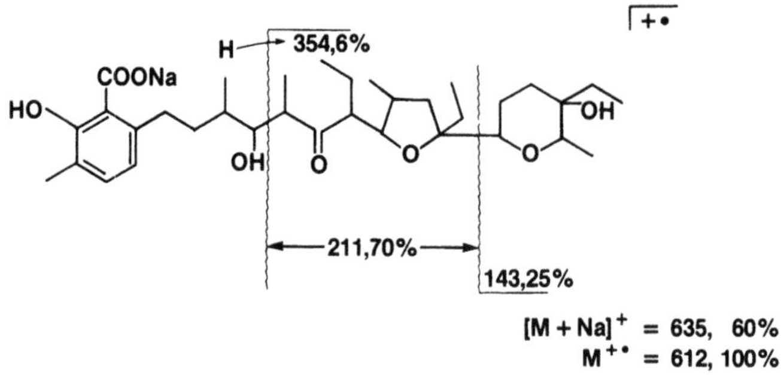

Scheme 8   FD fragmentation of sodium lasalocid A.

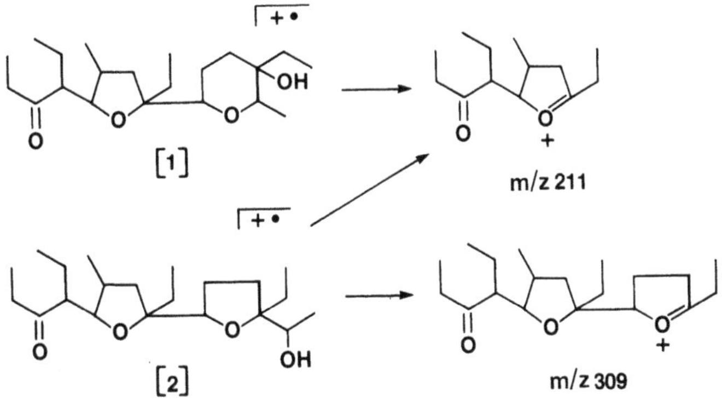

Scheme 9 Differentiation of the retro-Diels Alder reaction products
of lasalocid A[1] and isolasalocid A[2] using EI spectrometry. (Source:
Westley et ., 1974b. With permission from *The Journal of Antibiotics*.)

In a recent publication Bose et al. (1979) obtained the negative
chemical ionization (NCI) mass spectrum of lasalocid, using CF_2Cl_2 as
a reagent gas. The three most intense peaks in the spectrum were
m/z 589, $(M-H)^-$, m/z 571, $(M-H-H_2O)^-$, and m/z 553, $(M-H-2 \cdot H_2O)^-$.
These data indicate that the NCI technique would be useful for examin-
ing other polyethers which are not entirely suitable for EI examination.

VI. LYSOCELLIN GROUP

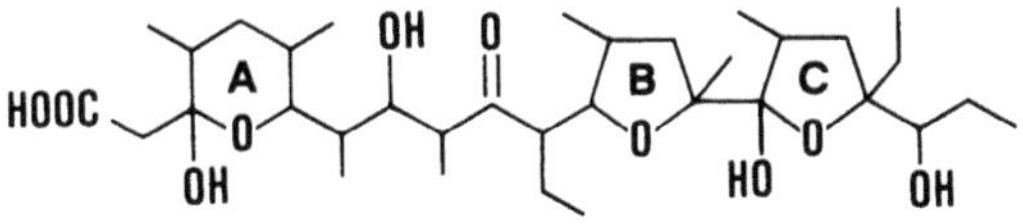

Lysocellin

Currently lysocellin is the only naturally occurring member of this
group. In the work-up of lysocellin by Koenuma and Otake (1977) two
artifacts were isolated:

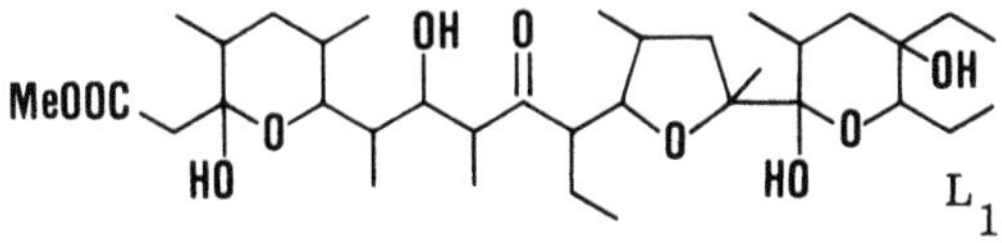

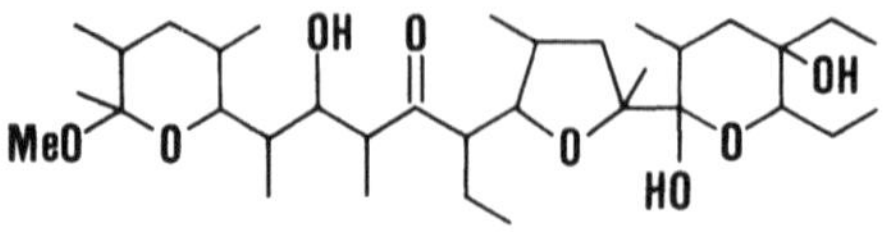

$$M_1$$

After lysocellin was treated with diazomethane L_1 was isolated along with lysocellin methyl ester and M_1 was isolated from methanolic mother liquors of lysocellin.

Alkaline-induced retroaldol cleavage of lysocellin, in a manner analogous to that discussed for the lasalocids, yields a product N_2

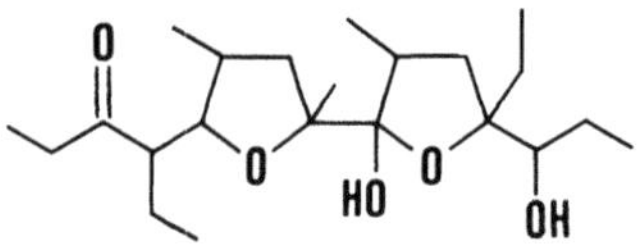

which gradually isomerizes to the compound N_3.

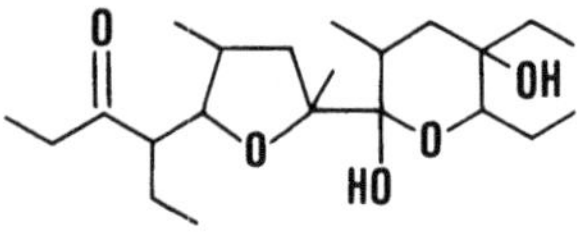

$$N_3$$

Although the mass spectrum of lysocellin has not been published nor discussed in the literature, mass spectrometry was used in the determination of the structures of L_1, M_1, N_2, and N_3 (Koenuma and Ōtake, 1977). As with lasalocid A and isolasalocid A (Group V), N_2 and N_3 could be distinguished by observing differences in the fragmentation of subsitutents on the C rings. Koenuma and Ōtake referred to the "ions A and ion B" as diagnostic peaks in differentiating the two isomeric C rings. The proposed genesis of these ions is illustrated in Scheme 10, which shows the fragmentation of N_2 and N_3. Ions A, m/z 59, 187, 225, and 325, which were present in the spectrum of N_2 but not in that of N_3, and ion B (m/z 125), which was exclusive to the spectrum N_3, serve to distinguish the two isomers.

The EI mass spectrum of L_1 had its highest mass ion at m/z 624 $(M-H_2O)^{+}\cdot$. A peak at m/z 125 with appreciable intensity and the correct elemental composition for ion B, a lack of ions analogous to the A series, and NMR evidence led to the assignment of the six-membered structure to the C ring. Similar evidence was used in establishing the structure of M_1.

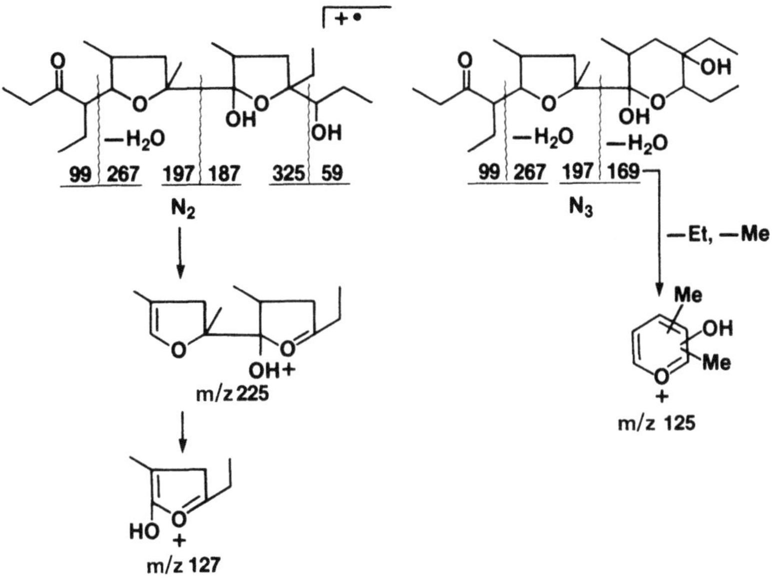

Scheme 10   EI fragmentation of ly̱socellin degradation products N$_2$ and N$_3$. (Source: Koenuma and O̱take, 1977. With permission from *The Journal of Antibiotics.*)

Reduction of lysocellin methyl ester with sodium borohydride followed by acetylation yielded lysocellin hexol tetraacetate. The EI spectrum of this compound contained a molecular ion at m/z 784 and fragments of structural significance (Scheme 11).

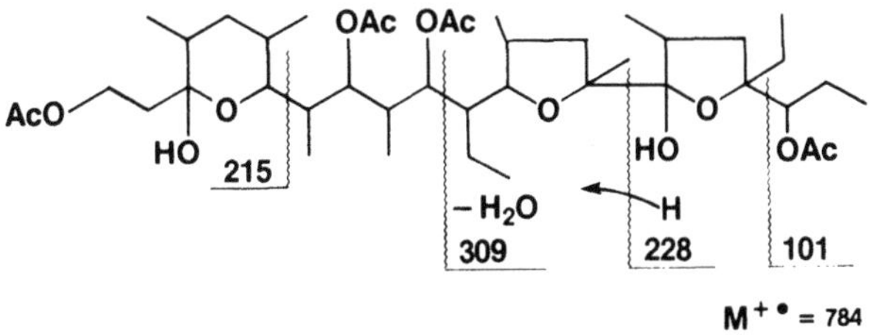

Scheme 11   EI̱ fragmentation of lysocellin hexol tetraacetate. (Source: Koenuma and O̱take, 1977. With permission of *The Journal of Antibiotics.*)

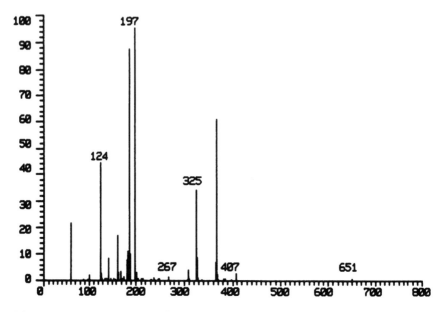

Figure 4   FD spectrum of sodium lysocellin beyond the BAT.

The EI and FR spectra of sodium lysocellin have been studied by
J. L. Occolowitz and R. L. Hamill (unpublished data, 1979). At the
BAT the FD spectrum showed a quasimolecular ion(m/z 651, 100%)
and a peak due to the loss of CO_2 (m/z 606, 15%). Beyond the BAT
extensive fragmentation is observed. The FD spectrum of sodium lysocellin beyond the BAT is shown in Figure 4 and rationalized in
Scheme 12.

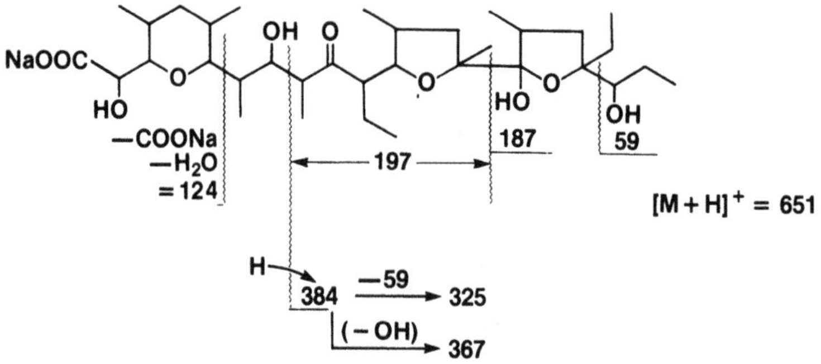

Scheme 12   FD fragmentation of sodium lysocellin beyond the BAT.

In the FD spectrum beyond the BAT only m/z 187 and 59 were re-garded as arising from simple fragmentations of the molecular ion; the other fragments likely arose by a combination of thermal and FD-in-duced fragmentations. Thus the retroaldol cleavage likely occurred prior to ionization to yield a compound of molecular weight 384 which abstracted sodium from the emitter to give m/z 407. The protonated ion m/z 385 lost H_2O to give m/z 367.

No molecular ions were observed in the EI spectrum of sodium lyso-cellin. The most prominent peak occurred at m/z 197 (see Scheme 12); m/z 141 was the second most prominent peak; it is the analog of m/z 155 in the spectrum of lasalocid A (see Scheme 7).

VII. MISCELLANEOUS GROUP

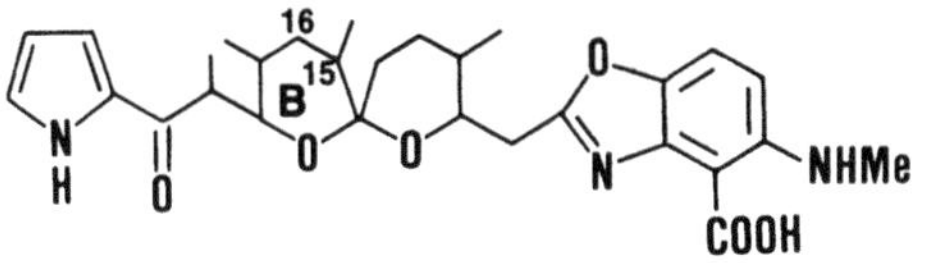

A 23187

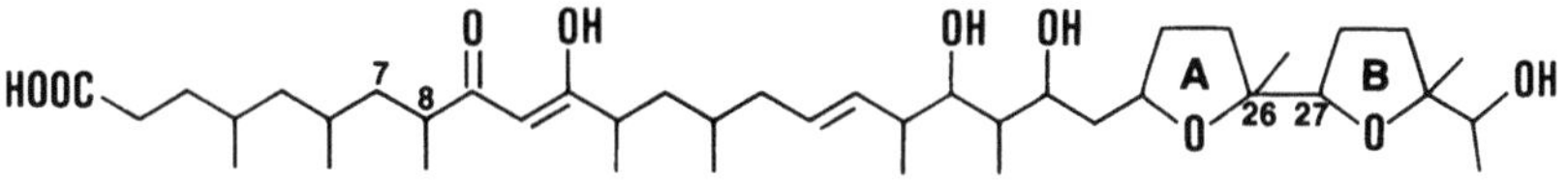

Ionomycin

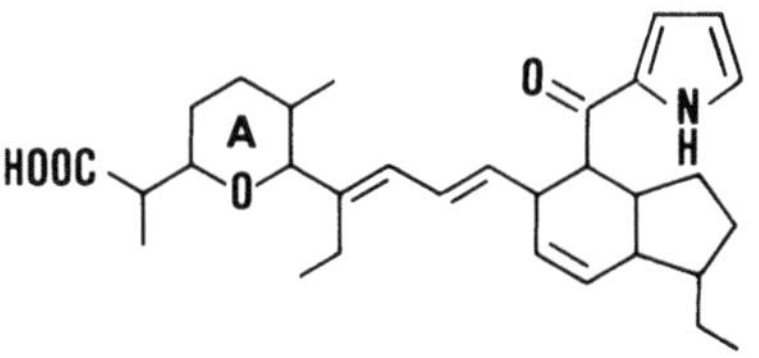

X-14547A

The members of this group are unique insofar as no like structures have thus far been found in nature. Strictly, X-14547A is not a poly-ether; however, its A ring is similar to that of many polyethers and it has the property of complexing and transporting divalent and mono-valent metal cations (Liu et al., 1979). For these reasons it has been included in this group.

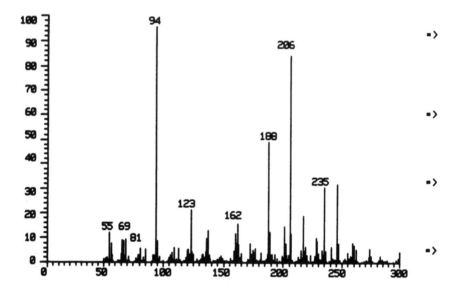

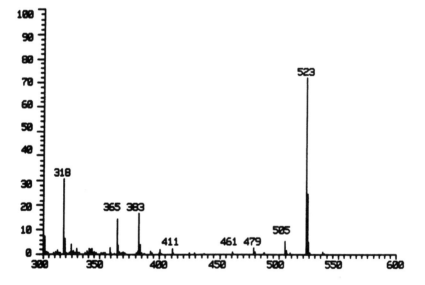

Figure 5   EI spectrum of A23187.

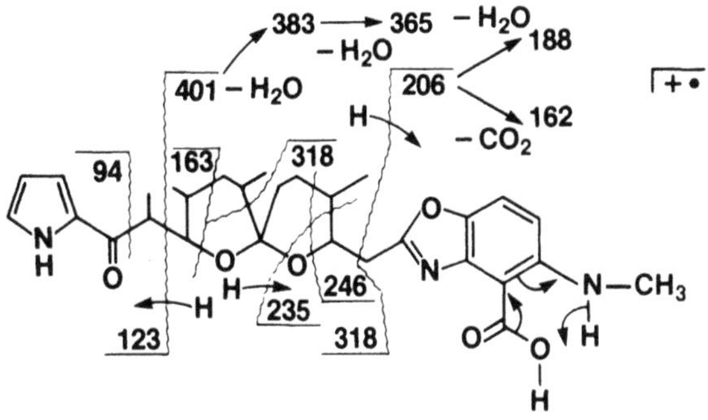

Scheme 13 EI fragmentation of A23187.

The structure of A23187 was determined by x-ray diffraction (Chaney et al., 1974). In the same paper the mass spectrometry of the acid, methyl ester, acetate, and methyl ester acetate were discussed briefly. All yielded molecular ions under EI conditions. The spectrum of A23187 is shown in Figure 5 and rationalized in Scheme 13.

In Scheme 13 the ratio of the intensity of the peak at m/z 318, which contains the pyrrole ring, to the intensity of the m/z 318, which contains the benzoxazole, is 3:2. All assignments are supported by accurate mass measurement.

The fragmentations of the B ring of A23187, which yield m/z 163 and 318, proved to be useful use in determining the structure of the microbial transformation products of A23187 methyl ester (Abbott et al., 1980). For example, the presence of peaks at m/z 163 and 332, of appropriate elemental composition, in the mass spectrum of a metabolite known to have one more oxygen than the substrate, showed that the oxygen in this metabolite was associated with C-15, the methyl attached to C-15 or to C-16. Final placement at C-16 was achieved by analysis of the NMR spectrum. Similar analysis of NMR and EI spectrometry showed that the two other microbial transformation products were N-demethyl A23187 methyl ester and 16-hydroxy-N-demethyl A23187 methyl ester.

The molecular ions $(2 \cdot acid - 2H + metal)^{+ \cdot}$ are the most intense peaks in the EI spectra of the calcium and magnesium salts of A23187, m/z 1082 and 1068, respectively. Other abundant species are $(M-264)^{+ \cdot}$ and the ion $(acid - H + metal)^{+}$.

Ionomycin differs from A23187 insofar as it chelates calcium and cadmium as a divalent acid, whereas A23187 complexes as a monovalent acid (Toeplitz et al., 1979). Both the calcium and cadmium salts yielded EI spectra containing molecular ions corresponding to (ionomycin $-2H$ + metal). Pertrimethylsilylation of the calcium salt yielded a mixture of calcium-free tetra- and pentatrimethylsilyl derivatives

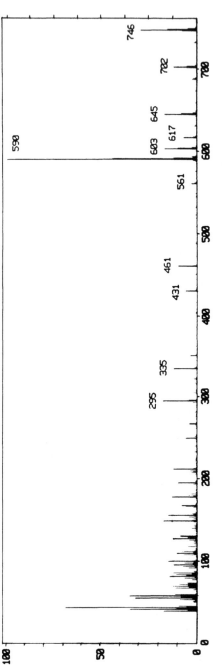

Figure 6 EI spectrum of calcium ionomycin. (Source: reprinted with permission from Toeplitz et al., 1979. Structure of ionomycin—A novel diacidic polyether antibiotic having a high affinity for calcium ions. *J. Am. Chem. Soc. 101*:3345. Copyright 1979, American Chemical Society.)

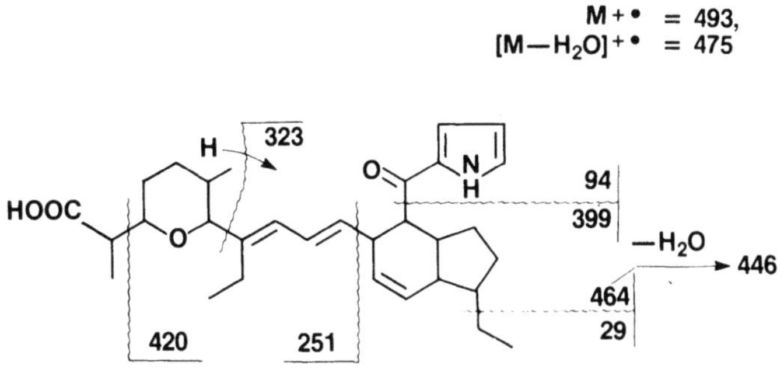

$$M + \bullet = 493,$$
$$[M - H_2O]^{+\bullet} = 475$$

Scheme 14   EI fragmentation of X-14547A. (Source: Westley et al.,
1979. With permission from *The Journal of Antibiotics*.)

which showed molecular ions at m/z 996 and 1068, respectively. The
EI spectrum of the calcium salt is shown in Figure 6.

Although they did not discuss the mass spectrum of the calcium salt
in detail, the authors of the paper listed elemental compositions for
the ions in the range m/z 562 to 746 ($M^+\cdot$). The most intense peak in
the spectrum, m/z 590, was due to the loss of $C_9H_{16}O_2$ from the molecular ion and presumably arose from simple fission of the bond between C-7 and C-8, with retention of the calcium on the frequent ion.
Other peaks in the range m/z 562 and above appear to result from fission of carbon-carbon bonds between the "west" end of the molecule
and C-8, as well as loss of the C_2H_5O substituent on the B ring and
fragmentation of the bond between C-26 and C-27.

The mass spectrum of X-14547A was discussed by Westley et al.
(1979). Its fragmentation is summarized in Scheme 14. As with A23187,
the peak at m/z 94 constituted strong evidence for the presence of the
pyrrole carbonyl moeity.

VIII. MONENSIN GROUP

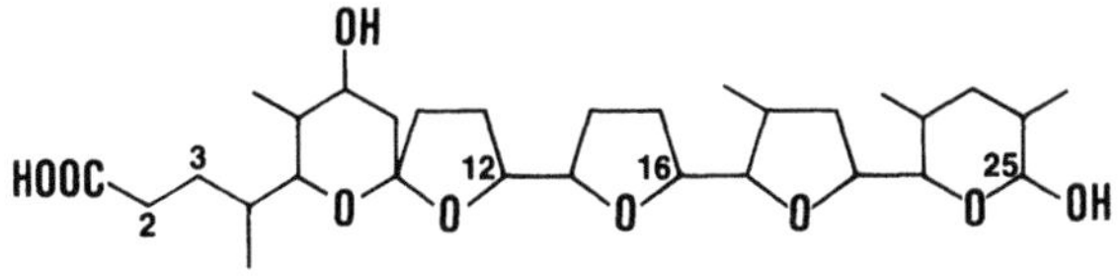

Compound	Substituent				
	2	3	12	16	25
Laidlomycin	Me	OCOEt	Me	Me	CH_2OH
Monensin	Me	OMe	Me	Et	CH_2OH
Monensin B	Me	OMe	Me	Me	CH_2OH
Monensin C	Et	OMe	Me	Et	CH_2OH
Monensin D	Me	OMe	Et	Et	CH_2OH
A712	Me	OCOEt	Me	Me	Me

The work of Chamberlin and Agtarap (1970) represents the first detailed description of the mass spectrometry of a group of polyether antibiotics. The publication describes the EI mass spectra of monensin, monensins B and C, their sodium, potassium, and rubidium salts, methyl esters, and acetates.

Monensin acid did not show a molecular ion in its EI spectrum, the highest mass peak observed occurred at m/z 634, $(M-2 \cdot H_2O)^{+\cdot}$. The methyl ester gave a spectrum showing an observable molecular ion at m/z 684. Molecular ions were also observed for diacetyl monensin methyl ester and sodium monensin at m/z 768 and 692, respectively. The tertiary hydroxyl at C-25 was not acetylated.

Of the acid and sodium salt of monensin, the sodium salt yielded an EI spectrum which was of the greater use in structure determination. The EI fragmentation of these compounds is summarized in Schemes 15 a and 15b. For monensin acid, Scheme 15a, the fragmentations shown represent a summary of the work of Chamberlin and Agtarap. For the salt, Scheme 15b, the fragmentations resulted from Chamberlin and Agtarap's work plus information from a study of monensin and its metabolites (Donoho et al., 1978).

In the paper of Chamberlin and Agtarap it was postulated that the peak at m/z 575 in the spectrum of sodium monensin arose by fission of the bond between C-3 and C-4. This involved the loss of $C_5H_9O_3$. The other fragmentation leading to m/z 575 in Scheme 15b also involves the loss of $C_5H_9O_3$. That both processes were operative in the EI spectrum is supported by the following observations. Firstly, in the spectrum of the monensin metabolite M-1 (Donoho et al., 1978), which has a hydroxyl at C-3 in place of the methoxyl of monensin, peaks at m/z 561 and 575 were observed. The composition of these ions corresponded to those expected if both processes were operating. Secondly, in the spectrum of sodium monensin C, which has an ethyl at C-2 in place of the methyl of monensin, peaks at m/z 575 and 589 were observed. Similarly observation of an intense peak at $(M-31)^+$ in

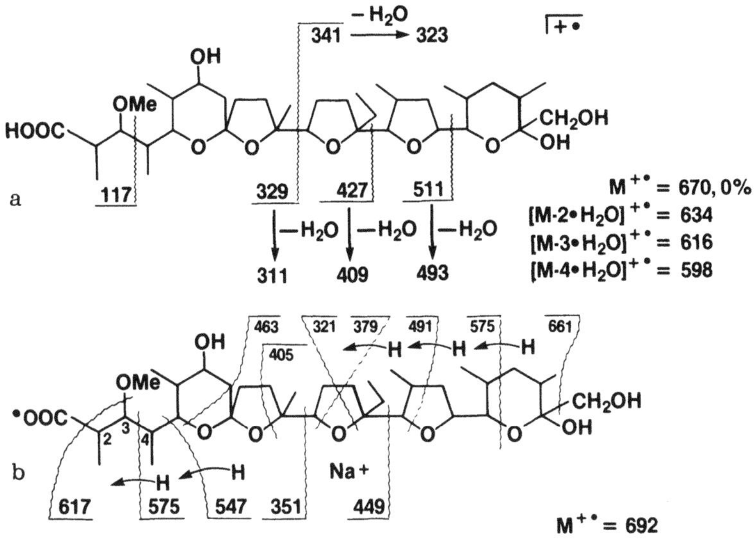

Scheme 15 (a) EI fragmentation of monensin. (Source: Chamberlain and Agtarap; 1970.) (b) EI fragmentation of sodium monensin. (Source: Chamberlain and Agtarap, 1970.)

the spectrum of metabolite M-1 indicated that loss of $-CH_2OH$ from C-25 of monensin is a likely process. This raises the possibility that m/z 617 in the spectrum of sodium monensin is at least partially due to the loss of $-CH_2OH$ and CO_2.

A combination of NMR and mass spectrometry was used to elucidate the structure of monensin D (D. E. Dorman, J. L. Occolowitz, and J. W. Paschal, unpublished data, 1978). Peaks critical to the structure determination of sodium monensin D were m/z 419 and 365, which occurred 14 MU higher than the corresponding peaks in the mass spectrum of sodium monensin (see m/z 405 and 351, Scheme 15b).

In the spectrum of diacetyl monensin methyl ester an intense peak occurred at m/z 131; this is an analog of m/z 117 in Scheme 15a. Observation of an intense peak at m/z 145 ($C_7H_{13}O_3$) in the spectrum of diacetyl monensin C methyl ester, together with NMR evidence, led to the proposal that monensin C differed from monensin in having an ethyl at C-2.

Prominent in the spectrum of diacetyl monensin methyl ester were peaks at m/z 423 and 325. These peaks are the analogs of m/z 409 and 311 in Scheme 15a, respectively. Ions m/z 423 and 325 resulted from the elimination of acetic acid and $CH_3COO\cdot$ from ions at m/z 483 and 384, respectively. The observation that m/z 483 was shifted to m/z 469 in the spectrum of diacetyl monensin B methyl ester, and that m/z 384 was not shifted, combined with NMR data, led to the proposal that monensin B has a methyl group at C-16.

Table 1 Peaks in the High-Mass Region of the Spectra of Sodium Laidlomycin and Sodium Monensin B

Peak	Laidlomycin m/z 720, $C_{37}H_{61}O_{12}Na$	Monensin B m/z 678, $C_{35}H_{59}O_{11}Na$
$M^{+\cdot}$	689	647
$[M-CH_3O]^+$	647	—
$[M-CH_3CH_2COO]^+$	—	603[a]
$[M-CH_3O-CO_2]^+$	603[a]	—
$[M-CH_3CH_2COO-CO_2]^+$	—	533
$[M-CH_3O-CO_2C_5H_{10}]^+$	533	—
$[M-CH_3CH_2COO-CO_2-C_5H_{10}]^+$	—	—

[a]Base peak.
Source: Kitame and Ishida, 1976. With permission from *The Journal of Antibiotics*.

Chamberlin and Agtarap (1970) also discussed the mass spectra of the potassium and rubidium salts of monensin. The spectra of these salts illustrated the alkali metal exchange reactions occurring in the mass spectrometer (see Section II). Also, by observing mass shifts in the spectra of the various salts, they were able to discern which ions retained an alkali metal atom.

Kitame and Ishida (1976) made use of mass spectrometry and NMR spectroscopy in deducing the structure of laidlomycin. In their study they noted common peaks in the spectra of sodium monensin B and sodium laidlomycin as well as peaks shifted 42 MU (CH_2CO) higher in the spectrum of laidlomycin. Table 1 summarizes the fragments occurring in the high-mass end of each spectrum. All assignments were supported by accurate mass measurement.

Ion m/z 603 in the spectra of the sodium salt of monensin B and laidlomycin is the analog of ion m/z 617 in the spectrum of sodium monensin (Scheme 15b). Similarly, the peak at m/z 533 is the analog of m/z 547. These data indicated that laidlomycin differed from monensin B in having a CH_3CH_2COO substituent at C-3. NMR and ir evidence added further support to this conclusion.

A712 (N. Tsuji, personal communication, 1978) differs from laidlomycin by having a methyl at C-25. By referring to Scheme 15b and Table 1, m/z 587 $(M-CH_3CH_2COO-CO_2)^+$ should be a prominent peak in the spectrum of sodium A712. It is the base peak in the spectrum of this compound. No $(M-CH_3O)^+$ peak was observed because of the absence of the methoxyl at C-2 and the hydroxymethyl at C-25. Other prominent peaks in the spectrum of sodium A712 which can be related to the fragmentation shown in Scheme 15b were the following: m/z 603 (575), 519 (491), 477 (449), 433 (463), 393 (351), 375 (405), and 291 (321), where the peaks in parentheses refer to the spectrum of sodium monensin.

IX. NIGERICIN GROUP

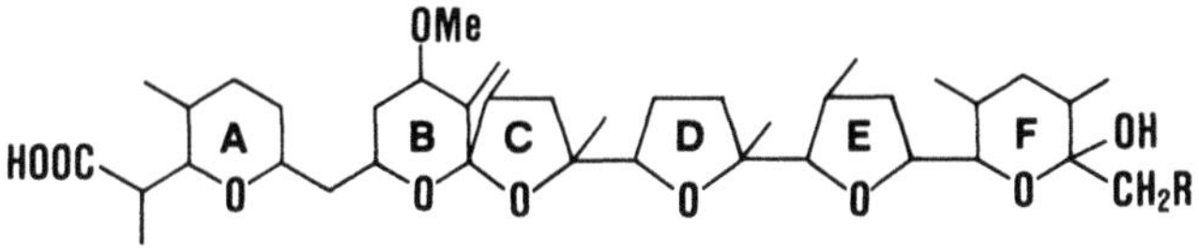

Nigericin R = OH
Grisorixin R = H

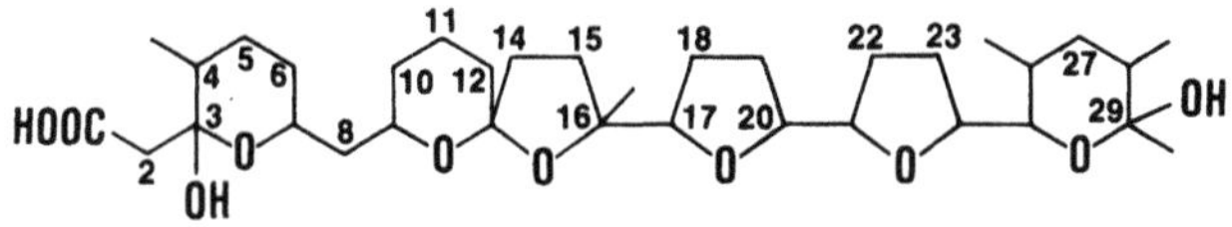

Substituent

Compound	2	5	6	8	10	11	12	14	15	18	20	22	23	27
BL580△	H	OMe	Sug Me	H	H	OMe	Me	Me	OMe	H	H	H	H	H
Carriomycin	Me	Sug	Me	H	H	OMe	Me	Me	OMe	H	H	H	H	H
Etheromycin	Me	OH	Sug Me	Me	H	OMe	Me	H	H	H	Me	H	H	OMe
Lonomycin A & B	Me	OMe	Me	Me	Me	OMe	H	H	H	H	Me	Me	OMe	OMe
Lonomycin C	H	OMe	Me	Me	Me	OMe	H	H	H	H	Me	Me	OMe	OMe
Mutalomycin	Me	OMe	Me	Me	Me	OH	H	H	H	H	Me	Me	H	H
A204A	Me	Sug	OMe Me	H	H	OMe	Me	Me	OMe	H	H	H	H	OMe
A204B	Me	Sug	OMe Me	H	H	OMe	Me	Me	OMe	H	H	H	H	H
A 6016	OH	OMe	Me	H	H	OMe	Me	Me	H	Sug	H	H	H	H
A 28695A	Me	OMe	Sug Me	H	H	OMe	Me	Me	OMe	H	H	H	H	H
A 28695B	Me	OMe	Sug Me	H	H	OMe	Me	Me	OMe	H	H	H	H	OH
K-41	OH	OMe	OMe Me	H	H	OMe	Me	Me	OMe	H	H	H	H	Sug
K-41B	OH	OMe	OMe Me	H	H	OMe	Me	Me	Sug	H	H	H	H	Sug

This group is distinguished by having the greatest number of members and by having the member with the highest molecular weight: K-41B, mol wt = 1060 (Tsuji et al., 1979).

Published EI data for acid and salt forms of this group of compounds are confined to nigericin, grisorixin, the three lonomycins, and mutalomycin, notably, those compounds not possessing the sugar moiety. In our hands, under EI conditions, the salts and acids of the sugar containing compounds fragmented extensively by elimination of the sugar moiety as Sug H, and the methoxyl groups as methanol. The spectra obtained were usually devoid of molecular ions and were complex. Methylation of the tertiary hydroxyl at C-29 and the carboxylic acid group yielded compounds which gave more useful EI spectra and FD spectra containing fragments of significance for structure determination.

The structure of nigericin was determined by Steinrauf et al. (1968) using x-ray diffraction. The mass spectra of nigericin, its methyl ester, sodium salt, and acetylmethyl ester were studied by Chamberlin and Agtarap (1970).

Nigericin acid did not yield a molecular ion in its EI mass spectrum. The highest mass peak observed was m/z 688 (M$-2\cdot$H$_2$O). Acetyl nigericin methyl ester gave an EI spectrum showing a molecular ion (m/z 780). The base peak of the spectrum of the acid occurred at m/z 481 and resulted from fragmentation between the D and E rings, with charge retention on the moiety containing the D ring. Cleavage between the C and D rings with charge retention on the moiety containing ring C yielded m/z 397. Ions m/z 481 and 397 lost a molecule of methanol to yield m/z 449 and 365, respectively. Fragmentation between C-7 and C-8 yields m/z 171, which contained the A ring.

Major fragments in the EI spectrum of sodium nigericin, which contained a molecular ion, are summarized in Scheme 16.

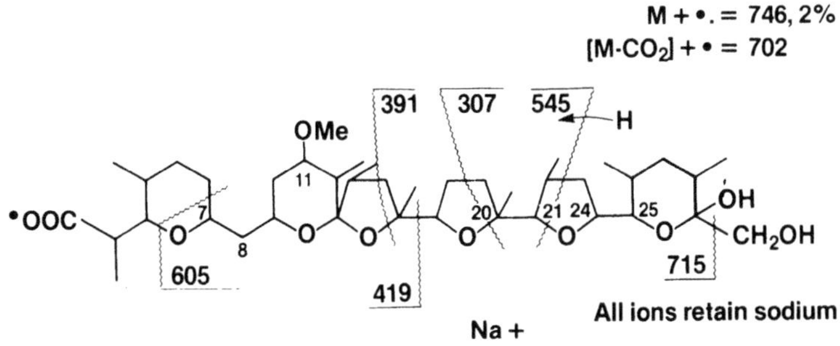

$M + \bullet . = 746, 2\%$
$[M\text{-}CO_2] + \bullet = 702$

Na +

All ions retain sodium

Scheme 16 EI fragmentation of sodium nigericin. (Source: Chamberlain and Agrarap; 1970.)

Chamberlin and Agtarap have pointed out the similarity of many of the fragmentations in the EI spectra of sodium nigericin and sodium monensin (Scheme 15b). The loss of the elements CH3O from the molecular ion could also arise from the loss of the methoxyl group at C-11. The fragmentation shown in Scheme 16 is proposed for reasons presented in the discussion of the EI fragmentation of sodium monensin (Group VIII).

Physical methods were used by Kubota and Matsutani (1970) to demonstrate the identity of polyetherin A and nigericin. In the course of this work the mass spectrum of nigericin methyl ester was obtained and analyzed. The EI fragmentation is summarized in Scheme 17.

The fragment ion resulting from fragmentation between the C and D rings, m/z 411 in Scheme 17, or its fragmentation products often given many intense peaks in the EI and FD spectra of the derivatives of other members of this group. Kubota and Matsutani (1970) also reported briefly on the EI spectra of a number of derivatives and degradation products of nigericin. Generally these gave a molecular ion or a $M-H_2O$ ion; no further fragmentation was reported.

The EI mass spectrum of grisorixin (Figure 7) was reported by Gachon et al. (1975). They noted that its fragmentation was similar to that of nigericin. The only difference mentioned was that fragmentation between the E and F rings of nigericin proceeded without hydro-

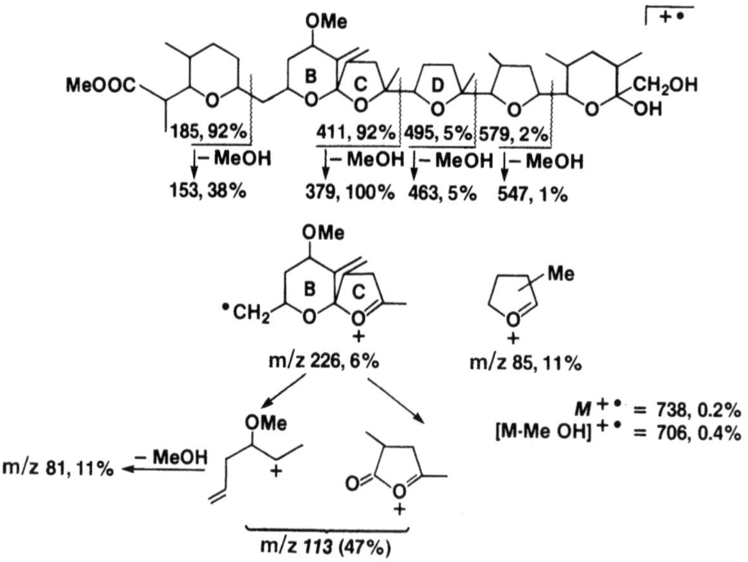

Scheme 17 EI fragmentation of nigericin methyl ester.

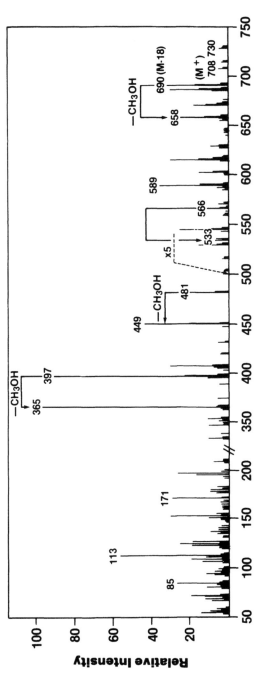

Figure 7 EI spectrum of grisorixin. (Source: Gachon et al., 1975. With permission from *The Journal of Antibiotics*.)

gen rearrangement to yield m/z 565 (see m/z 579, Scheme 17), whereas in the case of grisorixin the fission proceeded with a hydrogen transfer to yield m/z 566.

Gachon and Kergomard (1975) reported on the EI spectra of methyl grisorixin, potassium grisorixin, and several chromic acid oxidation products of methyl grisorixin which were esterified with diazomethane. The spectrum of the methyl ester was very similar to that of methyl nigericin. The spectrum of the potassium salt was similar to that of sodium nigericin. In addition to the fragmentations shown in Scheme 16, Gachon and Kergomard noted fragmentation of the C-7 to C-8 bond of potassium grisorixin to yield m/z 209 (7%), of the C-20 to C-21 bond to yield m/z 519 (4%), and of the C-24 to C-25 bond to yield m/z 603 (10%). Notably absent in the spectrum was an intense $(M-31)^+$ peak, indicating that the elimination of the C-11 methoxyl from $M^{+\cdot}$ is not a favored process for potassium grisorixin or, by analogy, for sodium nigericin.

Nigericin and grisorixin are the only members of the group which do not possess a hydroxyl at C-3. The presence of the C-3 hydroxyl accentuates fission of the C2—C3 bond via a McLafferty rearrangement.

This process is usually noted as a further fragmentation of the ion resulting from fission of the C16—C17 bond.

There appears to be no extensive analysis of the EI fragmentation of the Ionomycins in the literature. Otake and Koenuma (1975) reported that Ionomycin A methyl ester gave a peak in its EI spectrum at m/z 824 $(M-H_2O)$ and that the sodium salt gave a molecular ion at m/z 850. In a study of DE-3936, shown to be Ionomycin A, Yamazaki et al. (1976) reported ions at $M^{+\cdot}$, $(M-CH_3)^+$, $(M-OCH_3)^+$, and $(M-CO_2)^{+\cdot}$ for both the sodium and potassium salts of Ionomycin A. Ionomycins B and C were reported to give the peaks $(M-CO_2-H_2O)^{+\cdot}$ at m/z 766 and 752, respectively (Mizutani et al., 1980).

J. L. Occolowitz (unpublished data, 1977) has found that the FD spectra of Ionomycin A methyl ester and Ionomycin A methyl ester methyl ether showed structurally significant fragments (Scheme 18).

For mutalomycin the only mass-spectral datum reported in the literature was the determination of the molecular weight of the sodium salt (776) by mass spectrometry (Fehr et al., 1977).

There are no published mass-spectral data on etheromycin, carriomycin, and BL580Δ, possibly because the underivatized acids and

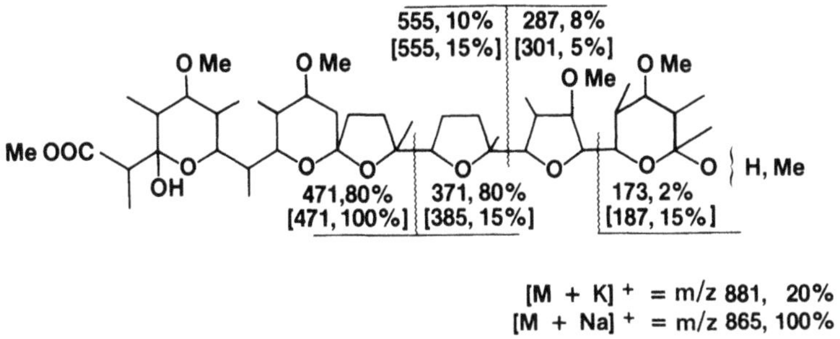

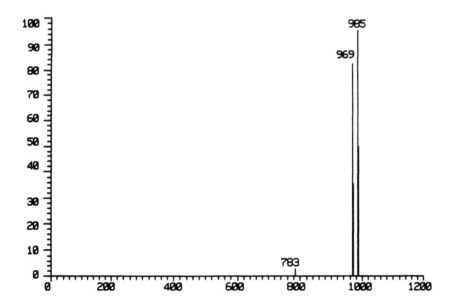

555, 10% | 287, 8%
[555, 15%] | [301, 5%]

471, 80% | 371, 80% | 173, 2%
[471, 100%] | [385, 15%] | [187, 15%]

$[M + K]^+ = m/z\ 881,\ 20\%$
$[M + Na]^+ = m/z\ 865,\ 100\%$

Scheme 18 FD fragmentation of Ionomycin A methyl ester and Ionomycin A methyl ester methyl ether. Peaks in brackets are for methyl
ester methyl ether. Cationized molecular ions are for methyl ester.

salts did not give satisfactory EI spectra. For the compounds discussed below, mass-spectral data were obtained in the authors' laboratories. Because etheromycin, carriomycin, and BL580Δ are similar to the compounds discussed below, it is likely that the following
approach can be extrapolated to the unexamined compounds.

Figure 8 FD spectrum of mixed sodium/potassium salts of K-41.

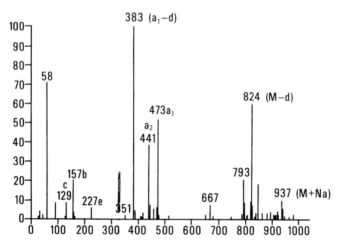

Figure 9   FD spectrum of A 6016 methyl ester methel ether.

In using mass spectrometry to examine the larger member of this group, the following approach has been useful.

1.   To determine the molecular weight the FD spectrum of the free acid or alkali metal salt is obtained. A typical spectrum, e.g., that of the mixed sodium/potassium salts of K-41, is shown in Figure 8. This spectrum was obtained at the BAT and shows m/z 969, M + Na)$^+$, and m/z 985, (M + K)$^+$. Spectra taken above the BAT showed also the ion (M + metal$-CO_2$)$^+$. FD/ FI peak matching at a resolution of about 8000, using a suitable reference compound, can be used to determine elemental

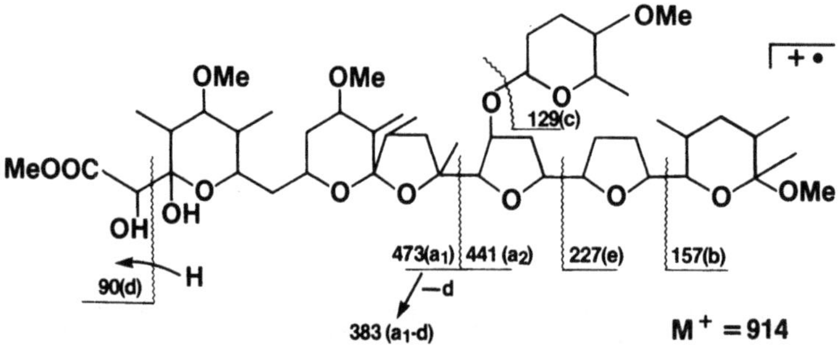

Scheme 19   FD fragmentation of A 6016 methyl ester methyl ether.

composition (Occolowitz et al., 1978). Because similar polyethers field-desorb at about the same emitter current, it may
be preferable to perform a FD/FD peak-matching experiment
using a known polyether as a mass standard (Dorman et al.,
1980).

2. To obtain structurally significant fragmentation it is necessary
to derivatize the polyether. Methyl ester formation with diazomethane and etherification of the C-29 hydroxyl by treating the
acid with methanol overnight at room temperature yield compounds of purity suitable for mass spectrometry without further
work-up. In the case of the etherification substitution of methanol with CD_3OH yields the trideuteromethyl ether. Observation of those peaks shifted 3 MU to higher mass in the deutero-
ether spectrum compared to the ether spectrum enables determination of those fragments containing the F ring.

As an example, the FD spectrum of A 6016 methyl ester methyl ether
is shown in Figure 9 and rationalized in Scheme 19.

This technique has been found applicable to the largest member of
the group, K-41B, whose methyl ester methyl ether gave a FD spectrum showing the significant peaks: $(M + Na)^+$, m/z 1111, 30%; a_1, m/z 647,

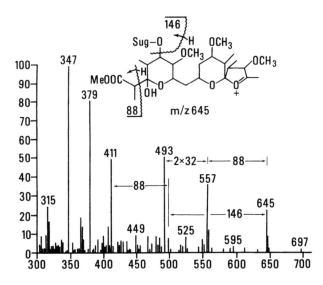

Figure 10 Portion of the EI spectrum of A204 methyl ester.

100%; a_2, m/z 441, 5%; b, m/z 301, 5%; a_1-d, m/z 557, 45%; and c, m/z 129, 6% (J. L. Occolowitz and R. L. Hamill, unpublished data, 1979).

A deficiency in using FD for generating structurally useful fragments is that there is only one observable fragmentation of the moiety a_1: elimination of the molecule d. In order to further define the moiety a_1, examination of the EI spectrum of a methyl ester can be useful. This is exemplified in Figure 10, which shows part of the EI spectrum of A204A methyl ester. In the figure, ion m/z 645 is the unfragmented moiety a_1: the mass and composition of the side chain are defined by m/z 557 (a_1-d), while the sugar moiety is indicated by m/z 499 (a_1-Sug H). Loss of both the sugar and the side chain yielded m/z 411, which sequentially lost its methoxyl groups as methanol to yield the series of ions m/z 379, 347, and 315. Information of this type resulted in the proposal of the correct structure of K-41 (Occolowitz et al., 1978). Using the spectrum of A204A as a model, it could be deduced that a_1 of K-41 did not possess a sugar moiety and had four methoxyl groups and a side chain whose composition was $C_2H_3O_3$.

A combination of NMR and FD mass spectrometry as outlined above was used to elucidate the structure of A28695B (Dorman et al., 1980).

X. NOBORITOMYCIN GROUP

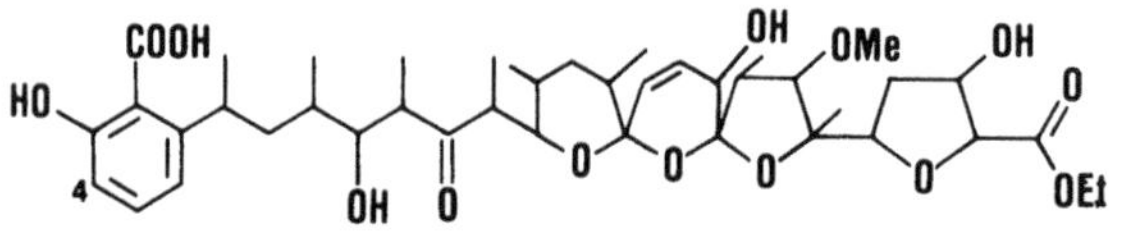

Compound	Substituent 4
Noboritomycin A	Me
Noboritomycin B	Et

The only published mass-spectral data for this group is a report by Keller-Juslén et al. (1978) that the sodium salts of noboritomycin A and B gave molecular ions at m/z 826 and 840, respectively. The following account of the mass spectra of the noboritomycins is derived from unpublished work performed in our laboratories (1979).

Under FD conditions the sodium salts gave molecular ions (100%) and peaks at (M + Na), 10%. Very little fragmentation was observed until most of the samples had been desorbed. At this emitter current

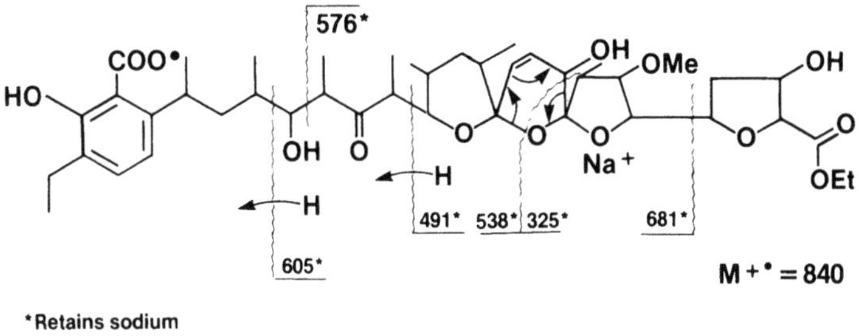

576*

COO• OH OMe OH

HO

OH O O O Na+ OEt

H

491* 538* 325* 681*

H

605* M+• = 840

*Retains sodium

Scheme 20 EI fragmentation of sodium noboritomycin B.

both compounds gave a peak at m/z 577. This peak is probably due to the protonated form of the ion shown in Scheme 20.

Similarities in the structures of members of the salinomycin (Group XI) and noboritomycin groups, notably, the presence of the β-hydroxy keto group in the acyclic portions of the molecules joining the A and B rings and the similar carbon skeletons of the B, C, and D rings, suggest similar modes of fragmentation. Fragmentation of the sodium salts of the noboritomycins under EI conditions are similar. The fragmentation of sodium noboritomycin B is illustrated in Scheme 20 and its spectrum is shown in Figure 11.

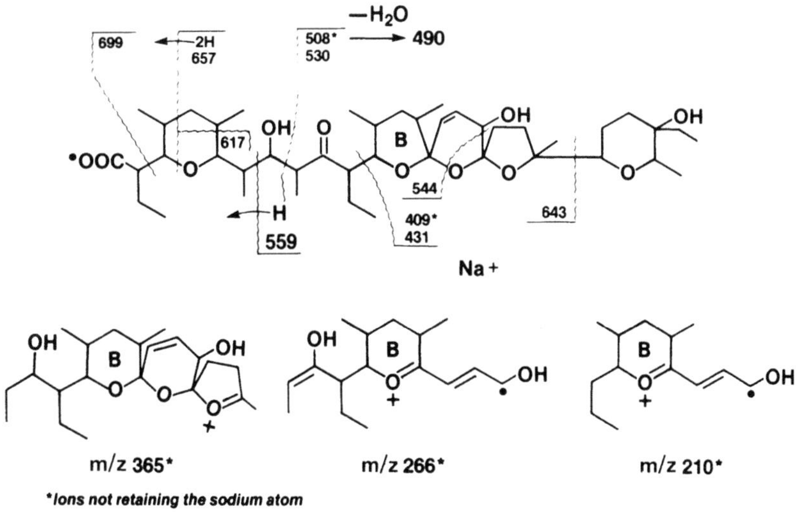

−H₂O

699 −2H 508* → 490
657 530

OH O OH OH

•OOC 617 B

544 O

H 409* 643
559 431

Na+

OH B OH OH B OH B OH

m/z 365* m/z 266* m/z 210*

*Ions not retaining the sodium atom

Scheme 21 EI fragmentation of sodium narasin.

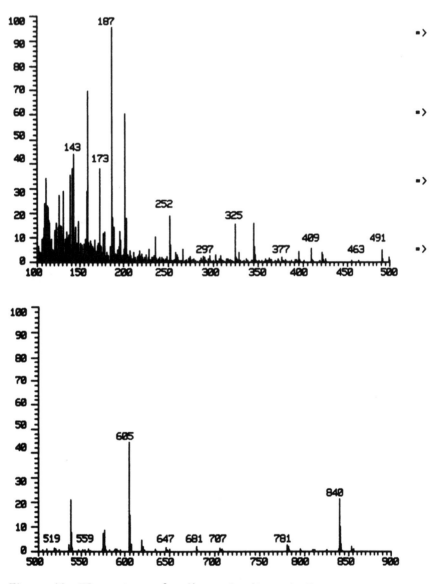

Figure 11 EI spectrum of sodium noboritomycin B.

In Scheme 20 all assignments were supported by accurate mass measurement (± 1 mMU).

Comparison of Scheme 20 with Scheme 21 shows the similarities between the EI fragmentation of sodium noboritomycin B and sodium narasin. In particular, the following pairs of peaks arise by analogous fragmentations: m/z 681, 643; 605, 559; 576, 530; 491, 493; and 538, 544 in the spectra of the sodium salts of noboritomycin B and narasin, respectively. An intense peak in the EI spectrum of sodium noboritomycin B above m/z 150 occurred at m/z 173 and had the composition $C_{12}H_{13}O$. This peak was also intense in the same mass range in the spectrum of sodium noboritomycin B. The composition of m/z 173 indicated that it contains the decarboxylated aromatic ring.

XI. SALINOMYCIN GROUP

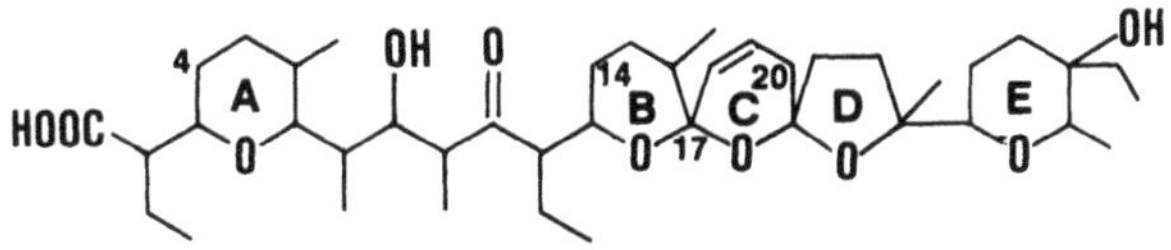

	Substituent		
Compound	4	14	20
Salinomycin	H	Me	OH
20-Deoxysalinomycin	H	Me	H
17-Epi-20-deoxysalinomycin	H	Me	H
Narasin	Me	Me	OH
Narasin B	Me	Me	=O
Narasin D	Me	Et	OH
20-Deoxynarasin	Me	Me	H
17-Epi-20-deoxynarasin	Me	Me	H

Determination of the structure of salinomycin by Kinashi et al. (1973) using x-ray diffraction provided the impetus for mass-spectral studies on this group of compounds. These studies resulted in the determination of the structure of narasin (Occolowitz et al., 1976; Seto et al., 1977), narasin B (Occolowitz et al., 1976), narasin D (Hamill et al., 1978), and 20-deoxynarasin and 17-epi-20-deoxynarasin (Nakatsukasa et al., 1979). Additionally, the structures of 20-deoxysalinomycin and 17-epi-20-deoxysalinomycin were determined by Westley et al. (1977) using x-ray diffraction. Mass spectrometry and other physical methods were used to show the equivalence of SY-1 and 20-deoxysalinomycin (Miyazaki et al., 1978).

From studies of the mass spectrometry of salinomycin and related compounds by Kinashi and Otake (1976) and studies of salinomycin, narasin, and related compounds by Occolowitz et al. (1976), a rationale for the EI and FD fragmentation was obtained for these compounds.

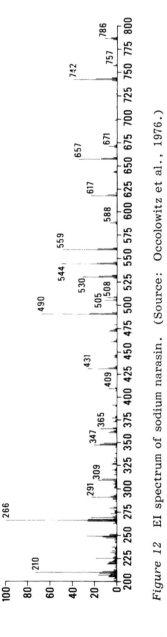

Figure 12 EI spectrum of sodium narasin. (Source: Occolowitz et al., 1976.)

EI-induced fragmentation of this group occurred mainly by two processes; fission between the rings, notably, α to the cyclic ether oxygens and β and γ to the keto group, and fragmentation of the C ring by a retro-Diels Alder mechanism. The mass spectrum of sodium narasin, Figure 12 is rationalized in Scheme 21 and is of general applicability to the other sodium salts.

Accurate mass measurements showed that m/z 657 in the spectrum of sodium salinomycin originated as depicted above and not as proposed by Kinashi and Otake (1976). Accurate mass measurements (Hamill et al., 1978) indicated that the B ring of sodium salts of compounds of this group also fragmented to yield the two ions shown in Scheme 22.

These ions were observed in the spectra of the sodium salts of narasin, narasin D, and salinomycin. This observation, together with appropriate shifts in the masses of the ions shown in Scheme 21, led to the conclusion that narasin D has an ethyl group at C-14.

Many of the fragmentations observed in the spectra of the sodium salts of this group also occurred in the spectra of the acids. In Scheme 21 the ion at m/z 544 has its analog at m/z 522 in the acid spectrum. The ions m/z 508, 490, 409, 365, 255, and 210 occurred in the spectra of both compounds. The free acid spectra did not show $(M-CO_2)^{+\cdot}$ peaks but, instead, intense peaks at $(M-H_2O)^{+\cdot}$.

Similarities between the fragmentation of the sodium salts of nobori-tomycin A and B and sodium narasin were discussed in Group X.

FD-induced fragmentation of narasin acid occurred by fission α to the cyclic ether oxygens and by the retro-Diels Alder mechanism. Fragments at m/z 199 and 143 explicitly defined the mass of the A and E rings and confirmed conclusions based on the EI spectrum. The FD fragmentation of narasin acid is depicted in Scheme 23.

Many of the fragmentations discussed above for the EI-induced fragmentation of narasin and its sodium salt were reported by Kinashi and Otake (1976) for salinomycin methyl ester. The molecular ion, m/z 764, had a relative intensity of 2%, and the M—H2O peak a relative intensity of 35%. Notably absent in the spectrum of the ester were the two fragmentations of the A ring analogous to those depicted in Scheme 21.

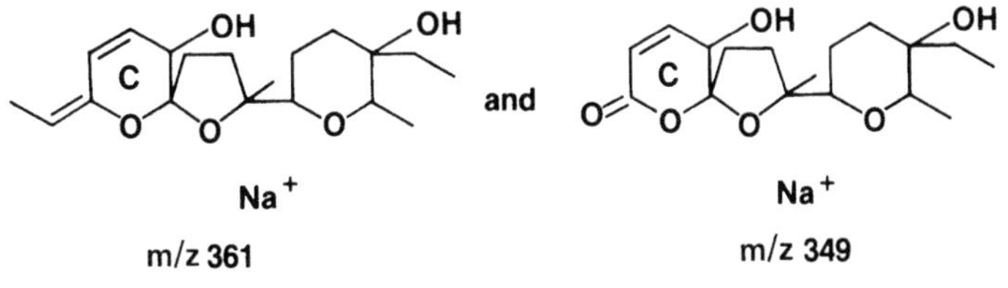

Scheme 22

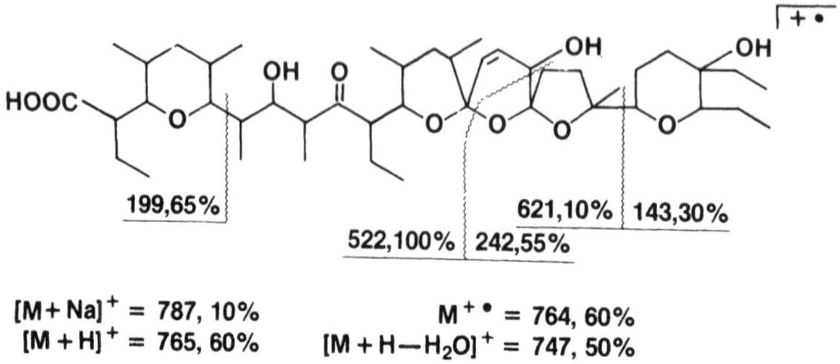

$[M+Na]^+ = 787, 10\%$ $M^{+\bullet} = 764, 60\%$
$[M+H]^+ = 765, 60\%$ $[M+H-H_2O]^+ = 747, 50\%$

Scheme 23   FD fragmentation of narasin.

Kinashi and Ōtake (1976) also discussed the EI spectra of two reduction products of salinomycin methyl ester and sodium salt: the
compounds where the 18-19 double bond had been reduced and the
compounds where the 11-keto group had been reduced to a hydroxyl.
For the methyl ester derivatives removal of the keto group or double
bond largely suppressed those fragmentations induced by these groups.
Thus in the 18,19-dihydrosalinomycin methyl ester spectrum the peak
at m/z 524 which arose by fragmentation of the C ring was weak, and
in the spectra of the epimeric 11-hydroxysalinomycin methyl esters a
peak at m/z 510 was absent. In the spectrum of sodium 18,19-dihydro-
salinomycin it is not clear whether reduction of the double bond suppresses the C ring cleavage, because the prominent peak at m/z 532
can arise by an alternate fragmentation (see m/z 530, Scheme 21).

The p-bromo- and p-iodophenacyl esters of narasin gave EI spectra
in which a number of relatively intense peaks arose by fission of the A
ring. The intensity of these peaks is presumably due to the low ionization potential of the phenacyl moiety which was retained in the
fragments. Scheme 24 summarizes these fragmentations.

Similar fragmentations of the A ring of the p-iodophenacyl ester of
narasin were used to show that narasin had a methyl group at C-4
(Occolowitz et al., 1976).

Westley et al. (1977) reported that the EI spectra of the C-17
epimers of 20-deoxysalinomycin were almost identical. Each gave a
molecular ion (m/z 734) and peaks due to the loss of 1 and 2 mol of
water from the molecular ion. Both spectra had their base peaks at
m/z 474. The authors proposed that this peak arose from the cleavage
of the C ring (see m/z 544, Scheme 21) followed by the elimination of
1 mol of water. Ion m/z 474 likely also arose by fission β to the aliphatic carbonyl followed by dehydration (see m/z 490, Scheme 21).
The ions resulting from these two processes are isomeric. Also reported was a small peak at m/z 591 due to the loss of the E ring from
the molecular ion.

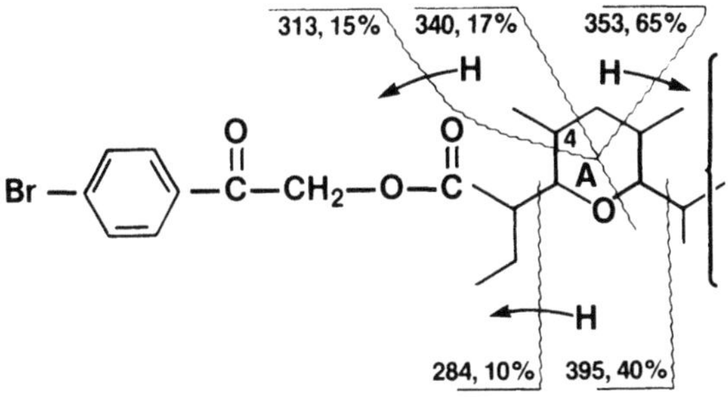

Scheme 24 EI fragmentation of the A ring of narasin p-bromophenacyl ester.

Miyazaki et al. (1978) compared the EI spectra of the methyl esters of salinomycin and 20-deoxysalinomycin. The mass spectrum of 20-deoxysalinomycin methyl ester included a molecular ion at m/z 748. By observing that a number of peaks in the spectrum of the deoxy compound occurred 16 MU lower than those in the spectrum of methyl salinomycin, the authors were able to deduce that the deoxy compound had one less oxygen associated with the B, C, or D rings. They did not observe the C ring cleavage in the spectrum of the deoxy compound, which strongly suggested that the hydroxyl attached to C-20 was absent. Final confirmation of the structure of the deoxy compound came by comparing the physiochemical properties of 18,19-dihydro-20-deoxysalinomycin prepared from the deoxy compound with the identical compound prepared by the hydrogenolysis of 20-O-acetylsalinomycin methyl ester.

The EI spectrum of sodium 20-deoxynarasin has been examined by J. L. Occolowitz (unpublished data, 1977). Except for m/z 266 and 212, analogs of all of the peaks enumerated in Scheme 21 for sodium narasin were observed in the spectrum of sodium 20-deoxynarasin. These data indicated that absence of the C-20 hydroxyl suppressed partially the retro-Diels Alder fragmentation of the C ring. However, m/z 528, the analog of m/z 544 in the spectrum of sodium narasin, was present in the spectrum of the deoxy compound.

Although 20-deoxynarasin exhibited the typical sodium scavenging in the ion source, which was discussed in Section II, epi-20-deoxynarasin acid did not.

XII. SUMMARY

The material in the foregoing sections has demonstrated that EI spectrometry can be used to obtain structural information for most of

the polyether antibiotics discovered to data. All of the known polyether antibiotics are amenable to examination by FD spectrometry.
As is true for all compounds, selection of a suitable derivative can
minimize undesirable pyrolytic reactions in the mass-spectrometer in-
let system and provide new fragmentations for structure determination.
The polyethers are unusual in that their salts often yield EI spectra
which are more informative than those of the acids. Formation of a
salt may be the only derivatization required.

ACKNOWLEDGMENTS

The authors thank J. M. Gilliam for obtaining much of the previously
unpublished data presented in this chapter and The American Chemical Society, The Japan Antibiotics Research Association, and Heyden
and Sons for permission to publish several figures. They also thank
Professor N. Otake and Dr. N. Tsuji for their generous gift of
compounds.

REFERENCES

Abbott, B. J., Fukuda, D. S., Dorman, D. E., Occolowitz, J. L.,
Debono, M., and Farhner, L. (1980). Microbial transformation of
A23187, a divalent cation ionophore antibiotic. *Antimicrob.
Agents Chemother.* 16:808-812.
Beckey, H. D. (1977). In *Principles of Field Ionization and Field
Desorption Mass Spectrometry*. Pergamon Press, Oxford, pp.
290-295.
Blount, J. F., and Westley, J. W. (1971). X-ray crystal and molec-
ular structure of X-206. *Chem. Commun. 1971*:927-928.
Blount, J. F., and Westley, J. W. (1975). Crystal and molecular
structure of the free acid form of antibiotic X-206 hydrate. *J.
Chem. Soc. Chem. Commun. 1975*:533.
Bose, A. K., Fujiwara, H., and Pramanik, B. N. (1979). Negative
chemical ionization mass spectra of multifunctional polar and under-
ivatized compounds of biological interest (1). *Tetrahedron Lett.
1979*:4017-4020.
Chamberlin, J. W., and Agtarap, A. (1970). Observations on the mass
spectrometry of monensin and related compounds. *Org. Mass
Spectrom.* 3:271-285.
Chaney, M. O., Demarco, P. V., Jones, N. D., and Occolowitz, J. L.
(1974). The structure of A23187, a divalent cation ionophore.
J. Am. Chem. Soc. 96:1932-1933.
Czerwinski, E. W., and Steinrauf, L. K. (1971). Structure of the
antibiotic dianemycin. *Biochem. Biophys. Res. Commun.* 45:1284-
1287.

Donoho, A., Manthey, J., Occolowitz, J., and Zornes, L. (1978). Metabolism of monensin in steer and rat. *Agric. Food Chem.* 26:1090-1095.

Dorman, D. E., Hamill, R. L., Occolowitz, J. L., Terui, Y., Tori, K., and Tsuji, N. (1980). The structure of polyether antibiotic A28695B. *J. Antibiot.* 33:252-255.

Fehr, T., King, H. D., and Kuhn, M. (1977). Mutalomycin, a new polyether antibiotic. Taxonomy, fermentation, isolation and characterization. *J. Antibiot.* 30:903-907.

Gachon, P., and Kergomard, A. (1975). Grisorixin, an ionophorus antibiotic of the nigericin group. II. Chemical and structural study of grisorixin and some derivatives. *J. Antibiot.* 28:351-357.

Gachon, P., Kergomard, A., Staron, T., and Esteve, C. (1975). Grisorixin, an ionophorus antibiotic of the nigericin group. I. Fermentation, isolation biological properties and structure. *J. Antibiot.* 28:345-350.

Gachon, P., Farges, C., and Kergomard, A. (1976). Alborixin, a new antibiotic ionophore: Isolation, structure, physical and chemical properties. *J. Antibiot.* 29:603-610.

Hamill, R. L., Nakatsukasa, W. M., and Occolowitz, J. L. (1978). Mass spectrometric structure determination of the ionophore A28086D. American Society for Mass Spectrometry, 26th Annual Conference on Mass Spectrometry and Allied Topics. St. Louis, Missouri, Paper RG8.

Keller-Juslén, C., King, H. D., Kuhn, M., Loosli, H. -R, and von Wartburg, A. (1978). Noboritomycins A and B, new polyether antibiotics. *J. Antibiot.* 31:820-828.

Kinashi, H., and Otake, N. (1976). An interpretation of the mass spectra of salinomycin and its derivatives. *Agric. Biol. Chem.* 40:1625-1632.

Kinashi, H., Otake, N., Yonehara, H., Sato, S., and Saito, Y. (1973). The structure of salinomycin, a new member of the polyether antibiotics. *Tetrahedron Lett.* 1973:4955-4958.

Kitame, F., and Ishida, N. (1976). The constitution of laidlomycin, a new antimycoplasmal antibiotic. *J. Antibiot.* 29:759-761.

Koenuma, M., and Otake, N. (1977). Studies of ionophorus antibiotics. XI The artifacts and the degradation products of lysocellin. *J. Antibiot.* 30:819-828.

Kubota, T., and Matsutani, S. (1970). Studies on the antibiotic nigericin (polyetherin A). *J. Chem. Soc. C 1970:695-703.

Kubota, T., Hinoh, H., Mayama, M., Motokawa, K., and Yasuda Y. (1975). Antibiotic A-130, isolation and characterization. *J. Antibiot.* 28:931-934.

Liu, C., Hermann, T. E., Lui, M., Bull, D. N., Palleroni, N. J., Prosser, B. LaT., Westley, J. W., and Miller, P. A. (1979). X-14547A, a new ionophorous antibiotic produced by *Streptomyces antibioticus* NRRL 8167. Discovery, fermentation, biological prop-

antibioticus NRRL 8167. Discovery, fermentation, biological properties and taxonomy of the producing culture. *J. Antibiot.* *32*:96-
106.

Miyazaki, Y., Shibata, A., Tsuda, K., Kinashi, H., and Ōtake, N
(1978). Isolation, characterization and structure of SY-I (20-
deoxysalinomycin). *Agric. Biol. Chem.* *42*:2129-2132.

Mizutani, T., Yamagishi, M., Hara, H., Omura, S., and Ozeki, M.
(1980). Lonomycins B and C, two new components of polyether
antibiotics. Fermentation, isolation and characterization, *J. Antibiot.* *33*:1224-1230.

Nakatsukasa, W. M., Marconi, G. G., Neuss, N., and Hamill, R. L.
(1979). Deoxynarasin antibiotics. U.S. Patent 4,141,907.

Occolowitz, J. L., and Hamill, R. L. (1979). Structure investigation
of higher molecular weight polyether antibiotics using field desorption mass spectrometry. American Society for Mass Spectrometry,
27th Annual Conference on Mass Spectrometry and Allied Topics.
Seattle, Washington, Paper MAMOB7.

Occolowitz, J. L., Berg, D. H., Debono, M., and Hamill, R. L.
(1976). The structure of narasin and a related ionophore. *Biomed.
Mass Spectrom.* *3*:272-277.

Occolowitz, J. L., Dorman, D. E., and Hamill, R. L. (1978). Structure of the polyether antibiotic K-41 by mass and nuclear magnetic
resonance spectrometry. *Chem. Commun.* *1978*:683-684.

Otake, N., and Koenuma, M. (1975). Studies on the ionophorous antibiotics. Part III. The structure of lonomycin, a polyether antibiotic. *Tetrahedron Lett.* *1975*:4147-4150.

Seto, H., Yahagi, T., Miyazaki, Y., and Ōtake, N. (1977). Studies
on the ionophorous antibiotics. IX. The structure of 4-methyl-
salinomycin (narasin). *J. Antibiot.* *30*:530-532.

Steinrauf, L. K., Pinkerton, M., and Chamberlin, J. W. (1968). The
structure of nigericin. *Biochem. Biophys. Res. Commun.* *33*:29-
31.

Toeplitz, B. K., Cohen, A. I., Funke, P. T., Parker, W. L., and
Gougoutas, J. Z. (1979). Structure of ionomycin—A novel diacidic
polyether antibiotic having a high affinity for calcium ions. *J. Am.
Chem. Soc.* *101*:3344-3353.

Tsuji, N., Nagashima, K., Terui, Y., and Tori, K. (1979). Structure
of K-41B, a new diglycoside polyether antibiotic. *J. Antibiot.*
32:169-172.

Tsuji, N., Terui, Y., Nagashima, K., Tori, K., and Johnson, L. F.
(1980). New polyether antibiotics, A-130B and A130C. *J. Antibiot.* *33*:94-97.

Westley, J. W., Benz, W., Donahue, J., Evans, R. H., Jr., Scott,
C. G., Stempel, A., and Berger, J. (1974a). Biosynthesis of
lasalocid. III Isolation and structure determination of four homologs
of lasalocid A. *J. Antibiot.* *27*:744-753.

Westley, J. W., Blount, J. F., Evans, R. H., Jr., Stempel, A., and Berger, J. (1974b). Biosynthesis of lasalocid. II X-ray analysis of a naturally occurring isomer of lasalocid A. *J. Antibiot.* 27:597-604.

Westley, J. W., Blount, J. F., Evans, R. H., Jr., and Liu, C. (1977). C-17 epimers of deoxy-(O-8)-salinomycin from *Streptomyces albus* (ATCC 21838). *J. Antibiot. 30*:610-612.

Westley, J. W., Evans, R. H. Jr., Sello, L. H., Troupe, N., Liu, C., and Blount, J. F. (1979). Isolation and characterization of antibiotic X-14547A, a novel monocarboxylic ionophore produced by *Streptomyces antibioticus* NRRL 8167. *J. Antibiot. 32*:100-106.

Yamazaki, K., Abe, K., and Sano, M. (1976). Structure of antibiotic DE-3936. *J. Antibiot. 29*:91-92.

chapter 5

STRUCTURE, CONFORMATION, AND MECHANISM OF ACTION AS REVEALED BY PROTON NMR

Marc J. O. Anteunis
NMR Spectroscopic Unit, Laboratory of Organic Chemistry,
State University of Ghent, Ghent, Belgium

I. INTRODUCTION

NMR spectroscopy offers the possibility of studying the conformational behavior of (bio)molecules in solution and eventually the dynamic aspects related to it (Dwek, 1973; James, 1975). In general, the architecture of biomolecules in the solid state does not differ greatly from that observed in solution, even for structures less conformationally defined than the pseudocyclic ionophores, despite the plethora of reasons one could advance against that idea. In addition, solution studies of ionophores enable one to look at the uncomplexed species which lack the "heavy" cation preferred for x-ray studies (Chapter 3), although some ionophores, such as monensin (Lutz et al., 1971), the bromo derivative of A23187 (Chaney et al., 1974), X-206 (Blount and Westley, 1975), and the C^{17} epimer of deoxy salinomycin (Westley, et al.) have been x-rayed in the free acid form as well as derivatives of lasalocid (Bissel and Paul, 1972) and the esters of septamycin (Pretcher and Weber, 1974; Kinashi et al., 1975) and of salinomycin (Kinashi et al., 1973).

The slight differences that may be uncovered between the three-dimensional structure of the free acid and the cation-charged species give a hint to the possible mechanism by which the metal ions may be trapped at the boundary of the membrane bilayer and transported to the other aqueous-membrane interface. NMR spectroscopy offers, in addition, other possibilities. Different environments (e.g., hydrophilic and lipophilic in nature) may be used, mimicking biological conditions. Dynamic aspects such as exchange phenomena (e.g., of the cations between complexed and uncomplexed species) may also be monitored relatively easily by NMR techniques under a variety of circumstances (Degani, 1978a,b).

Thus it has been found by ^{1}H NMR studies that in chloroform, lasalocid transfers its barium cation directly from the complex to the acid form $[\Delta G^{\ddagger}(CDCl_3) = 10.2$ Cal/mol; Patel and Shen, 1976], while in protic solvents the rate of exchange is independent of the reactant concentration and hence the rate-determining step consists in the dissociation of BaX^+ $[\Delta H^{\ddagger}(CD_3OD) = 6.5$ Cal/mol, $\Delta S^{\ddagger}(CD_3OD) = -20$ e.u.; Shen and Patel, 1976.]. We have found (M. Anteunis and N. A. Rodios, unpublished data) by monitoring appropriate proton signals in the ^{1}H NMR specta that the rate of exchange of Na^+ between monensin free acid and the complex in mixed surroundings (toluene: CD_3OD) is at least of the fourth order in the protic cosolvent. Similar results were observed for lonomycin (see Rodios and Anteunis, 1978b). This is in accordance with a mechanism whereby the solvation shell of the cation in water is dismantled stepwise in a consecutive, competitive way by the ionophore (Burgermeister and Winkler-Oswatitsch, 1977; Urry et al., 1975). Using ^{23}Na NMR spectroscopy, Degani (1977) has been able to measure the thermodynamic dimensions for the sodium-binding process of monensin in CD_3OD $[k_{assoc} = 6.3 \times 10^7$ sec^{-1}

$(\Delta H_a^{\ddagger} = -0.8 \text{ Cal/mol}; \Delta S_a^{\ddagger} = -3.9 \text{ e.u.}); k_{dissoc} = 63 \text{ sec}^{-1}$
$(\Delta H_d^{\ddagger} = 10.3 \text{ Cal/mol}; \Delta S_d^{\ddagger} = -15.8 \text{ e.u.})].$

Scope and Limitations of ^{1}H NMR Spectroscopy

^{1}H NMR studies of polyether antibiotics became conceivable only when at the beginning of the 1970s high-field spectrometers at frequencies of 270 MHz (magnetic field strength of 6.34 T) or more were marketed. The simplest member, lasalocid, already possesses 54 protons, and some have more than 80 protons. An illustration of a dramatic spectral simplification with increasing field strength is shown in Figure 1. With the further introduction of pulse techniques, several advantages

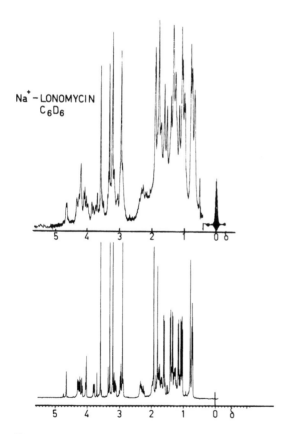

Figure 1 Comparison of resolutions achieved for K$^+$-lonomycin at field strengths of 90 MHz (2.11 T; top) and 360 MHz (8.44 T; bottom).

have since been added. The sensitivity enhancement achieved by
working in the time domain allows smaller sample sizes to be studied.
Filtering (e.g., resolution or sensitivity enhancement) can be easily
achieved mathematically, since convolution in the frequency domain
reduces to a multiplication of the free induction decay with a suitable
weighting function. Additionally, pulse NMR is particularly suited to
measure dynamic effects as, e.g., relaxation times.

Although no studies on ionophores using two-dimensional spectroscopy (Freeman, 1980) or multiplet selection (Campbell et al. 1975)
have been reported yet, these techniques will in the near future considerably increase the utility of ^{1}H NMR spectroscopy for the study of
macrobiomolecules in solution. In the beginning ^{1}H NMR spectroscopy
was only rarely applied to ionophores, and for fragmentary analytical
purposes only, e.g., for the determination of aromatic and olefinic
functionalities, to detect the presence or absence of methoxy groupings, for the identification through deuterium exchange of hydroxyl
protons, etc. (salinomycin at 100 MHz: Kinashi et al., 1973; Miyazaki
et al., 1974; grisorixin at 100 MHz: Gachon and Kergomard, 1975;
alborixin at 270 MHz: Gachon et al., 1976; ionomycin at 100 MHz:
Wen-Chih Liu et al., 1978; narasin at 100 MHz: Berg and Hamill,
1978; carriomycin at 90 MHz: Imada et al., 1978; laidlomycin: Kitame
et al., 1974; lasalocid at 220 MHz: Schmidt et al. 1974). Some more
advanced studies were achieved with nonactin at 220 MHz, determining
the formation constants for the K$^+$ complex (Prestegard and Chan,
1969) and comparing the Na$^+$, K$^+$, and Cs$^+$ complexes of it (Prestegard
and Chan, 1970). The earliest most complete studies that also disclosed by relaxation times measurements the dimeric nature of lasalocid
A-Na$^+$ in nonpolar solvents, but the monomeric nature in methanol solutions, were only reported in 1976 (270 and 360 MHz) (Shen and Patel,
1976; Patel and Shen, 1976).

It has since been demonstrated at these laboratories that ^{1}H NMR
spectroscopy remains a unique method, giving a plethora of structural
and conformational information despite or, rather, by virtue of its
complexity, both in the appearance of the proton patterns and their
complicated dependence on a multitude of structural parameters.

^{1}H NMR spectroscopy must be considered as a powerful adjunct to
other heteronucleic studies, the latter undoubtedly having a promising
future (^{18}O, ^{15}N, ^{37}Cl; Bystrov et al., 1977; Levy and Lichter, 1979;
Axenrod and Webb, 1974). Among these, special attention should be
paid to ^{203,205}Tl (Srivanavit et al., 1977; Briggs and Hinton, 1979)
and ^{23}Na NMR spectroscopy (Degani, 1977; Degani and Elgairsh, 1978;
Haynes et al., 1969; Haynes et al., 1971; Grandjean and Laszlo, 1979)
and other alkali or alkali earth nuclei, and, last but not least, to ^{13}C
NMR spectroscopy (Chapter 6). ^{13}C NMR spectroscopy offers certain

advantages that ^{1}H NMR does not have. It provides direct information on the number of carbons and their directly bonded protons. Shifts are hardly influenced by the solvent systems used (even for aromatic solvents), so that they are directly related to the structural and spatial environment of each of the carbons themselves. This allows the simulation and prediction of spectra (sticked spectra) and a reliable comparison between different ionophoric spectra. Rapid recognition and structural determination may therefore be achieved using ^{13}C NMR. The natures (axial or equatorial) of frequently encountered methyl and ethyl groupings are easily discerned by typical shift increments, and ^{13}C NMR provides information particularly about those carbon atoms that lack protons. Finally, biosynthetic studies have successfully demonstrated their polyketide-type pathway (Chapters 1 and 3, Volume 1; White et al., 1973) by the use of ^{13}C-enriched substrates. These studies are undertaken in addition to mass spectroscopy (Chapter 4).

For more detailed information about the behavior of biomolecules, one should not be discouraged by the complexity of proton spectra. ^{1}H NMR spectroscopy demands only small samples. Any spectral characteristic that in principle can be extracted from NMR phenomena has in the past been used in ^{1}H NMR to gain maximal information, such as shifts, couplings (mostly interproton proton coupoing, but also carbon-proton couplingfor ^{13}C-enriched samples), relaxation phenomena (T_1) caused by overall tumbling (giving access to, e.g., aggregation phenomena and segmental rotational features) or chemical exchange broadening effects under different conditions of hydroxyl protons, and, last but not least, specific solvent effects [e.g., aromatic solvent-induced shifts (ASIS) or even changes in molecular state caused by varying the polarity of the environment, etc]. Several of these criteria are typical for ^{1}H NMR. To give some examples, the nature of the anomeric configuration of the desoxy sugar fragments to which ionophores are frequently conjugated is easily assigned by inspection of the vicinal coupling constants of the anomeric (acetalic) proton. Another typical advantage of ^{1}H NMR concerns the nature and character of hydroxyl protons. Disclosing their behavior [ease of isotope exchange phenomena; broadening by temperature jump; temperature shift gradients $d\delta/dT$ (see Kopple et al., 1969, and Ohnishi and Urry, 1969) solvent titrations; extent of saturation transfer while irradiating the residual water peak or other hydroxyl proton partners, etc.] gives information on the direct structural environment and/or hydrogen-bridge mechanism they are involved in. Alternatively, the detection of (slowly) exchangeable hydroxyl protons can be identified in proton-decoupled ^{13}C spectra because the isotopic substitution from [13]C−OH to [13]C−OD causes dedoubling of the newly formed [13]C(OD) species (Gagnaire and Vincendon, 1977; Gagnaire et al., 1978).

Still other advantages could be added and should perhaps in the future be looked for, as they have been successfully applied in other biochemical fields (e.g., peptides).

In the Tl complexes of ionophoric substances geminal couplings $^2J(^{203,205}Tl, ^{13}C)$ via a coordinating oxygen path $Tl---O-^{13}C$ are diagnostic not only to assign coordination sites (Lallemand and Michon, 1978), but also because these $Tl-^{13}C$ couplings represent spin-spin interactions between nuclei separated by a noncovalent bond. Corresponding couplings $^3J(Tl, H)$ can be detected (see Lehn et al., 1970) and their size may be related with the strength (length) of the coordination bonds involved.

The use of lanthanide ion-induced shift reagents (LIS reagents; Hofer, 1976) has in the case of the ionophores not been explored as fully as it has been for peptides (Nieboer and Falten, 1977) but may in certain cases be helpful. Usually the potential coordination sites are not exposed to an accessible region for La^{3+}, as they participate already in ligand formation for the cation or are directed away into the cavity of the pseudocyclic structure. But accessibility (or non-accessibility) of, e.g., certain oxygens is a major point of interest. Some of the ionophores do possess hydroxyl and alkoxy groups at their surface (X-206), or they expose in the monomeric form a non-screened polar face. These pecularities should be studied by LIS reagents, together with convolution-deconvolution techniques.

Also, relaxation reagents either caused by paramagnetic lanthanide-type (see Bradbury et al., 1974; Morris and Dwek, 1977) or nitroxyl radical reagents should be used in order to detect regions of solvent exposure. Protons that can come in close contact with these reagents show line broadening concomitant with upfield shift displacements (see Kopple and Schamper, 1972; Kopple and Go, 1977; Morishima, Endo and Yonezawa, 1971, 1973).

Finally, it should be realized that most of the hitherto reported intensive proton studies at high field have used instruments that operate in the continuous wave mode (CW). Nuclear Overhauser effects (NOE) (Noggle and Schiemer, 1971; Bell, 1973) have rarely been examined as a result of the overlapping nature of many patterns. At present, NOE difference spectroscopy is standard. Therefore it can be expected that the application of NOE phenomena, even under high-frequency conditions, will become routine, as it has been successfully used in the protein field (see Glickson et al., 1976). Advantages and disadvantages of high-field NMR have been reviewed by Anet (1974).

Some believe that for molecules with an appreciable electrical dipole moment, extra peak splitting by quadrupole mechanisms will occur at (very) high magnetic fields as a result of molecular orientation effects because of the anisotropic susceptibility of such species (see Lohman and MacLean, 1978).

II. STEREO NOTATION AND CODING

A. Symbols

In order to represent the structural and stereochemical features as complete as possible in the projection formulas of the ionophores, the following coding system will be used.

1. For the numbering of the (carbon) skeleton, oxygen atoms, nitrogen atoms, and side chains, we follow the numbering system introduced by Westley (1976): in numbering the oxygen heterocycles the ring oxygen takes precedence over any oxygen substituent such as hydroxyl or methoxyl (J. W. Westley, private communication, 1978). Rings may be coded A, B, . . . , X, starting at the carboxylic head along the principal backbone.
2. Oxygens that participate in the coordination of the trapped metal ion are encircled; others like nitrogen bear a broken line.
3. Hydrogen bondings are visualized by dotted lines.
4. Flattened pyranoid rings may be indicated by an open circle (double broken line) that is drawn inside the ring and in the region where flattening occurs (e.g., A23187, ring C).
5. The following symbols will be used as reported next to the appropriate bond to indicate torsion angles (see Bucourt, 1974) (Figure 2).

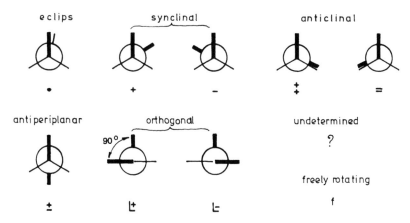

Figure 2 Symbols used to indicate master torsion angles along the principal backbone. (Source: Anteunis and Rodios, 1981.)

The torsions are *not* defined according to the Cahn-Ingold-Prelog sequence rules but, rather, as is the case in peptide chemistry, they are
defined along the longest carbon backbone skeleton ("master torsions").
    Alternatively, torsions along side chains are defined and visualized
by following the path along the principal chain bearing the atoms with
the highest numbers and bifurcating toward the side chain under consideration, e.g., in etheromycin (Figure 3). Incipient heterogeneity
in conformational character along rotors (called hinges; see Section
IV) are symbolized by 🞘 .
    Note that, alternatively, ring torsions inside the ring are not
necessarily identical with master torsions [e.g., C(45)−C(46)].
    With the proposed representation one can remap the entire spatial
structure, taking a variability of about ±30° around each torsion.
Eventually the exact torsion values could be determined (as, e.g., extracted from solid-state data). For most purposes, however, and certainly from determinations obtained in solution, the uncertainties introduced above are a more or less realistic reflexion of the proposed values for these solution conformations obtained by NMR spectroscopy

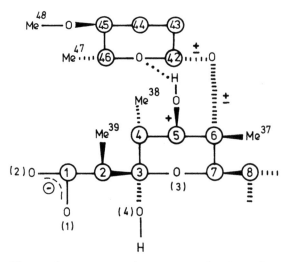

Figure 3 Fragment in stereoprojection of etheromycin with indication
of master torsion angles and side-chain torsions as C(6)C(5)−OH and
C(7)C(6)−OC(42) as proposed in Figure 2.

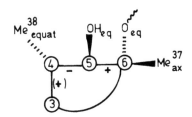

Figure 4　Ring A of etheromycin showing the equatorial and axial sub-
stitutions as deduced from their spatial indication (α or β bonds) and
from the clockwise sequence in the +,− sign of the ring torsion angles.

(e.g., from vicinal coupling constants). This is not a serious drawback for the ionophores that occur as pseudocycles by head-to-tail
hydrogen bonding, because by handling the molecular models many
ambiguities that might remain from the original conformational notation
vanish.

There is an advantage to introducing the nature and signs of ring
torsions. It is known that when the clockwise sequence of signs is
+,−, then a β bond bears (quasi) axial character. Hence in ring A of
etheromycin (Figure 4) the substituents at C(2),C(8), Me(38),O(5),
and O(6) are all equatorial, but Me(37) is axial.

This will simplify the discussion of, e.g., the size of exocyclic
coupling constants and its relation to the axial-equatorial character
of the exocyclic methyl group (see below).

B.　Structural Representations of Some
　　Carboxylic Acid Ionophores

Schemes 1 to 15 represent the projection formulas in the stereocoding
of the solution conformation of carboxylic ionophores that will be discussed in subsequent chapters. They are arranged in alphabetical
order. (Source: Anteunis, 1981.)

C.　Stereoviews

Stereoviews of some ionophores are presented in Figures 5 to 11. They
contain quantitative information on observed aromatic solvent-induced
chemical shifts that will be discussed in Section III.F.

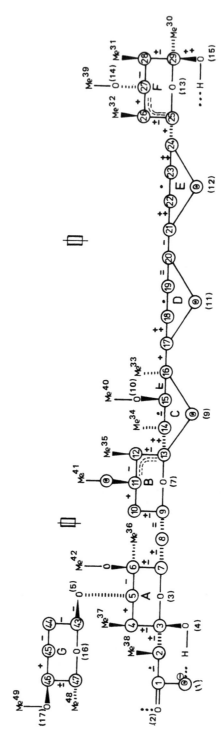

Scheme 1: Antibiotic A204A.

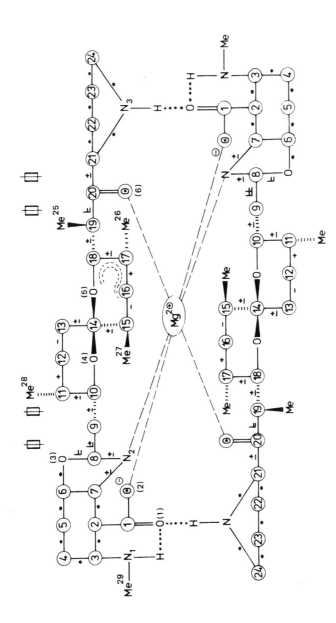

Scheme 2 :   Antitiotic A23187, magnesium salt.

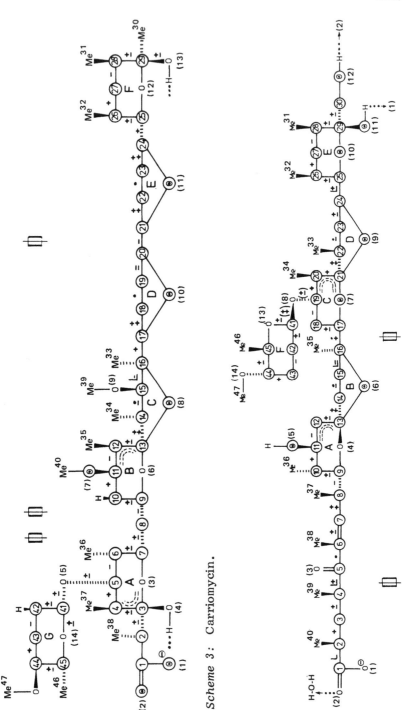

Scheme 3: Carriomycin.

Scheme 4: Dianemycin.

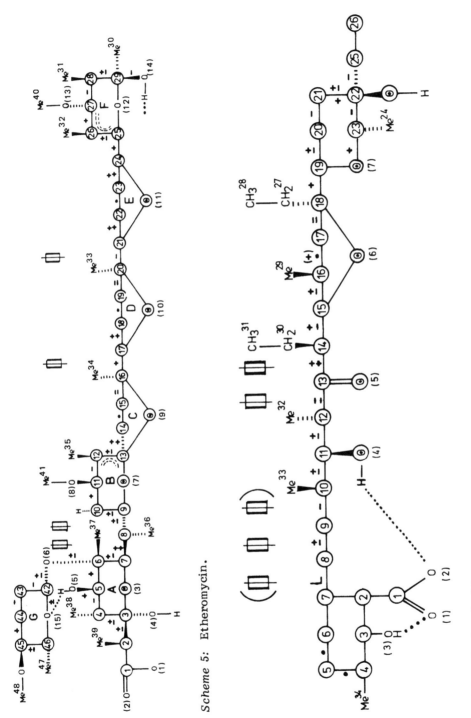

Scheme 5: Etheromycin.

Scheme 6: Lasalocid.

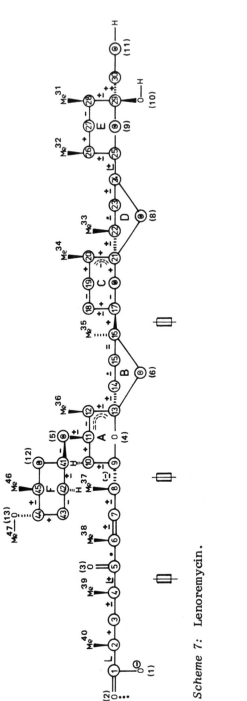

Scheme 7: Lenoremycin.

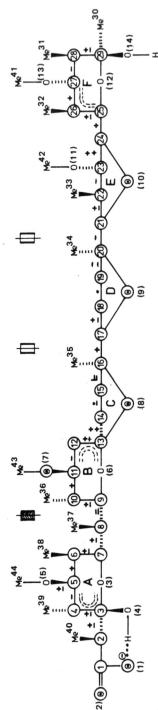

Scheme 8: Lonomycin.

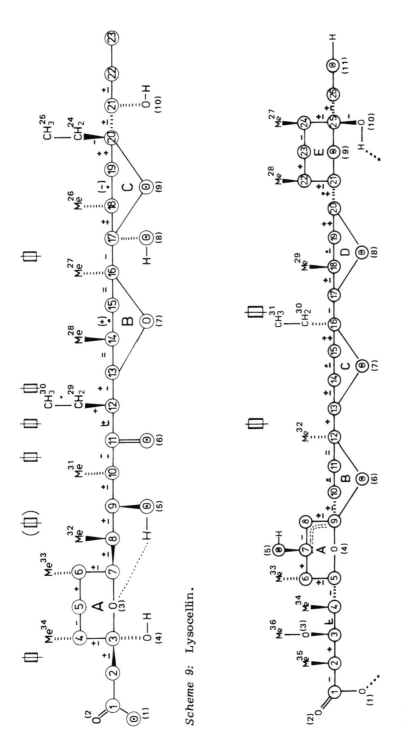

Scheme 9: Lysocellin.

Scheme 10: Monensin.

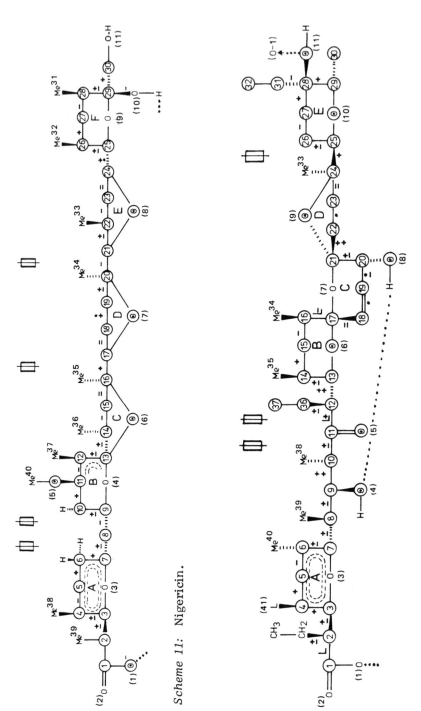

Scheme 11: Nigericin.

Scheme 12: Salinomycin (L = H). Narasin (L = Me).

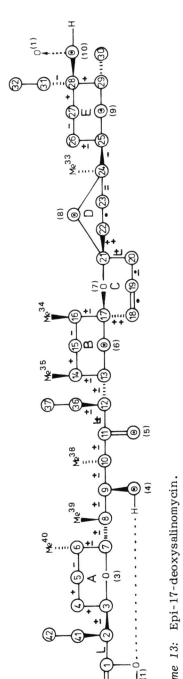

Scheme 13: Epi-17-deoxysalinomycin.

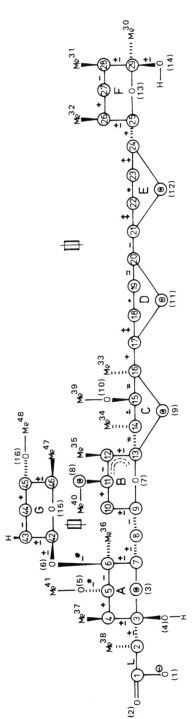

Scheme 14: Septamycin.

262

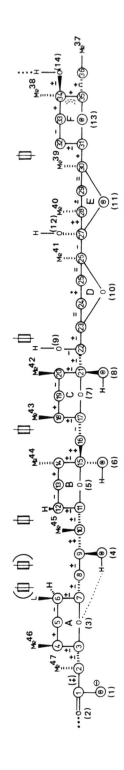

Scheme 15: Antibiotic x-206 (L = H). Alborixin (L = Me).

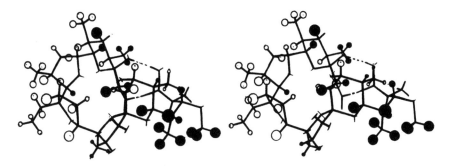

Figure 5 Stereoview of Na^+-monensin (without a water molecule mediating the head-to-tail hydrogen bonds) illustrating the typical distribution of hydrophilic (●) and lipophilic (○) regions, respectively. The pronouncedly hydrophilic region is distributed within the most polar part of the molecule, that is, at the head (carboxylate grouping) and tail (alcoholic functions) of the covalent structure. The middle part of the molecule constitutes the lipophilic part. The sizes of the circles correspond to the importance of the observed Δ(ASIS) $\times$ 10^{-2} values; ○——, from −5 to +5; ○ ——, from 5 to 15; ○ ——, from 15 to 25; ◯ ——, from 25 to 35; ◯ ——, from 35 to 45; ◯ ——, from 45 to 55; and ◯ ——, larger than 55. ├── indicates that no Δ(ASIS) was measured. (Source: Anteunis, 1981.)

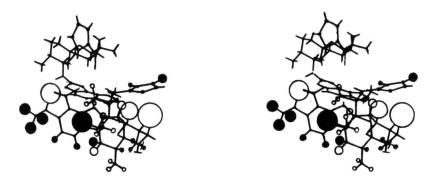

Figure 6 Stereodrawing of the sandwichlike dimeric superstructure of [A23187]$_2$Mg showing for one subunit the relatively high lipophilic parts achieved after aggregation. The lipophilicity fraction increases from 0.27 in the free acid to 0.49 in the dimeric salt.

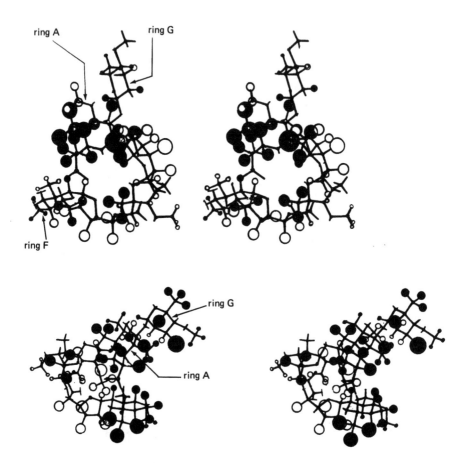

Figure 7 Distribution of hydrophilic and lipophilic regions in Na⁺-septamycin (top) and in Na⁺-A204A (bottom), shown in stereodrawing. In both cases (as in lonomycin and carriomycin) ring A possesses increased hydrophilicity as a result of the presence of alkoxy and hydroxy groupings. This is also the case for ring F in Na⁺-A204A (see Na⁺-etheromycin in Figure 8). The differences in overall character for the sugar fragments G are noticeable: the sugar is more "polar" in Na⁺-A204A. (Source: Anteunis, 1981.)

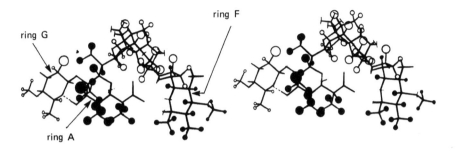

Figure 8 Distribution of lipophilicity and hydrophilicity in Na⁺-etheromycin represented in stereodrawing. Note the hydrophilic character of rings A and F as the result of the presence of polar substituents. The sugar ring G has a low hydrophilic character, in contrast to septamycin and A204A (Figure 7). This can be explained by a hydrogen bridge mechanism occurring in apolar solvents between O(5)H and O(15) (see also Scheme 5).

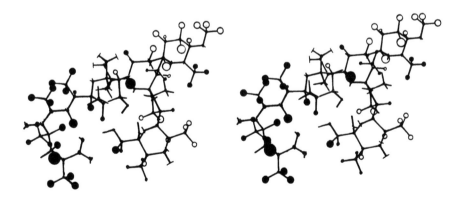

Figure 9 Stereodrawing of Na⁺-dianemycin. The relatively long acyclic chain at the head is pronouncedly hydrophilic, as in Na⁺-lenoremycin (Figure 10).

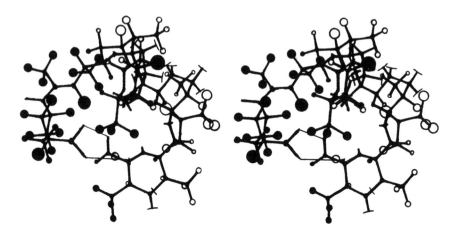

Figure 10 Stereodrawing of Na⁺-lenoremycin showing the hydrophilic nature of the acyclic head chain. (Source: Anteunis, 1981.)

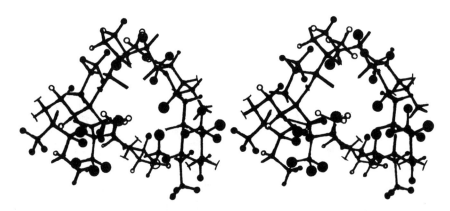

Figure 11 Stereodrawing of Na⁺-X206 viewed from the side which is probably the zone for releasing the cation. The almost equally distributed hydrophilicity is remarkable. The low fractional lipophicity [f(−) = 0.13; Table 5] is probably overestimated, as many protons for which ASIS effects could not be obtained (e.g., H-5a, H-5e, H-19a, H-19e, H-33a, and H-33e; represented by strokes in the present representation) are situated in or near the (not very pronounced) lipophilic regions.

D. Spectral Representations

Figures 12 to 23 display 360-MHz FT ^{1}H NMR spectra (quadrature detection, resolution 0.226 Hz per point; resolution enhancement by Gaussian multiplication) of some ionophores arranged in alphabetical order. See also Figure 1 for Na^+-Ionomycin in C_6D_6.

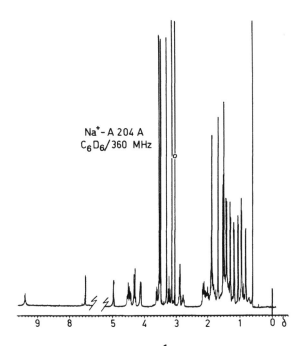

Na^+- A 204 A
C_6D_6/360 MHz

Figure 12 360-MHz FT ^{1}H NMR spectra of some ionophores in alphabetical order (Na^+-A204A in C_6D_6, H^+-A23187 in C_6D_6, Na^+-carriomycin in C_6D_6, Na^+-dianemycin in C_6D_6, Na^+-lenoremycin in $CDCl_3$ and C_6D_6, Na^+-lysocellin in $CDCl_3$, Na^+-monensin in C_6D_6, Na^+-nigericin in $CDCl_3$, H^+-salinomycin in $CDCl_3$, H^+-septamycin in $CDCl_3$, and Na^+-X-206 in $CDCl_3$.

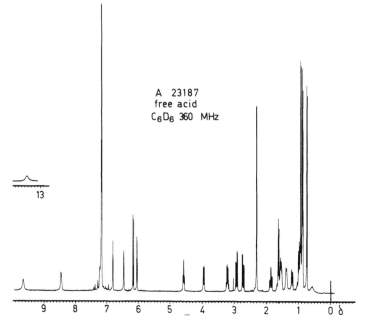

A 23187
free acid
C_6D_6 360 MHz

13

Figure 13

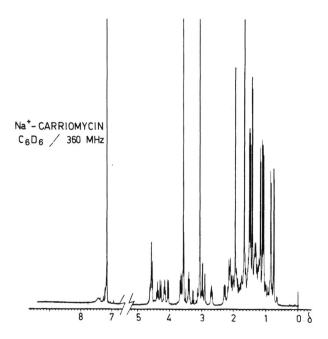

Na^+- CARRIOMYCIN
C_6D_6 / 360 MHz

Figure 14

268

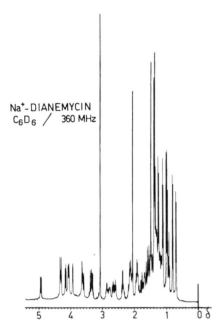

Figure 15

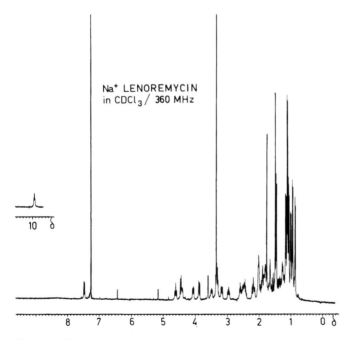

Figure 16

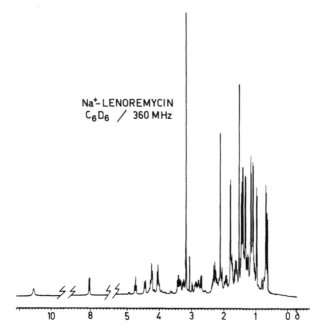

Figure 17

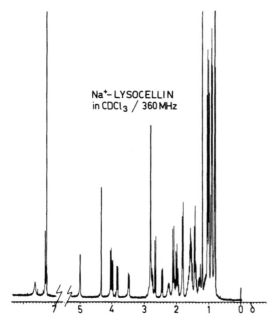

Figure 18

270

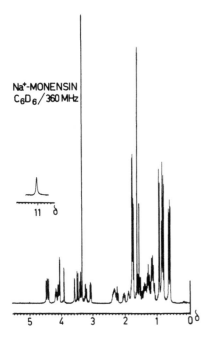

Figure 19

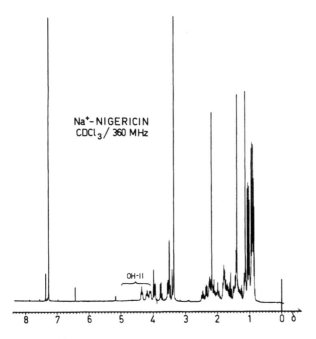

Figure 20

271

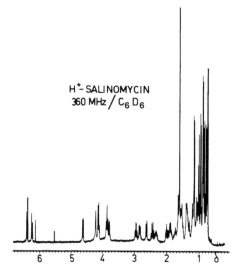

Figure 21

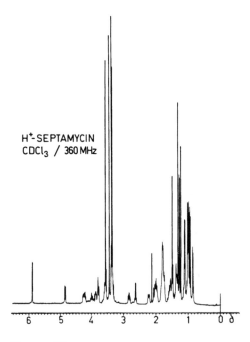

Figure 22

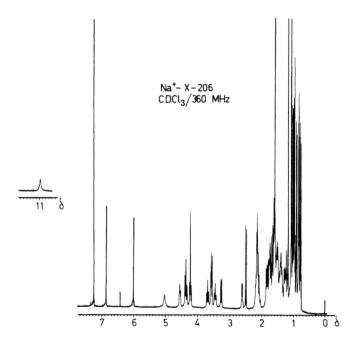

Figure 23

III. APPLIED METHODOLOGY AND CRITERIA

A. General Considerations

Neither the free acids nor the salts of the ionophores are soluble in water. We have systematically studied their ^{1}H NMR spectra and often at different temperatures in different solvent systems, such as chloroform, carbon disulfide, acetone, benzene, or toluene, but rarely in CD_3OD. Usually there are no large solvent shifts, except for aromatic solvents. They rarely exceed 0.2 ppm. If they differ by more, e.g., in comparison to those obtained in polar solvents (acetone-d_6, $CD3OD$), this is a clear indication for aggregation (dimer formation), as demonstrated in Na^+-lasalocid, which exists as a head-to-tail dimer in apolar solvents, thus avoiding unfavorable solvent-solute interactions with the polar face of the (relatively small and insufficiently wrapped) ionophore. The monomeric form is the preferred form in acetone and methanol (Schmidt et al. 1974; Patel and Shen, 1976; Shen and Patel, 1976). In dimeric packing, therefore, several protons shift by as much as 0.3 ppm due to their new location in the diamagnetic screening region of the aromatic chromophore of the second lasalocid molecule.

The complexity of the spectra is usually pronounced and the number of mutually coupling protons is appreciable. Especially for the aliphatic protons, it may be predicted that many coupling constants extracted directly with first-order approximations are only apparent values. They may differ considerably from the real values.

Aromatic solvents, on the contrary, do often cause large ASIS effects: from paramagnetic shifts of a maximum 1.0 ppm to diamagnetic shifts as large as 0.6 ppm. With such large shifts, especially substantial for the aliphatic protons, a possible violation of the real coupling-constant value may be detected. If extracted coupling constants remain unchanged within 0.1 Hz (and for badly resolved patterns of 0.2 Hz) when changing the solvent, it may be safely assumed that the first-order interpretation is a fairly realistic one.

As at the time of our measurements we had no access to FT facilities on our instrumentation, we were not able to apply any of the resolution-enhancement techniques. Therefore we used all methods available in order to gain more confidence in the interpretation of badly resolved patterns. Sometimes NMDR techniques were successful only in one particular solvent. Often minor changes in the spectral appearances of multiplets, caused by changes of the solvent system, were very helpful. As expected, resolution was usually better at the higher temperatures, and especially hydroxyl protons shifted their position or collapsed under these circumstances.

A rather peculiar experience and one typical for the probe geometry of our VARIAN CW 300-MHz apparatus (magnetic field direction along the axis of the sample tube) was the sometimes dramatic enhancement of resolution on aging, especially for aromatic solutions and when the sample was left in the magnetic gap. Subsequent filtering of the solution removed definitively the cause of this unpleasant phenomenon.

In order to force the ASIS effect we also used α- bromonaphtalene (at higher temperatures), recognized previously as a super-ASIS solvent (see Danneels and Anteunis, 1974, unpublished results). Unfortunately, only the nondeuterated compound is commercially available and the solvent, therefore, can practically only be used for CW registration or correlation spectroscopy (Dadok and Sprecher, 1974; Gupta, et al., 1975). One should wish also for a less viscous solvent.

An extreme example of spectral degeneracy in certain solvents was encountered during a spectral registration of Na^+-lysocellin in C_6D_6:CD_3OD (50:50). It was found that the C(20)-C(21)H(OH)-C(22)H_2-Me(23) fragment under these circumstances must represent an $A.MX.X_3'$ spin system: one of the methylene protons is isochronous with the methyl protons (accidental shift, but not coupling equivalence). Therefore the Me signal appears as an apparent doublet (Figure 24). Simulations with the same J values as those extracted from spectra run

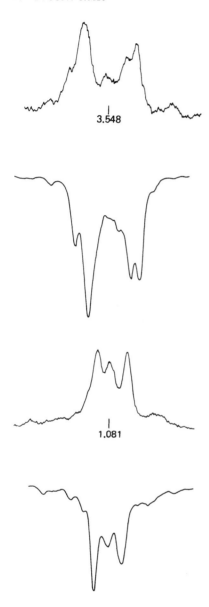

Figure 24 Experimental and simulated patterns A and X of a degenerated A.MX.X$'_3$ spin system in Na$^+$-lasalocid [C$_6$D$_6$:CD$_3$OD 50:50; C(20)−C(21)H(OH)−C(22)H$_2$−Me(23) fragment with ^{3}J(A,M) = 2.0, ^{3}J(A,X) = 20.0, ^{3}J(X,X') = 7.2, and ^{2}J(M, X) = ^{2}J(X', X') = −12.5 Hz].

in other solvents, showed satisfying agreement for the degenerated patterns.

Another illustration is found in dianemycin free acid, where in CDCl$_3$ both $^3J(17a, 18a)$ and $^3J(17a, 18e)$ are equal (6.0 Hz) because 18a and 18e are isochronous. However, in other solvent systems they are well differentiated, as they are in the salt (e.g., 10.0 and 1.2 Hz!) (Anteunis et al., 1977). The reader is referred to Section III.D for the consequences that degeneracies have on the correct interpretation of spectral data.

Polar solvents (CD$_3$OD, CF$_3$CD$_2$OD, etc.) were less frequently used. These solvent systems could offer certain interesting features (hydrogen-bridge-breaking solvents, mimicry of the cytoplasmatic and intercellular surroundings); however, here one is faced with additional artifacts (?), especially when looking at the free acid species.

Free acid species often are (chemically?) unstable in protic solvents. Transformation to other species (believed to result in nonclosed derivatives) has been proposed (Rodios and Anteunis, 1980). Therefore a thorough study of the original cation-uncharged ionophore is rendered difficult (but not always impossible for certain ionophores, because the half time of "deterioration" at 38°C was found to amount to about 6 hr for monensin, although considerably smaller for nigericin free acid). The presence of labile hemiacetal functions and/or spiro acetal functions may be at the origin of these molecular changes. This lability in aqueous solvents is well known by (bio)chemists and this property demands special precautions during the preparation of the free acid species. This is usually performed by acidic aqueous treatment at some stage of the procedure. [An alternative recipe that avoids destructive conditions makes use of an aqueous dichloroacetic acid treatment of a chloroform solution of the salt (D. E. Dorman, J. W. Paschal, and M. A. Bogan, personal communication, 1979).] In contrast, the complexed species are stable in CD$_3$OD (for over a year).

Only small *concentration* shifts occur, usually less than 0.1 ppm, except for some (but not all) hydroxyl protons. Thus the same spectral appearances are found for 1-2 M solutions (obtained at CW at 300 MHz) as for <0.1 M samples (obtained in FT at 360 MHz). In lasalocid and lysocellin and in certain solvent systems of a structure-disrupting nature one may find larger concentration-dependent shift differences, which is again an indication of the presence of multiple forms (monomer $\longleftrightarrow$ dimer) in equilibrium with each other.

A final remark should be made. The ionophores are sometimes produced in the form of mixed salts (Na$^+$, K$^+$, . . .). Due to the slow chemical exchange (T/2 > 10^{-3} sec) between two different species, *composite* spectra are obtained and are very confusing. Similar superposed spectra may be obtained during the preparation of the complex starting from the free acid form and for the same reasons (see Anteunis et al., 1977; Anteunis, 1977c; Patel and Shen, 1976). Either *prolonged* contact shaking, sonification with saturated aqueous solutions or brine or the addition of an excess of, e.g., solid NaSCN, KSCN, shifts the equilibrium between the different species entirely to a single form. By this, good-quality spectra may finally be obtained.

B. Operational Strategies

Although possible strategies are manifold and may vary a lot, depending on the technical possibilities that the hardware offers (see Section I), the strategy outlined in these sections is limited to our own experience, whereby a noncomputerized high-field spectrometer operating in CW has been used most of the time (VARIAN HR-300); the only (indispensable) periphery that was available being a decoupling unit (SC 8525-2).

The general appearance of a ^{1}H NMR spectrum of a carboxylic ionophore (Figure 1) is such that more or less well-differentiated patterns are found in the region below δ 2.0. In addition, a region between δ 0.8-1.5 offers access to the direct observation of doublets and/or triplets originating from methyl and/or ethyl groupings. ASIS effects for the latter are usually large [see Me(46) in X-206 at δ 0.4 in C_6D_6], so that accidental overlap may easily be avoided by taking the appropriate solvent.

Starting by observing each low-field pattern individually and following its collapse to a simpler pattern while sweeping the saturation field H_2 over the remaining spectral region and approaching as close as possible the pattern under observation (usually a 30-Hz distance from the observation field on the HR-300) allow one to find the spectral connections. It may be necessary to vary the irradiating field strength in order to obtain clear-cut decoupling. In performing NMDR experiments, one should be aware of the Bloch-Siegert effect (Anderson and Freeman, 1962) that tends to bring the resonances of perturbed (X) and observed (A) protons in the direction X to A. This effect is proportional to the square of the applied field strength and inversely proportional to the original separation of X from A (this effect may result in shifts of 30-50 Hz for nearby separations of 250 Hz and strengths (γ,H$_2$) of 100 Hz.

Other instrumental difficulties on the HR-300 apparatus (in CW) were quite often very disturbing. Secondary (electronic) effects caused the appearance of wiggle-beats at regular 50-Hz intervals from the H$_2$ position. Some regions, moreover, were unaccessible because the receiver coil was not able to pick up enough energy without a concomitant bad signal/noise ratio. This drawback mainly arose when the strong RF field came close to the (huge) TMS peak (or, alternatively, huge solvent peaks, e.g., α-bromonaphtalene) and could be circumvented by locking on an added second reference substance (e.g., CH_2Cl_2) or using a heteronuclear lock. Finally, erroneous responses were noticed when the irradiating field was positioned at a distance from a *strong* absorption (Me, *Me*O) corresponding to the spinning side band of that strong peak. (Changing the spinning speed allowed the recognition of that phenomenon. Alternatively, the same responses are noticed when H_2 is positioned equally far above and below the principal bond). We never observed spoiling effects due to electrical current leakage, which often occurs in crossed-coiled instruments and for solutions of high conductivity.

Once coupling connections are found by consecutive double irradiations, the inverse procedure may be done. As most partners of the low-field protons are situated in the complex aliphatic region (δ 0.5-2.0), only close comparisons in that region between irradiated and non-irradiated spectra allow the confirmation of the previously detected connection. At the time of our measurements double resonance difference spectroscopy could only be achieved indirectly through registrations, mediated by time-averaging computer (e.g., TAC model C-1024 from VARIAN). Evaluation of changes in spin patterns can presently easily be done by subtracting procedures.

If the interconnected patterns are of excellent resolution—mostly belonging to AB, ABX, and at the most ABMN subspectral parts (they may additionally be connected to Me)—homonuclear INDOR spectra (Baker, 1962) may be run with the advantage of applying low field strengths, thus inproving the selectivity of perturbations to about 1 Hz. The higher-order character of the latter two spin systems allows the determination of the relative signs of related interproton couplings, enabling the discrimination between, e.g., geminal ($-$) and vicinal ($+$) interactions. Also, INDOR (Kowalewski, 1969) allows a very close approach between irradiating and observing positions (as close as 10 Hz). In pulsed excitation NMR two (pseudo) INDOR techniques are feasible: double resonance difference spectroscopy (Feeney and Partington, 1973) and selective populations inversion (Chalmers et al., 1974; Sorenson et al., 1974).

The interconnections between methine protons (for Me) and/or methylene protons (for Et) with the high-field doublets and triplets are also easy to realize. They are very informative with respect to the recognition of structural fragments of the type AMX_3 (e.g., $-O-CH-CH-CH_3$ or $-CO-CH-CH-CH_3$ etc.). This is indeed a frequently encountered structural unit in ionophores as a result of their biosynthetic pathway (Chapters 1 and 3, Volume 1). The recognition of low-field patterns consisting in a repetition of subspectral quartets is straightforward, as is the case for $-O-CH(Me)$ fragments. It is of primary importance to determine the apparent coupling constants involving the Me groups in widely differing solvent systems (see the nature of Me groups in Section III.D). In judging qualitatively the spectral proximity of mutually interacting patterns, an inspection of the "roof effect" is very helpful. A simple example of this effect is represented by the appearance of an AB quartet, giving rise to a ratio of intensities between the intense and small peaks which is equal to the ratio of the distances between the inner and outer peaks (Figure 25). Similar considerations are applicable for a qualitative judgment of the spectral locations of protons which are strongly coupled.

Except for "accidentally" zero interproton couplings, the outlined NMDR procedures allow one to follow the constitutional connections of protons along parts of the backbone (e.g., Anteunis and Verhegge, 1977). Often the spectral (and corresponding constitutional) track is lost in a complex aliphatic region. The information lost is, however, of minor importance, except in relation to the correct assignment of certain methyl (ethyl) positions and if one is dealing with ASIS measurements (Section III.F).

In a few cases a trail is lost because the interproton coupling is too small, e.g., when the torsion angle in an ethano-fragment is near $90°$. This happens four times in X-206! [$^3J(7, 8B) = {}^3J(9, 10) \leq 1.0$ Hz; $3J(8B, 9) = {}^3J(22, 23) \sim 0$ Hz: Anteunis, 1977b.] An optimal resolution is essential in order to detect small residual couplings. Careful comparison of spectra obtained in different solvents and especially between the free acid and/or salt are helpful, although it is true that differences are minor but sometimes sufficient to solve the problem.

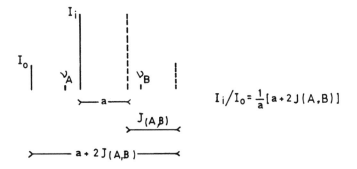

$$I_i/I_0 = \frac{1}{a}[a + 2J(A,B)]$$

Figure 25 Relative intensities of a pattern of an AB spin system showing the roof effect.

Also, comparisons between very similar structures are essential (see H-22 in respectively alborixin and X-206; Rodios and Anteunis, 1979b). Another typical case that offered a pitfall, because an extensive trail was lost, is exemplified by the originally wrong (interchanged) assignments of H-14 and H-20 in X-206 (Anteunis, 1977b). In alborixin the path of the C(6) to C(14) could be tracked (at 360 MHz), albeit not without difficulties (accidental nearby zero couplings), thus allowing one to locate H-14 (and the corresponding connected Me) with certainty (Rodios and Anteunis, 1979b).

Consecutive NMDR and/or homonuclear INDOR are interrupted for a path that is isolated by a quaternary C unit. The sole solution left for gaining more information in these cases may be Overhauser enhancement experiments. Here NOE difference spectroscopy is a reliable prerequisite. It should be kept in mind that NOE experiments are best performed on degassed samples (removal of residual paramagnetic oxygen) in solvents having nuclei with low magnetic moments and that the "nonirradiated" spectrum taken for comparison should, in fact, not be obtained by cutting off the decoupler but, rather, by *displacing* the position of H_2 outside any absorption region, e.g., somewhere near δ 8. We have encountered only one occasion of such an effect. (The impossibility to detect NOE was mostly due to instrumental (electronic) side effects making some subtle observations in intensity changes unreliable.) With more modern instrumentation such experiments, uncovering structural proximity in some indeed overcrowded molecular regions, become of greater importance.

In Na^+-lysocellin the doublet at δ 0.96 in C_6D_6:CD_3OD, attributable to either Me(33) or M3(34), showed increased intensity (no collapse) while irradiating H-8 (Anteunis, 1977d). This must be the result of a proximity effect, making an assignment to Me(34) less probable. Also, the reverse procedure (irradiating Me and observing the methine or methylene NOE partner) should be better (Laszlo and Stang, 1971), because in the original upset the relaxation of the Me has a greater chance to proceed more efficiently via other neighbors by dynamic nuclear coupling.

In the above-mentioned case presumably the relaxation of Me(33) was mediated via Me(32), the coupling partner of H-8, while Me(32) and Me(33) are indeed close to each other.

Some nicely structured doublets {occasionally triplets, e.g., Na^+-lenoremycin: $^3J[O(11)H, 30A] = 5.9$ and $^3J[O(11)H, 30B] = 7.7$ Hz in $CDCl_3$; Anteunis et al., 1977} belong to hydroxyl protons and they could easily be confused by their spectral appearance with signals from carbon-bearing backbone protons. They may often be distinguished by their higher sensitivity to changes in either temperature, solvent (ASIS!), or chemical exchange capability (catalysis through Et_3N is most effective). These criteria may fail, however, for solvent-screened hydroxylic groups, but for these, noticeable shift differences are often encountered in comparing the free acid form with the corresponding salts (complexation shift) or even among the salts derived from different cation species {e.g., $\delta[O(4)H]$ = 7.57 (Na$^+$) and 9.2 (K$^+$) in Ionomycin; Rodios and Anteunis, 1979a}.

The reader is referred to Section III.E for a further discussion of the spectral behavior of O*H* groups.

C. ^{1}H Chemical Shifts and Their Predictability

1. *Conformational impacts*

Typical shift values for specific kinds of protons are greatly compromised by their reliance on many secondary effects, resulting in appreciable overlap of the representative spectral regions, where a certain type of proton may absorb. This is to a first approximation a greater disadvantage, compared to ^{13}C spectroscopy (Chapter 6). However, a scrupulous analysis of the data makes the picture less discouraging and deviations from a mean value may result in valuable conclusions with respect to diagnostic structural environments. Dramatic shift alterations may originate from conformational pecularities often encountered in biomolecules of some complexity, such as in peptides and proteins, and they are well recognized. This is, for example, the case for unusual high- or low-field spectral locations of protons exposed to local magnetic ring currents caused by aromatic rings (e.g., respectively coaxial to, or coplanar with, the ring). Shifts as large as 2 ppm may occur (e.g., Wüthrich, 1976). Thus chemical shifts of (methyl) protons around 0.5-0.6 ppm or lower in nonaromatic solvents (!) definitively disclose a (methyl) group situated above an aromatic system. Typical examples are found for Me(28) in Na$^+$-lasalocid located at high field (δ 0.54) in CDCl$_3$ (internal aromatic induced shift through dimer formation) but at δ 0.87 in CD$_3$OD, because in the latter solvent the ionophore exists as a *monomeric* species (Schmidt et al., 1974; Patel and Shen, 1976; Shen and Patel, 1976). Proton H-18 is 1.0 ppm more shielded in the (dimeric) Mg^{2+}_(A23187)$_2$ packed structure than it is in the freely rotating monomeric free acid species. For the same reasons screening effects by diamagnetic ring currents are observed in the same ionophore for H-17 (Δ = +0.53 ppm), H-16 (Δ = +0.55 ppm), H-15 ($\Delta \sim 0.25$ ppm), and H-10 ($\Delta \sim 0.3$ ppm) (Anteunis, 1977c).

2. *Shift predictions*

We have statistically treated the observed shifts for the α-carbinol (OC*H*−) and β-carbinol protons (OCC*H*−) in the six- and five-membered rings of 17 ionophores by computer fitting (Borremans and Anteunis, 1981). The following multiparameter equation was used:

$\delta^i = \delta_0 + \Sigma_j \delta_j \cdot n_{ij}$, where δ^i is the chemical shift of the ith proton, δ_0 is the basic value independent of i and j, and the δ_j are the increment parameters that may influence the basic shift and multiplied by the number of appearances.

1. $\Delta\delta(g)$: the presence of a gauche substituent that is known to result in a shielding, irrespective of the nature, e.g., oxygen or carbon. Thus an axial proton suffers constitutionally from at least two gauche interactions.
2. $\Delta\delta(a)$: the presence of an antisubstituent, again without consideration of its kind. Thus an equatorial proton possesses automatically two antisubstituents.
3. $\Delta\delta(sd)$: the presence of a syndiaxial substituent. Quasi-syndiaxial situations (five-membered rings) were *fully* counted, and if acyclic fragments were inspected, the several allowed rotameric states (avoiding those with syndiaxial strain) were equally weighted for contribution.
4. $\Delta\delta(\beta)$: the presence of a β-oxygen; thus this increment value is automatically present in $(-CHC\diagdown-O)$ fragments.
5. $\Delta\delta(\beta^4)$: a correction term for the presence of a geminal β-*dioxy* grouping (acetalic or hemiacetalic). This increment concerns $(-CH-C\diagdown-O)$ fragments only.
6. $\Delta\delta(OMe)$: this correction was needed to bring the experimental values for $(\diagup CH-OMe)$ fragments into the correct range of prediction with similar confidence as the remaining $(\diagup CH-O-)$ moieties.

Table 1 shows the best values obtained by computer fitting (Borremans and Anteunis, 1981). We mention here some relevant observations:

1. Most predictions can be made to the nearest 0.25 ppm or better.
2. Except for some typical cases (see Section III.C.3), there are no differences in shift behavior between salts and free acids. This is illustrated in the separate data handling of CHO protons in six-membered rings (CHO6H and CHO6Na).
3. Increments concerning the five-membered rings are smaller than those for six-membered rings as a result of the overestimation of the effects, for example, in idealizing the furans in biased conformations with a pucker equalizing that in typical chairs. This is, however, not the case for $\Delta\delta(g)$.
4. In 45 of a total of 308 points (15%) the deviations between the calculated and experimental values exceed the RMS value but fall within twice that value, while for 11 cases (3.6%) the error is indeed larger (see also Section III.C.3).

5. We are unable to give a physicochemical meaning for $\Delta\delta$(OMe), all the more because the sign is opposite when operating for six- and five-membered rings.

6. The main effects on the β protons belonging to $-CH(Me)C\diagdown-O$ fragments in the six-membered rings are $\Delta\delta$(g) and $\Delta\delta(\beta^2)$ followed by $\Delta\delta$(sd). In the five-membered rings the factors contributing the most are $\Delta\delta$(sd) and $\Delta\delta(\beta)$. The fact that all potential contributions were estimated for furanoses with exaggerated pucker (60°) is certainly at the origin of the observed differences. Predictability is nevertheless unexpectedly good. It must be remembered that in the selection of the preferred conformations those obtained in the solid state were taken for granted, but the total range of shifts for prediction (from 1.9 to 2.6 ppm) is rather narrow.

3. Complexation shifts and shift anomalies

Usually no large deviations for shifts between protons in the free acids and complexes are noticed (complexation shifts). Some differences, as noticed in lasalocid, lysocellin, and A23187 result from the fact that these ionophores dimerize in apolar solvents. By doing so, some protons come in the screening zone of aromatic fragments [e.g., H-10a, but expecially H-18 in $Mg^+(A23187)_2$]. In general, it remains difficult to pinpoint the exact origin of most discrepancies, that is, to define real complexation shifts as the result of the proximity to the metal ion with their linkage to oxygen ligands.

The ether proton at the first corner of the penultimate (five-membered) ring usually resonates at a field lower than predicted, but the effect is particularly visible in the salts (mean deviation in free acids, +0.25 ppm; in salts, +0.45 ppm), suggesting a complexation shift effect of +0.20 ppm (downfield).

The ether protons of the last ring often resonate at a field higher than predicted (-0.27 ppm as a mean). This is especially so when this proton is solvent accessible (H-19a in Na^+-lasalocid; H-25a in Na^+-salinomycin, Na^+-narasin, and H^+-episalinomycin; H-31a in X-206 and H^+-alborixin). For those protons that are less solvent accessible the opposite tendency (mean "extra" deshielding of 0.20 ppm) is noticed (H-21a in H^+-monensin; H-25a in H^+-nigericin, lonomycin, Na^+-A204A, Na^+-etheromycin, Na^+-lenoremycin, and dianemycin). Perhaps this observation may be indicative of a "cavity effect." We are unable at the present time to explain still other anomalies (Borremans and Anteunis, 1981) such as the unexpected screening of H-35e in H^+-X-206 and alborixin opposed to a pronounced deshielding in Na^+-X-206, while this observation is not paralleled in ionophores bearing the same structural fragments (H-29e in salinomycin, narasin, etc.). These and other examples show that shift predictions are still to be made with caution.

Table 1 Basic Values δ_0 and Increments $\delta_j{}^a$ in ppm for the Prediction of Shift Values in $CDCl_3$ of Ring Protons in the α and β Positions of Oxygen in Carboxylic Acid Ionophores

Identification[b]	Number of points	δ_0	$\Delta\delta(g)$	$\Delta\delta(a)$
CHO6H	65	3.61_6	-0.07_3	0.19_5
		(± 0.017)	(± 0.001)	(± 0.002)
CHO6Na	76	3.66_8	-0.11_0	0.20_2
		(± 0.011)	(± 0.001)	(± 0.001)
CHO5NaH	55	5.31_6	-0.48_0	0.06_5
		(± 0.015)	(± 0.001)	(± 0.002)
CHCO6NaH	89	1.79_4	-0.20_7	0.05_2
		(± 0.059)	(± 0.013)	(± 0.013)
CHCO5NaH	22	1.96_4	0.06_0	0.05_5
		(± 0.053)	(± 0.007)	(± 0.003)
O$-$CH$-$O	6	4.72	-0.15	0.10
		(± 0.12)		

[a] δ_0, $\Delta\delta(g)$, $\Delta\delta(a)$, . . . represent δ_j of the equation discussed in Section III.C.2.
[b] Coding is as follows: CHOxH, carbinyl proton in x-membered ring (free acids or salts, or both).

D. Coupling Constants and Conformation

1. Vicinal interproton coupling constants

In the interpretation of coupling constants a major problem arises from the fact that one could extract only apparent values from first-order interpretations of the ^{1}H NMR patterns. This value can differ greatly from the true value if the nuclei that interact are further *strongly* coupled to other partners, e.g., if the spectral appearance possesses higher-order character. Thus the value $^3J(A, B)$ between two nuclei A and B will become admixed if either A or B is further strongly coupled with other spins, e.g., A with C, whereby the counterpart (B) does not interact directly. This admixture will in that case result in

$\Delta\delta(\beta)$	$\Delta\delta(sd)$	$\Delta\delta(\beta^2)$	$\Delta\delta(OMe)$	RMS error	Experimental region[a] (ppm)
0.0	0.21_1	—	-0.54_9	0.17_2	2.8-4.3
—	$(\pm0.000_8)$	—	(±0.004)		
0.0	0.24_6	—	-0.49_8	0.15_3	2.8-4.3
—	$(\pm0.000_5)$	—	(±0.002)		
0.00_7	0.18_1	—	$+65_0$	0.13_4	3.4-4.5
(±0.004)	$(\pm0.000_6)$	—	$(\pm0.004_5)$		
0.04_8	0.18_5	0.24_7	—	0.18_8	1.2-2.3
(±0.012)	$(\pm0.001_2)$	$(\pm0.004_7)$	—		
-0.14_2	0.21_4	0.01_0	—	0.13_1	1.9-2.6
(±0.004)	(±0.005)	(±0.007)	—		
0.22	—	—	—	—	4.4-4.6

a lowering of the apparent value. Alternatively, in an AXY spin system where X and Y become isochronous, the apparent values $J(A, X)$ and $J(A, Y)$ will tend to become equal.

In many cases higher-order character was always present and could not be avoided. This is illustrated by the fact that extracted coupling constants could vary a lot with field strength or by changing the solvent system (resulting eventually in changed spectral positions). This is strongly the case for aliphatic fragments, e.g., $-C\gamma H- C^\beta H- C^\alpha H_3$, if shifts of β and γ protons are similar. Because $^4J(\gamma, CH_3)$ is almost zero, the apparent coupling $^3J(H^\beta, H^\alpha)$ will be lower when

$\delta(H^\gamma) \simeq \delta(H^\beta)$ and will even be halved when $\delta(H^\gamma) = \delta(H^\beta)$. Concomitantly, a broadening of the Me signal (higher-order appearance) by unresolved additional splittings may occur. Thus in Na^+-septamycin the value $^3J[26a, Me(32_{eq})] = 5.6$ Hz is certainly falsified in $CDCl_3$, as in benzene it increases to 6.3 Hz (at 300 MHz). We have therefore used the best apparent coupling values in our statistical treatments, either by taking the most realistic value extracted from the spectrum in the best solvent (usually the largest that was measured among different solvent systems), or we (M. J. O. Anteunis, unpublished) have taken values recently obtained from spectra obtained at higher field strengths (360 MHz) than originally published. No large discrepancies, however, were found when these values were compared with the "best choice" obtained from 300-MHz spectra.

Finally, a major problem was also met for multiplets originating from several weak interactions. Even with resolution-enhancement procedures, overlap results in an apparent equalizing of the different coupling constants involved. This "mixing" by overlap may result to apparent equal values that can in fact differ by more than 1 Hz, even under the best conditions of registration.

2. Endocyclic coupling constants

It is a well-known fact that vicinal coupling constants are related periodically with the torsional angle formed between two nuclei separated by three bonds (Karplus-Conroy dependency). The practical problem is related to the best choice of the parameters used in such periodic expressions. I will not insist on the countless propositions that can be found in the literature. A major point, however, is that coupling-constant values are greatly influenced by the presence of electronegative substituents and especially by their relative orientation with respect to the vicinal proton. The case of oxygen deserves special attention in relation to the ionophores in which $O-CH_A-CH_B$ fragments are so common.

Antiperiplanarity of oxygen to H_B lowers the coupling by almost 2.0 Hz (Anteunis, 1966; Anteunis et al., 1966) and empirical sets of values for several other dispositions developed for carbohydrates at these laboratories (De Bruyn and Anteunis, 1976) have been verified by an extensive statistical treatment of the literature data, leading to a generalized Karplus equation (Haasnoot, et al., 1980; Altona and Haasnoot, 1980; Haasnoot et al., 1981; for $^3J(^{13}C, H)$ see Spoormaker and de Bie, 1978, 1979).

According to a recent statistical treatment by Altona and Haasnoot (1980), of 327 conformationally pure and undeformed pyranoses and related compounds, a prediction within 0.3 Hz would be possible for vicinal interproton coupling constants in sugarlike structures.

In analogy to this, Borremans and I (F. Borremans and M. J. O. Anteunis, unpublished) followed a statistical least-squares treatment of the coupling constants J^i to be predicted as described by the linear equation $J^i = J_0 + \sum_j J_j \cdot n_{ij}$, where the J_j are additive coupling parameters corresponding to the jth structural element and n_{ij} is the number of times the structural element j occurs for a particular J^i. The following contributions were taken into account:

1. When CH_2CH fragments were considered together with $CH-CH$ fragments, an increment value $\Delta J(f) = 1$ was used for the former. If these fragments were treated separately, the $\Delta J(f)$ term was omitted.

2. $\Delta J^\alpha(g)$ and $\Delta J^\alpha(a)$ were introduced for each oxygen atom that stays respectively gauche and anti to one of the coupling protons and that is implanted onto the ethano fragment under consideration (α effects). $\Delta J^\alpha(a)$ can only operate for gauche couplings.

3. $\Delta J^\beta(g)$ and $\Delta J^\beta(a)$ express corrections to be made for the presence of an oxygen, adjacent to, and respectively in gauche and anti relation with one of the coupled partners (β effects).

4. $\Delta J(sd)$ was used for the presence of a syndiaxial substituent, either oxygen or alkyl. This increment has perhaps the least physicochemical meaning. It expresses, rather, contributions arising from ring-deformation effects, e.g. (local) flattening when syndiaxial strain is present. The introduction of this parameter was essential to bring typical structural elements in comparable ranges. It has use, therefore, only for predictability purposes in ionophores, where multisubstitution and resulting ring deformations are frequently present and for substitution patterns that are often common to many of them.

It is questionable whether the determined increments have any physicochemical meaning. The only purpose of the present treatment was to assist empirically in the identification of certain structural features that may be present along typical coupling paths. Table 2 lists the computed results. The following coding system was adopted: (1) the $J(a, a)x(CH_2CH)$ and $J(a, a)x(CHCH)$ are antiperiplanar coupling constants for CH_2CH fragments and CHCH fragments, respectively, in a x-membered ring; (2) the $J(g)x$ are the gauche couplings (either axial-equatorial or equatorial-equatorial) in six-membered rings (x = 6), five-membered rings (x = 5), or acyclic fragments (x = Ac).

The following comments should be considered:

1. Predictions made with the well-established parameters of Altona and Haasnoot (1980) developed for undeformed pyranoses were systematically too high. Applied to 53 cases of $^3J(a, a)$ values and 14 cases of $^3J(e, e)$, the overestimation amounted to 0.6 Hz,

Table 2 Basic Values J_O and Increments J_j[a] (Hz) for the Prediction of Coupling-Constant Values in Pyranoid, Furanoid, and Acyclic Fragments of Carboxylic Acid Ionophores

Type[b]	Number of points	J_O	$\Delta J(f)$	$\Delta J^{\alpha}(g)$
$J(a,a)6(CH_2CH)$	26	12.5_4 (±0.071)	c	-1.6_1 (±0.025)
$J(a,a)6(CHCH)$	36	11.0_6 (±0.025)	c	-1.0_2 (±0.011)
$J(a,a)Ac$	31	10.5_3 (±0.033)	$+0.77$ (±0.10)	d
$J(a,a)5$	19	10.2_2 (±0.35)	$+0.6_4$ (±0.26)	d
$J(a,a)$[e]		12.4	$+0.5$	-1.4
$J(g)6$	48	4.3_9 (±0.042)	f	-0.60_4 (±0.020)
$J(g)Ac$	32	1.4_4 (±0.15)	$+0.3_2$ (±0.73)	$+0.8_3$ ($\pm0.05_2$)
$J(g)$[e]		4.4	f	$+0.5$

[a] $\Delta J(f)$, $\Delta J^{\alpha}(g)$, etc. represent the J_j of the equation discussed in Section III.D.1.
[b] For coding see text.
[c] The increment, distinguishing $-CH_2CH-$ from $-CHCH-$ fragments, has not been used because the data points belonging to these fragments have been treated separately.
[d] Introduction of $\Delta J^{\alpha}(g)$ was irrelevant and therefore omitted, because in each case one gauche substitution was always present.
[e] Data for sugar analogues, reported by Altona and Haasnoot (1980).
[f] This increment was not considered in gauche couplings except for acyclic fragments.

$\Delta J^{\alpha}(a)$	$\Delta J^{\beta}(g)$	$\Delta J^{\beta}(a)$	$\Delta J(sd)$	RMS error	Experimental range (Hz)
—	-0.16_3 (± 0.032)	$+0.5_0$ (± 0.011)	$+0.2_0$ (± 0.004)	0.23	9.2-12.0
—	0.4_6 (± 0.046)	$+0.1_3$ (± 0.010)	-0.0_3 (± 0.007)	0.24	8.7-11.5
—	$+0.2_5$ (± 0.10)	-0.5_2 (± 0.061)	$+0.07_3$ (± 0.032)	0.63	9.9-12.5
—	-0.13_3 (± 0.18)	-1.0_3 ($\pm 0.26_4$)	$+0.5_2$ (± 0.25)	0.96	8.8-11.3
—	—	$+0.5$	—	0.3	—
-1.7_0 (± 0.025)	$+0.37$ (± 0.008)	-0.66 (± 0.008)	-0.46 (± 0.003)	0.27	1.5-4.5
-0.0_3 (± 0.10)	-0.3_8 (± 0.03)	-0.3_6 ($\pm 0.07_5$)	$+0.3_1$ ($\pm 0.05_4$)	0.47	0-3
-1.8	—	—	—	0.3	—

and in 44 cases of $^3J(a, e)$ it amounted to 0.2 Hz. Thus, although the discrepancy is certainly due to deformation effects in the present cases, other unrevealed factors must be present. Pure deformation effects should result in overestimation for certain types [e.g., $J(a, a)$ for flattening] but underestimation for others within the same fragment [e.g. $^3J(e, e)$]. The reader is referred to point (3) for typical examples. After fitting the present cases with specifically adapted increments (Table 2) the trend of overestimation is found in comparing the resulting basic values J_0 with those for undeformed pyranoses [e.g., $J_0(a, a)6(CHCH) = 11.0_6$ Hz against 12.4 Hz].

2. Predictions are only reasonably good for pyranoses. They may fail completely for floppy fragments, for example, five-membered and acyclic fragments, and should therefore not be used here.

3. The RMS value is somewhat larger for $J(g)$ than for $J(a, a)$ values, despite the fact that an additional parameter has been used [e.g. $\Delta J^\alpha(a)$]. This is expected, as these couplings are not in the extremum of the periodical Karplus-Conroy curve and will thus be most sensitive toward ring deformation. When coupling constants obtained from protons belonging to ring B, bearing the typical substitution pattern shown in Figure 26, were used, much worse predictions than those tabulated were made. The reason is twofold. Proton H-11 is usually very badly resolved in most spectra, its pattern invariably consisting in a multiplet with small band width. Furthermore, the substitution of that ring (Figure 26) will certainly cause puckering at C(10) and flattening at C(12). This would partially explain the low values for $^3J(9a, 10e)$ and $^3J(10e, 11e)$ but large values for $^3J(10e, 11e)$ and especially for $^3J(11e, 12a)$ [nigericin, carriomycin, septamycin, A204A, etheromycin; see equivalent

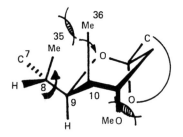

Figure 26   Substitution pattern of ring B common to many ionophores.

$^3J(18e, 19a)$ and $^3J(18e, 19e)$ in dianemycin]. Additional strain between Me(35) and Me(36) incluidng the acyclic rotor $C(8)-C(9)$ complicates the picture [$^3J(8, 9a) \leqslant 0.8$ Hz].

4. Some of the computed increments are of the expected sign and importance: (a) $\Delta J(f)$ amounts to +1.5 for $J(a, a)6$ and is about +0.7 for $J(a, a)5$ and $J(a, a)Ac$. The threefold increase in comparison to Altona and Haasnoot's value is especially due to the too low basic value of 11.0_6 Hz for $J(a, a)6(CHCH)$. This concerns fragments that are the most substituted, hence suffering from deformation; (b) $\Delta J^\alpha(g)$ are well reproduced in comparable sets. This contribution is very important and negative for $J(a, a)$ predictions and moderately important (and positive) for $J(g)$; (c) $\Delta J^\beta(g)$ and $\Delta J^\beta(a)$ are now always of the same sign. The normal and expected values (about -0.2 and +0.5 Hz, respectively) are again observed for the least-substituted fragment $-CH_2CH-$.

3. *Interproton vicinal couplings involving methyl groupings (exocoupling)*

The sizes of proton vicinal coupling constants involving methyl protons on a ring (exocoupling) are typically larger for axial than for equatorial methyl groups, and this can be used within certain limits for solving constitutional problems (Anteunis, 1971). An increase of methyl coupling constants is, however, a general phenomenon if steric congestion occurs (Samek, 1971). Therefore not only axial Me groups but also highly sterically hindered equatorial Me groups show larger exocyclic couplings. Usually the distinction in kind is also more critical, as expected, in five-membered rings (quasiaxial and quasiequatorial).

Finally, one should realize that there is an artificial decrease of the apparent value $^3J(\alpha, \beta)$, when in a propano-fragment $-C^\gamma H-C^\beta H-C^\alpha H_3$ shifts of the β and γ protons become similar (isochronism) because $^4J(\gamma, CH_3)$ is very small and contributes to $^3\overline{J}(\beta, CH_3)$. The apparent coupling constant $^3\overline{J}(\alpha, \beta)$ would equal $\frac{1}{2}|^3J(\beta, CH_3) + ^4J(\gamma, CH_3)| \simeq \frac{1}{2}{}^3J(\beta, CH_3)$ if β and γ became fully isochronous. Concomitantly, broadening of the Me signals may occur as a result of additional unresolved splitting. This is especially experienced for aliphatic fragments $-C^\gamma H_2-C^\beta H(C)-C^\alpha H_3$ involving axial methyl groups, because the antivicinal (axial) proton is shifted downfield, that is, in the direction of H^β (and its geminal partner). In the interpretation of $^3\overline{J}(H, Me)$ couplings one should pay much attention to (1) possible steric congestion (for Me equatorial) and (2) the second-order character of the spin system [$\delta(\beta) \simeq \delta(\gamma)$]. The former effect gives additional information about the constitutional neighborhood of the methyl group. The latter phenomenon may be detected by running spectra in different solvents (CS_2, $CDCl_3$ and aromatic) or by comparing the coupling constants in different forms (free acid and salt). Comparison of values extracted from spectra obtained at different fields is, of course, the most unambiguous method. If differences are noticed, it is an indication of second-order character. Also, unusual broadening effects are suspicious.

I will first illustrate the above artifacts by some examples.

1. In A23187 we have $^3\bar{J}[17e, Me(26_{ax})] = 6.1$ Hz for the free form taken in $CDCl_3$; this low value results from $\delta(16a) \simeq \delta(15a) \simeq \delta(17e) \simeq 1.6_5$. This isochronism is avoided in C_6D_6 ($^3\bar{J}[17, Me(26)] = 6.8_5$ Hz), but only partly so in the salt [$^3\bar{J} = 6.5 - 6.7$ Hz], with broadening of the Me(26) signal.

2. In Na^+-septamycin the value of $^3\bar{J}(26a, Me_{eq}^{32}) = 5.6$ Hz is anomalous (Rodios and Anteunis, 1978a). Although the spectral locations of adjacent methylene protons H-27 could not be determined, their aliphatic nature makes it probable that at least one of these absorbs near H-26a. This is a typical situation met in such fragments (dianemycin, carriomycin, etc.), but these protons are fortunately sensitive to ASIS effects. Hence $^3\bar{J}(26a, Me_{eq}^{32})$ amounts to 6.3 Hz when the spectrum is taken in C_6D_6.

3. Also, in septamycin $^3\bar{J}[12, Me(35_{eq})] \simeq 7.2$ Hz is much too high for an *equatorial* Me group. Here this group suffers from appreciable steric strain, being orientated over the adjacent spiro-furanose, among other things. Such high solvent-independent (sic) values are encountered for all ionophores, either in free or salt form and bearing the same constitutional fragment (carriomycin, A204A, lenoremycin, etc.).

Borremans and I have averaged the observed $^3\bar{J}(H, Me)$ values for 20 axial and 50 equatorial Me groups implanted in a pyranoid fragment and for 40 acyclic and for 14 methyl groups inplanted on furanoid fragments, and have found the following typical values: $^3\bar{J}(H, Me_{ax}) = 7.0 \pm 0.1_5$ Hz (number of cases = 20) and $^3\bar{J}(H, Me_{eq}) = 6.5_5 \pm 0.2_5$ Hz (number of cases = 50). In our selection of $^3J(H, Me)$ of a specific Me group we have used only the *largest* coupling value among those obtained under different circumstances (free acid, salt, different solvents, 300- or 360-MHz spectra, etc.).

It is difficult to set out the furanoid methyls in axial/equatorial groupings, because five-membered rings are certainly mobile systems in solution. Two groups are nevertheless clearly distinguishable: those possessing $^3\bar{J}(H, Me_{eq}) = 6.4 \pm 0.2_5$) Hz (quasiequatorial) and those having $^3\bar{J}(H, Me_{ax'}) = 7.0 \pm 0.2_5$) Hz (*quasiaxial* or *quasiequatorial* with steric congestion). As an overall mean we found in the ionophores $^3J(H, Me) = 6.6_5 \pm 0.3_5$ Hz for furanoid methyls.

Table 3 Mean Apparent Vicinal Exocouplings $^3\bar{J}$ (Hz) for (Quasi)-Axial and (Quasi)Equatorial Alkyl Groupings

Nature	$^3\bar{J}$	σ Error	Number of data points
$>$CH$-$Me$_{ax}$			
Pyranoids	7.0	0.1_5	20
Furanoids	7.0	0.2_5	7
$>$CH$-$Me$_{eq}$			
Pyranoids	6.6_5	0.2_5	50
Furanoids	6.4	0.2_5	7
$>$CH$-$Me acyclic	7.0	0.3	40
$-$CH$_2$$-$Me	7.4	0.2	21

For freely rotating ethyl groupings, generally $^3\bar{J}(CH_2, CH_3) \simeq 7.4_0 \pm 0.2$ Hz (n = 21), but here again values tend to be higher for constraint groupings [e.g., 7.6 Hz for $^3\bar{J}(30, 31)$ in monensin and for $^3\bar{J}(25, 26)$ in lasalocid, or 7.5 Hz for $^3\bar{J}(22, 23)$ in lysocellin, etc.].

Methyl groups substituted on acyclic fragments couple with their methine proton to an extent of 7.00 ± 0.3 Hz (n = 40). In four cases the deviation was somewhat larger:

1. $^3\bar{J}[8,Me(32)]$ (Na$^+$-lysocellin) = 6.2 to 6.4 Hz. It is remarkable that a nuclear Overhauser effect was detected on Me(33) while irradiating H-8 (Anteunis, 1977a; Section III.B), raising the question if relaxation of Me(32) has affected the spatially close Me(33).
2. $^3\bar{J}[2,Me(39)]$ = 7.4 Hz in nigericin free acid (C$_6$D$_6$).
3. $^3\bar{J}[2,Me(40)]$ = 6.4 Hz in Na$^+$-lenoremycin.
4. $^3\bar{J}[2,Me(40)]$ = 6.2 Hz in Na$^+$-dianemycin.

For these cases there is no reason that higher order is at the origin of the statement. One notices that the latter three are α to a carboxyl(ate) group. Table 3 reports the typical values for exocoupling constants involving methyl groups for the different structural environments as discussed in this chapter.

3. Geminal proton coupling constants

Geminal coupling constants ^2J may be influenced by several factors, but two among these attract attention: (1) when a methylene grouping is adjacent to a π system (aromatic, ethylenic, carbonyl, carboxylate), the magnitude of ^2J is influenced by the relative positioning of the protons with respect to the nodal plane of the π system (Barfield and Grant, 1963; Barfield et al., 1976; Abraham and Bakke, 1978); (2) the absolute value ^2J is lowered when adjacent free orbitals (e.g., a free electron pair of oxygen) stay parallel with the carbon hydrogen bond(s) of the methylene grouping under consideration (Anteunis, 1966; Anteunis et al., 1971a, 1971b; Chivers and Crabb, 1970).

Barfield-Grant effect

For "freely" rotating methylenes next to a π system an average value of $^2J = -14.4$ Hz may be used. If the nodal plane of the π cloud bisects the methylene bond angle, the lowering effect is the largest ($^2J = -18.4$ Hz). The π effect vanishes ($^2J = -12.4$ Hz) when the π nodal plane is perpendicular to the bisector of the methylene proton angle. Thus the rotation around $N=C(8)(O)-CH_2(9)$ in A23187 is not entirely free in the acid [$^2J(9) = -15.2$ Hz] and is different in the Mg^{2+} salt [$^2J(9) = -12.8$ Hz] (Anteunis, 1977c; Pfeiffer and Deber, 1979).

Parallelity effect

When θ defines the angle between the bisector of the two p electron lobes of oxygen and the bisector of the methylene $C-H$ bonds, then a periodical dependence between θ and the additivity contribution $\triangledown J$ on ^2J may be sketched. Extreme values of ^2J for a $-O-CH_2(C)$ unit are -5.8 ($\theta = 0°$) and -11.8 Hz ($\theta = 90°$) (Anteunis et al., 1971b; Davies and Hudec, 1975). These considerations allow insight into the rotational state of the $(C)CH_2-OH$ fragment as present in, e.g., nigericin (free, -11.2 Hz; salt, -12.0 Hz), monensin (free, -14.5 Ha; salt, -12.5 Hz), lenoremycin (salt -11.9 Hz), and dianemycin (free, -11.1 Hz; salt, -12.0 Hz). Geminal couplings also depend on electronegativity contributions and the spatial orientation of β-electronegative substituents (Davies, 1975), and therefore coordination of the OH function with the metal ion and/or H bond formation may have an influence. Therefore $^2J(CH_2O)$ is used only an as indication and in conjunction with other criteria (see Section III.E), and it is not expected that for the time being these geminal coupling constants constitute a very reliable criterion.

4. Long-range coupling constants

Most of the long-range constants that were observed are related to hydroxyl protons. The reader is referred to Section III.E for a further discussion of these. Long-range interactions are the most important if the two protons that couple are connected by a σ framework that follows a planar zigzag path. Only in a few cases have we been able to demonstrate $^4J(e, e)$ in a pyranoid system, as in X-206 with $^4\overline{J}(e, e) = 1.0$ Hz [e.g., $^4J(e, e)$ was originally wrongly reported as $^4J(35e, OH\text{-}14)$: Anteunis, 1977b] and in 17-epi-deoxy-(O-8)-salino-mycin with $^4J(27e, 29e) = 1.5$ Hz (Anteunis and Rodios, 1981).

E. Hydroxy Groups

The spectral behavior of hydroxyl protons is complex and not yet en-tirely understood, but obviously characteristics may be correlated with their chemical and physical natures. As expected from their hy-drophilicity (see Section III.F), ASIS effects for OH protons are usually strongly positive (paramagnetic shift), especially when they are near an ionic center. If the hydroxyl proton is in an otherwise lipophilic zone or pointing inward but not close to an ionic center, the ASIS effect, however, becomes small [e.g., O(9)-H in X-206 free acid]. Several other important criteria may be handled. Paramagnetic shift becomes appreciable when hydroxyl protons are involved in H-bridge bonding mechanisms. In the ionophores the strongest-bridged protons absorb at δ 12 to 14, but in other compounds these absorp-tions may be as low as δ 19 (De Keukeleire et al., 1971).

Mutual chemical exchange is revealed by broadening of the absorp-tion peak, especially if the individual OH resonances are close together in the ^{1}H NMR spectrum. Inversely, peaks that absorb in the spec-trum close to each other and that do not collapse to a single (broad) peak disclose a low rate of chemical exchange. Thus the protons giving rise to a (very broad) absorbance (mutual exchange) at $\delta \frown 6.0$ in monensin free acid [COOH + H_2O + O(11)H] do not chemically exchange rapidly with O(10)—H located at δ 6.3, although the latter is also appreciably broadened by some other independent exchange phenom-enon. An increase in temperature, however, or the addition of a powerful catalyst for proton exchange, such as Et_3N, will cause the collapse of signals which belong to protons that can mutually exchange.

We have used Et_3N as a powerful catalyst since the early 1970s, even when strongly H-bridged protons are involved (e.g., absorbing at δ 19!). One condition, however, is that the OH species under con-sideration are solvent accessible. Thus in nigericin free acid COOH, O(9)H, and O(10)H interchange moderately well [one very broad peak with $W/2 \frown 300$ Hz(!)], yet they do *not* narrow by addition of Et_3N.

More interesting information can be obtained from NMDR experi-ments. If exchange is appreciable between a typical OH and residual H_2O in the solvent [located at $\delta \frown 1.5$ (CDCl$_3$) or $\delta \frown 1.7$ to 1.9 (C_6D_6), even if not visible under CW procedures], one may observe an appreciable decrease in the intensity of the OH signal on irradiation of the residual water peak at δ 1.5 to 1.8. Eventually all couplings that would be present between the OH in question and other protons disappear under these circumstances. In this way the other protons to which this OH couples can also be detected. Irradiation of one OH signal causes a decrease in intensity of all other OH-signals of protons involved in chemical exchange phenomena with the former.

One may obtain an idea of the accessibility to an OH proton by studying the rate of exchange H↔ D (disappearance of the OH signal) after adding CD_3OD or shaking the solution with D_2O. As long as protic solvents do not initiate different conformations (e.g., lasalocid), alternatively, CD_3OD may be added as a cosolvent and the rate of disappearance of the OH signals monitored.

The couplings that exist between O*H* protons and the carbinol protons [$^3J(CH-OH)$ and $^4J(CH-C-OH)$] are diagnostic. Apparent coupling constant $\bar{J}$ are the true ones, as long as hydroxyl protons are involved that do not exchange too fast. If the half times of chemical exchange (T/2) exceeds 1/J, the apparent coupling constant, however, is lowered and may eventually vanish. Therefore, if $\bar{J}$ remains unaffected by changes in temperature or the solvent, it is reasonable to accept that the observed value approaches the real one; otherwise one knows only a lower-limit value.

We will now discuss the nature of OH signals for the individual cases of the ionophores in light of the foregoing criteria. This was not done at the beginning of our investigations, as we were originally mostly interested in only the backbone conformation of the carriers. In addition, the present discussion will for some cases deviate from the original published data where these data have been found to need some revision. Table 4 gathers the data obtained from 300-MHz ^1H spectra. For a stereoscopic inspection of some of the cases the reader is referred to Sections III.C and III.F discussing lipophilicity.

Monensin

Free acid (Anteunis and Rodios, 1978)
The broad signal at δ ~ 6.2 in $CDCl_3$ is a composite of an envelope integrating for four protons (assigned to H_2O + COO*H* + O*H*-11) and a broadened envelope resulting from one proton {assigned to O*H*-10 [$^4J(24,O(10)H) < 1.5$ Hz]}. The proximity of both patterns, although themselves broadened and indicating chemical exchange processes, excludes rapid reciprocal equilibration. They disappear only slowly by treatment of the sample with D_2O. As for the sharper *doublet* at δ 4.46 $^3J(7,OH-5) = 8$ Hz, assigned to O(5)H one can saturate each of the patterns by irradiation of the other. Therefore all of the mobile protons grouped in the three signals observed do exchange mutually, but at a lower rate than H_2O, COO*H*, and O*H*-11 do internally. The apparent long-range coupling observed for O(10)*H* and the vicinal

one for O(5)H disclose, respectively, a planar /\/\ arrangement with
H-24 for the former [e.g., realized when O(10)H is the H donor in
bridging with O(5)H; see Figure 27], while a torsion of <150° may be
estimated for the HC(7)−O(5)H fragment (if the apparent couplings
are true couplings). Accepting the presence of an encapsulated molecule of H_2O mimicking the position of the ion in the salt, the complete
H-bridge mechanism can be depicted as in Figure 27. This is at variance with an earlier proposition of Anteunis and Rodios (1978), but
closer to the proposition of Lutz et al. (1971) obtained from solid-state
data, except that the O(5)H−O(6) bridging is not well explained by
the vicinal coupling constant, which must result from an average of
different positionings of the O−H bond (e.g., with H_2O). This scheme
explains all the observed characteristics of the ^{1}H NMR patterns.
Salt (Anteunis, 1977)
The signal reported to absorb at δ 9.6 contains two protons, assigned
to OH-10 and OH-11. Both protons shift appreciably downfield in
C_6D_6 [Δ(ASIS) + 240); (see Figure 19 for a spectrum obtained at 360
MHz] and are therefore both involved in the head-to-tail hydrogen
bonding. The OH−5 absorption is located at δ 3.55. There is a very
slow exchange for it with D_2O, even slower than was already the case
in the free acid. The OH peaks could not be suppressed by irradiation
of the residual H_2O peak in C_6D_6 (δ 1.6), but they could in $CDCl_3$.
The faster chemical exchange does not alter the J̄ values obtained for
the free acid, and they therefore represent real values: $^3J(7,OH-5)$ =
1.5 Hz *and* $^4J(8a,OH-5)$ = 2.7 Hz disclosing a different rotameric

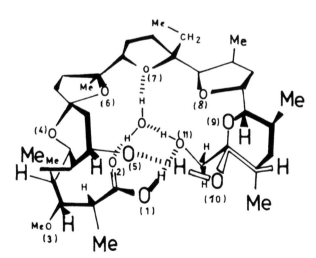

Figure 27 Schematic representation of the monensin pseudocycle with
indication of the newly proposed H-bridge bonding mechanism. (Source:
Anteunis and Rodios, 1978).

Table 4   Characteristics of OH Signals in the 300-MHz ^{1}H NMR Spectra of the Ionophores

Ionophore	Assignment	δ [a]	Appearance[b]	Δ(ASIS)[c]	Internal exchange[d]
Na$^+$-lysocellin	H$_2$O (extra)	3.84	sl.br.		
	OH-4	5.0	sl.br.		With all
	OH-5	4.31	sh.		With all
	OH-9	7.31	sh.		With all
	OH-10	7.62	br.		With all
H$^+$-monensin	COOH + H$_2$O + OH-11	~6.0	v.br.		With all
	OH-5	4.46	sl.br.		With all
	OH-10	6.3	br.		With all
Na$^+$-monensin	OH-5	3.5$_5$	sh.	+35	+
	OH-10 + OH-11	9.6	v.br.	+240	+
H$^+$-nigericin	COOH + OH-10 + OH-11	5.3	e.br.		
Na$^+$-nigericin	OH-10	10.3	e.br.	+123	+
	OH-11	5.5$_4$	br.	+31	+
H$^+$-Ionomycin	COOH	Not found	e.br.		
	OH-4	5.3	sh.	+45	
	OH-14	Not visible	e.br.		
Na$^+$-Ionomycin	OH-4	7.5$_7$	sl.br.		
	OH-14	8.3$_3$	br.	+100	
K$^+$-Ionomycin (in C$_6$D$_6$) at 360 MHz	OH-4	8.6$_3$	br.		
	OH-14	9.0$_6$	e.br.		
H$^+$-X-206	COOH + OH-8 + OH-14 (+ H$_2$O?)	~3.5	e.br.		?
	OH-4	3.4$_2$	sh.	+54	-
	OH-6	6.4$_5$	sh.	+30	-
	OH-9	2.4$_4$	sh.	+8	-
	OH-11	6.0$_2$	sh.	+30	-
Na$^+$-X-206 (in CS$_2$)	OH-4	3.93	sh.	(+47)	
	OH-6	6.80	sh.	(+38)	
	OH-8	4.64	br.	(+77)	+
	OH-9	2.06	sh.	(+54)	
	OH-11	5.98	sh.	(+43)	
	OH-14	11.9	br.	(+43)	+
Na$^+$-lenoremycin	OH-10	8.3$_3$	br.	+95	
	OH-11	9.9$_2$	sl.br.	+56	
H$^+$-dianemycin	COOH + OH-5 OH-11 + OH-12	~5.3	v.br.		

$\{H_2O\}^e$	^3J (Hz)	^4J (Hz)	Metal ion[f] ligand	Remarks
+			−	Assignments of OH-4 and OH-5
+			+	may be inter-
+			+	changed
+	(21, OH) ≈ small		+	
+	(7, OH) ≈ 8.0			Only slow exchange between δ ~ 6.0
		(24, OH) ⩽ 1.5		& δ 6.3
− (In C_6D_6)	(7, OH) = 1.5	(8a, OH) = 2.7	+	Mutual saturation
− (In C_6D_6)			+	by NMDR in $CDCl_3$
−				No enhancement of rate exchange when +Et$_3$N
		(30B, OH) or	−	^2J(30A, 30B) by 1 Hz lower than in the free acid
		(30B, OH) ≈ 2	−	form; see text for $3\bar{J}$ or $4\bar{J}$.
+		(4, OH) = 1.6		OH-14 at δ 6.9 in C_6D_6 at 60°C (e.br.)
			+	
			−	
?				All assignments of OH can be done
+	(9, OH) = 0.0	(10, OH) small		because of diag-
−		(14, OH) = 0.6		nostic coupling
−	(22, OH) = 12.5			phenomena
−		(28, OH) = 1.4		
	(9, OH) = 0.0	(10, OH) = 1.0	+	
		(14, OH) = 0.8	+	
+			+	
	(22, OH) = 11.8		−	
		(28, OH) = 0.9	+	
+			−	
+			−	
	(30A, OH) = 5.8		−	^2J(30A, 30B) = 12
	(30B, OH) = 7.8			
				Position strongly concentration dependent

Table 4 (Continued)

Ionophore	Assignment	δ [a]	Appearance[b]	Δ(ASIS)[c]	Internal exchange[d]
Na^+-dianemycin	OH-5 + OH-11 OH-12 + H_2O	~5.3	v.br.		
Na^+-A204A	OH-4	6.3_6	sl.br.	+126	+
	OH-15	8.7_7	br.	+73	+
Na^+-etheromycin	OH-4	7.25	sl.br.	+75	−
	OH-5	4.78	sh.	+56	+
	OH-14	8.50	br.	+150	+
H^+-carriomycin	COOH + OH-13	~9	e.br.		
		5.8_5	sh.	+46	
Na^+-carriomycin	OH-4 + OH-13	6.2		+123	
	OH-13				
H^+-septamycin	COOH + OH-14	6.4	e.br.		
	OH-4	5.8_8	sh.	+61	
Na^+-septamycin	OH-4	6.22	sl.br.	+113	
	OH-14	~8.9	v.br.	+75	

[a] In ppm from TMS internal in $CDCl_3$ unless otherwise stated.
[b] Sh. = sharp; sl.br. = slightly broadened (W/2 < 10 Hz); br. = broadened; v.br. = very broad; e.br. = extremely broad (>100 Hz).
[c] Δ ASIS = $[\delta(C_6D_6) - \delta(CDCl_3)] \times 10^2$; positive value if paramagnetic shift in C_6D_6.
[d] Internal exchange is indicated as positive if saturation of {OH_A} decreases the intensity of OH_B.
[e] Is indicated as positive if irradiation of the residual water peak of the solvent (usually at δ 1.5 to 1.7) causes the OH peak to become spin saturated.
[f] Is indicated + if the OH participates in metal ion coordination.

state of O*H*-5 in comparison with the free acid form. Now O*H*-5 has become perhaps the H donor to OH-10, the reversed situation from the free acid, and both OH-10 and OH-11 are H bridged to COO⁻, the latter not participating in ion coordination. Bridging of O(5)H to O(6) cannot definitively be excluded, however. This would rationalize all the NMR observations but stays at variance with the x-ray data of the Ag^+ salt, where O(5)H was found to be bound to O(10)H via a H_2O molecule, its presence otherwise being presumably the result of crystal packing only (Lutz et al., 1971).

$\{H_2O\}^d$	^3J (Hz)	^4J (Hz)	Metal ion^f ligand	Remarks
			OH-5 + OH-11- OH-12+	One proton can be separated by addition of Et_3N; in C_6D_6 two bands are found at 360 MHz; $\delta \sim 4.9$ (v.br.) and $\delta \sim 8.8$ (e.br.)
+		(4, OH) $\lesssim$ 2	+ —	Newly determined long-range coupling from 360 MHz
+	(5, OH) = 1.3		+ — —	
		(4, OH) = 1.5	+	All peaks collapse by heating or adding Et_3N
		(4, OH) = 1.6		All peaks collapse by heating or adding Et_3N
		(4, OH) = 0		

2. Nigericin (Rodios and Anteunis, 1977)

Free acid

Only one signal representing three mobile protons is found at δ 5.3 as an extremely broad envelope ($W/2 > 300$ Hz at 300 MHz). The mutual chemical exchange but solvent-screened character of the protons is revealed by the unchanged aspect of the pattern after addition of Et_3N. Furthermore, $^2J(30)$ of the -C(30)H_2OH fragment is in the free acid about 1 Hz lower than in the salt, indicating a changed disposition along the O—H rotor, e.g., by a concomitant rotation along C(30)—O from "outward" position (gauche) in the salt to an

"inward" position (antiperiplanar), thus becoming bridged with
—COOH (see below).

There is a possibility that in the free acid form a molecule of water
is trapped, as is the case for grisorixin in the solid state (Alléaume,
1975). This would explain the rotational preference for the primary
alcoholic fragment. Although it is extremely difficult to obtain correct
integrations for very broad bands, Rodios and I concluded that an H_2O
molecule is probably absent.

Salt

The two OH signals have become differentiated, one being strongly hydrogen bridged (δ 10.3 very broad) and displaying a long-range interaction with H-30B [$^4J(30B,OH) = 2$ Hz]. This must therefore be
OH-10, whereby the O—H bond is disposed in a planar $\wedge\wedge$ arrangement with H-30B. A head-to-tail cyclization by OH-10/COO⁻ bridging
[Δ(ASIS) = +12.3] as in the crystal (Steinrauf et al., 1971) seems
logical. The absorption of the secondary alcohol O*H*-11 is found as a
broadened signal at a not too low field (δ 5.54). Therefore, and in
contrast to the Ag⁺ salt as reported by Steinrauf et al. (1971) but
in agreement with the findings of Shiro and Koyama (1970), O*H*-11
would not participate in the pseudocyclic closure by H bridge to the
carboxylate function. This could be expected, while in the parent
grisorixin (in which CH_2OH has been substituted for CH_3) such a
participation is excluded. The moderate ASIS effect on O*H*-11 is somewhat surprising. It may be explained by a reorientation [$^2J(30)$ increased by 1 Hz] which brings the OH group close to a strong shielding (lipophilic) zone that ends sharply at H-23 (see Section II.F). Hence
for some reason the proton is oriented toward C-28 (at variance with
the original proposal of Rodios and myself) rather than towards COO⁻
(Figure 28).

Rodios and I are not able to exclude, however, a reversed spectral
assignment for OH-10 and OH-11. If the observed coupling with H-30B
is vicinal in character (lowered from the true value because of the

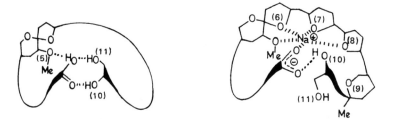

Figure 28 Hydrogen-bonding mechanism in H⁺- (left) and Na⁺-niger-
icin (right). (Source: Steinrauf et al., 1971.)

chemical exchange phenomenon), then we should conclude that it is OH-11 that is participating in the H bridging with COO⁻. This would explain the absence of a pronounced ASIS effect (for OH-10 this time). It would mean that the buttoning shut differs with that in Ag^+- and Tl^+-grisorixin (Alléaume and Hickel, 1970; 1972). The decreased accessibility of the H-bridge bonding zone with respect to monensin may be explained by the better fit of nigericin (see Section IV.C.3).

3. Lonomycin (Rodios and Anteunis, 1978b, 1979a)

Free acid
Both COOH and OH-14 protons are not visible in the $CDCl_3$ spectrum, while OH-4 at δ 5.3 (broad) is identified by its long-range coupling to H-4 [$^4J(4,OH) = 1.6$ Hz]. A ⋀⋀-mode arrangement by the bridging of OH-4 with O(8) is probable while OH-14 becomes engaged in the H-bridge bonding mechanism with COOH. Being an axial group, OH-4 points toward the periphery and displays proton chemical exchange.
Salt
The two OH-groups are differentiated in the Na^+ salt: OH-4 at δ 7.57 and OH-14 nearby δ 8.33. The patterns collapse by raising the temperature. Their low-field position indicates H-bridge bonding with COO⁻, as observed in the crystal of the Tl^+ salt (Otake et al., 1975). In the K^+ salt they are not differentiated (δ 9.3).

4. Ionophore X-206 (Anteunis, 1977b) and alborixin (Rodios and Anteunis, 1979b)

Free acid
Note that the assignments of OH-8 and OH-6 have been revised (Rodios and Anteunis, 1979b). This rather hydrophilic ionophore offers a very interesting set of *seven* mobile protons. Three of them are gathered under one very broad band, as they exchange mutually (COOH, OH-8, and OH-14). All others show separated signals and are identified through the assessment of either long-range couplings (revealing a planar zigzag disposition with their coupled partner) or a vicinal coupling. A large ^3J is found here, e.g., for OH-9 (12.5 Hz in X-206 and 13.0 Hz in alborixin, wrongly reported as 3 Hz), uncovering the antiperiplanar disposition of H-22 toward O(9)H. This OH is orientated inward, is solvent inaccessible, and does not participate in H-bridge formation. Hence it is a sharp, high-field signal with a negligible Δ(ASIS) effect. The nonexistence of a ^3J for OH-4 but long-range coupling with H-10 reveals a nonperipheral O(3) orientation (buried and with no {H₂O} effect) (see Section IV.B). The long-range coupling between H-14 and OH-6 and absence of {H₂O} effect can only be explained by a H-bridge mechanism involving O(5). Radios and I note that the disposition with respect to H-14, although near

a planar zigzag, is *not* of the classical /\/\ mode. The OH-11 must be bridged to OH-6, with the former being the donor. By this rationale a /\/\-mode path is realized between OH-14 and H-35$_{ax}$; hence the observed long-range interaction. This orientation is also expected from the exoanomeric effect (Section IV.B).

Salt

Similar features are found, except for the OH-8 that is bridged in the free acid with the carboxylate group. This is no longer so in the salt. As the carboxylate group is now involved in ion trapping, OH-8 finds its bridging partner in O(10) (exoanomeric effect!; see Section IV.B), the latter not participating in coordination. The nearby position of OH-14, through H-bridge bond formation with COO⁻, allows chemical exchange between OH-8 and OH-14. Another point deserves comment. Undoubtedly OH-14 bridged to COO⁻. Yet the ASIS effect is not large (but reported against CS_2 as the reference solvent). A reported long-range interaction (Anteunis, 1977b) tentatively ascribed as ^4J(35e, OH-14) but detected by inspecting the H-35e signal during an irradiation in the region where both residual water and H-33e are usually found (δ 1.6 to 1.7), was presumably wrongly assigned, as it may well have been confused with a long-range coupling existing between H-35e and H-33e.

One notices that the hydrogen bridges O(8)H—O(10) and especially O(11)H—O(6)H reinforce the tennis-ball seam conformation typical for these ionophores (Alléaume et al., 1975; Blount and Westley, 1971). The latter bridge is situated in a zone that is somewhat hydrophilic (see Section III.F.2 and IV.C.2), e.g. at a site for cation access (Figure 29). It is probable that OH-6 and OH-11 are two functions among others that are involved in stripping off the solvation shell of the cation during capture.

5. *Lenoremycin and dianemycin (Anteunis et al., 1977)*

These ionophores represent a couple of very similar structures behaving, nevertheless, differently. Lenoremycin bears the deoxy sugar fragment in a way such that its pyranoid oxygen participates in the metal coordination. In dianemycin this function is taken over by an OH grouping at a somewhat different distance from the cavity. This represents also an additional mobile proton. In the crystal of the salt the buttoning shut is mediated by an extra H_2O molecule in dianemycin (Steinrauf et al., 1971). Although this could not be ascertained in solution, there is indeed only one broad OH envelope. But OH-5 in dianemycin may be separated out of this broad band by adding Et_3N. Also, in the salt, two separated broad bands in C_6D_6 are noted (δ ~ 8.8 and 4.9). Thus it is very probable that only OH-11 and OH-12 are intimately involved in an accessible H-bridge bonding mechanism (as, e.g., would be especially the case if H_2O participates), while OH-5 is farther away (Figure 30). The x-ray data are in perfect con-

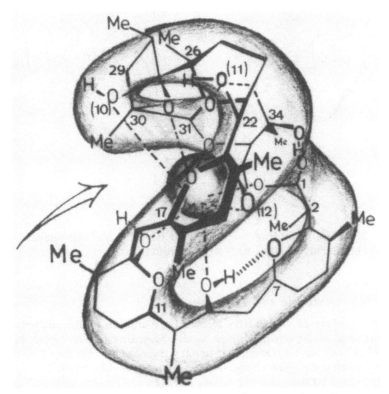

Figure 29 Schematic representation of the tennis ball-seam conformation of X-206 and alborixin, showing the easiest access for water-
solvated ions (from the rear back at the left) as follows from ASIS
studies. The opened zone is further characterized by the presence
of boundary-accessible OH groupings (OH-4, OH-6, and OH-11).
(Source: Anteunis, 1977b.)

cordance with this statement (Czerwinski and Steinrauf, 1971) if
OH-5 is, e.g., bridged to O(6), thus stabilizing the otherwise
strained conformation of ring A (see Section IV.B.). The different
behavior of the terminal hydroxylic groupings OH-10 and OH-11 in
Na⁺-lenoremycin (equivalent to OH-11 and OH-12 in dianemycin) is
remarkable. They form *distinct* patterns, albeit both at low field
[OH-10 at δ 8.33 (very broad) and OH-11 at δ 9.92], indicating strong
hydrogen bonding. Nevertheless, OH-11 still couples with the adjacent
methylene protons and to a large extent (5.8 and 7.8 Hz). We propose,
therefore, that OH-11 is involved in H bridging to COO⁻, while the
tertiary OH-10 is less strongly bound and more involved in an ex-
ternal chemical exchange.

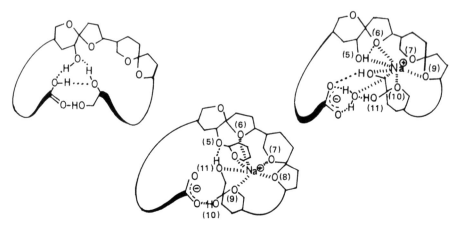

Figure 30 Hydrogen-bonding mechanism in H$^+$- and Na$^+$-dianemycin-
H$_2$O and of the closely related Na$^+$-lenoremycin.

6. *Na$^+$-A204A* *(Anteunis and Verhegge, 1977)*

A new study performed at 360 MHz (M. J. O. Anteunis, unpublished)
has revealed that while irradiating H-4, the peak due to OH-4 at δ 6.4
narrows [^{3}J(4, OH-4) ≤ 2] and its intensity decreases. Shifts of H-4
and of the residual H$_2$O are therefore very nearby. The most deshielded hydroxyl proton, as expected, belongs to the OH-15 that
fixes the backbone in the pseudocyclic conformation by H bridging with
COO$^-$. Both mobile protons collapse to one signal at higher temperatures, indicating mutual exchange. The observed long-range coupling
would indicate that the O(4)H bond pointing inward is weakly hydrogen
bonded to COO$^-$.

7. *Na$^+$-etheromycin* *(Anteunis and Rodios, 1978)*

With respect to A204A, an additional OH function is present in etheromycin, and this is indeed found at δ(OH-5) = 4.78, identified through
^{3}J(5, OH) = 1.3 Hz. Its sharp appearance, not influenced on irradiation of either of the two other OH signals (which themselves are mutually influenced) indicates that the observed coupling constant must
be the real one. Hence the torsion around C(5)H—OH is gauche.
Rodios and I conclude from ASIS studies that OH-5 may be H bridged
with the deoxy sugar ring oxygen O(15) (Section III.F) and is thus
far removed from the others.

8. *Carriomycin* *(Rodios and Anteunis, 1978)*

In the salt only one collapsed signal at δ ⁓ 6.2 is observed, showing
that the three mobile protons are mutually exchangeable. In the free

acid, OH-4 is orientated inward, the O—H bond being coplanar and in
⌒⌒ fashion to H-4. Here OH-13 closes the cycle with COO⁻, and the
slow exchange between OH-4 and OH-13 can be speeded up by an increase in temperature or by adding Et_3N.

9. Septamycin (Rodios and Anteunis, 1978a)

Similar features as for carriomycin are found. In the free acid OH-4
is orientated toward the inner cavity [$^4J(4, OH) = 1.6$ Hz]. Although
at room temperature no fast exchange can be observed, this orientation
of O—H must have been changed in the salt, while ^4J vanishes. If
O(8)Me was originally a (weak) proton acceptor for OH-4, this oxygen
becomes a coordination site in the salt, explaining the change in rotation of OH-4.

F. ASIS Effects and Lipophilicity Index

Since Ledaal (1968) has proposed a rationale for the interpretation of
ASIS (aromatic solvent-induced shift) effects on proton shifts its
utility for structural elucidations has been overwhelmingly demonstrated. The observed specific shifts may be visualized as the result
of a mean (time-averaged) orientation of the plane of the aromatic
ring perpendicular to bond-dipole vectors in the molecule, and preferentially at the positively charged side. Although this simplified
Ledaal model handles discrete solvation, in fact a multitude of collision
complexes occur (Engler and Laszlo, 1971). Alternatively, the solute-
solvent interaction may be of a specific type with localized effects,
e.g., occurring with complexes involving strong interaction terms such
as hydrogen-bond bridging or equivalent mechanisms (Schwyzer and
Ludescher, 1969; Pitner and Urry, 1972; Urry, et al., 1974; Llinás
and Klein, 1975). In medium-sized biomolecules a time-averaged collision complexation will enable the recognition of extended boundaries
possessing lipophilic or hydrophilic character. (I will avoid the term
of hydrophobicity; see Cramer III, 1977.) It is indeed a frequently
observed feature that biomolecules often possess well-defined but
rather extended regions of different polarities which play a major role
in their mode of action.

Aromatic solvent structuralization is exceptionally high around ionic
species (see Schwetlick, 1971; see also Cox, 1921), and a molecule like
benzene will collide on a polar surface in a direction which is parallel
with its plane, i.e., in the direction of its most polarizable tensor. It
will, however, offer its plane perpendicular to lipophilic structural
fragments. From this one expects protons in the neighborhood of ionic
and highly polar regions to become deshielded in aromatic solvents
(positive ASIS effect) but screened when situated at lipophilic surfaces
(negative ASIS effect). This, in principle, must allow a mapping of the
surface character. In our conceptualism ASIS includes both long-range

(ionic, polar) and short-range effects (polarization, van der Waals; see Burgermeister and Winkler-Oswatitsch, 1977). Ionophorous antibiotics are ideal models for a test of this concept. They are neither too large nor too spherical, making most of their protons solvent accessible. Protons that are not in close contact with the surface will display low ASIS effects, and the experimental results should therefore be restricted to surface protons only, a fact that should be considered in studies of macromolecules (e.g., globular proteins, etc). In relatively small spherical molecules this is not a problem, as solvent-buried protons are relatively scarce and may strengthen anyway the character of the zone wherein the solvent-accessible protic neighbors are embedded. Thus Me(34), H-18a, and H-19a in lenoremycin, although situated in a pronouncedly lipophilic region, show no ASIS effects, being sterically screened off by other fragments, e.g., H-11 for Me(34), Me(36) for H-18a, and Me(33) for H-19a (see also further). I will define the ASIS effect as the difference between the observed shift of proton i measured in benzene against that found in chloroform and expressed in 10^2 ppm: $(ASIS)_i = 10^2 \times [\delta_i(C_6D_6) - \delta_i(CLCl_3)]$. This definition raises the problem of the nature of the reference solvent to be used. An ideal "inert" solvent should be apolar with an isotropic reaction field but still have enough solubility. For practical reasons chloroform seems to be the best choice, especially for the study of membrane-affecting substances. One can determine the ASIS effect for each individual proton. The sign will define the character of the zone in which it is embedded [ASIS(+) when hydrophilic, ASIS(−) when lipophilic], while the size of the effect reflects the importance of that character. These effects are represented in Figures 5 to 11 in stereo-drawings by using open circles (lipophilic in nature) and filled circles (hydrophilic in nature), the size of the circles reflecting the importance of the effect. The ASIS effect cannot be measured for all protons. (Those that were not accessible are indicated in the stereo-drawing by a stroke). The number of accessible protons [n(+) and n(−)] are indicated in Table 5, and also the number of protons for which ASIS effects could be obtained. I have also indicated the mean ASIS effect, both for shielding [ASIS(−)] and deshielding [ASIS(+)]. Finally, the fractional lipophilicity f(−) or fractional hydrophilicity f(+) of the biomolecule can be defined as the relative importance of its global lipophilic or global hydrophilic character, respectively, by dividing the summated specific effects by the total effect: $f(\pm) = \Sigma ASIS(\pm)/[\Sigma ASIS(+) + \Sigma ASIS(-)]$.

When less than 80% of the total amount of protons could be studied, one should interpret the results with some caution. The fractional lipophilicity will express the relative ease for the biomolecule to occur in a specific surrounding (the membrane?).

1. *Fractional lipophilicity and ease of cationic transport*

Turnover numbers or rates of cation carriage are determined at two stages of the physical process (Lindenbaum et al., 1979; Krasne and Eisenman, 1976). A first kinetic barrier is to be surmounted at the membrane aqueous interface. Here mainly conformational implications will control the speed in this "equilibrium domain." A second barrier is to be surmounted during the translocation of both the charged and discharged carrier across the membranic bilayer itself. Either both or one of the two barriers will restrict the speed of the overall cation conveyance. Perhaps the fractional lipophilicity will help in understanding the relative ease of translocation across the lipophilic bilayer zone. For this one needs the $f(-)$ values (normalized, e.g., per unit volume in comparing carriers of different size) for both the free acid and the complexes. The values have not been determined systematically for both the free and complexed ionophores (e.g., Table 5), and relatively little kinetic and thermodynamic data were available until now for polyether antibiotics (Burgermeister and Winkler-Oswatitsch, 1977). With the increasing possibilities of different techniques, including NMR spectroscopy of heteronuclei such as ^{23}Na (Degani and Elgavish, 1978), we may expect that such problems can soon be tackled efficiently. Some qualitative aspects will now be discussed (Table 5).

Fractional lipophilicity is normally highest for ionophores in their free acid form, as expected, except for those that form aggregates after trapping, giving rise to superstructures (dimers) with high and increased lipophilic coating (A23187, Figure 6; lasalocid, etc.). It can be predicted that in these cases the equilibrium domain, characterized by increasing conformational rigidity and entropically unfavorable aggregation, will represent at least one of the rate-determining steps for the overall process.

Some carboxylic ionophores possess almost identical f values in both the salt and free acid forms. For carriomycin it is the result of increasing $\overline{ASIS(+)}$ concomitant with an increasing $\overline{ASIS(-)}$ in the salt, i.e., the different zones both become more intensified in character. For septamycin it is mainly due to spreading of a weak lipophilic zone.

Pronounced decreases in fractional lipophilicity are found in the salts of lonomycin, nigericin, and X-206. We may expect, therefore, that the translocation of a cation across the bilayer itself ("kinetic domain") will be the energetic restriction in these cases.

The fractional lipophilicity seldom amounts to more than 0.5. The most lipophilic carriers seem to be H^+-nigericin, $(A23187)_2Mg$, Na^+-etheromycin, H^+- and Na^+-salinomycin, Na^+-carriomycin, Na^+-monensin, and H^+- and Na^+-septamycin [$f(-) > 0.4$].

Table 5   Lipophilicity Fractions f(−) for Carboxylic Acid Polyethers

Ionophore	State	Formula	Number and percentage of protons
A204A	Na^+	$(C_{49}H_{83}O_{17})Na$	81 (97.6%)
A23187	H^+	$C_{29}H_{37}N_3O_6$	36 (97.3%)
	Mg^+	$(C_{29}H_{36}N_3O_6)_2Mg$	34 (94.4%)
Carriomycin	H^+	$C_{47}H_{80}O_{15}$	77 (96.3%)
	Na^+	$(C_{47}H_{79}O_{15})Na$	76 (96.2%)
Dianemycin	Na^+	$(C_{47}H_{77}O_{14})Na$	68 (88.3%)
Etheromycin	Na^+	$(C_{18}H_{81}O_{16})Na$	75 (92.5%)
Lasalocid	H^+	$C_{34}H_{54}O_8$	45 (83.3%)
	Na^+	$(C_{34}H_{53}O_8)_2Na_2$	37 (69.8%)
Lenoremycin	Na^+	$(C_{47}H_{77}O_8)Na$	67 (87%)
Lonomycin	H^+	$C_{44}H_{76}O_{14}$	69 (90.8%)
	K^+	$(C_{44}H_{75}O_{14})K$	69 (92.0%)
Monensin	Na^+	$(C_{36}H_{61}O_{11})Na$	57 (96.7%)
Nigericin	H^+	$C_{40}H_{68}O_{11}$	57 (83.8%)
	Na^+	$(C_{40}H_{67}O_{11})Na$	56 (83.5%)
Salinomycin	H^+	$C_{42}H_{70}O_{11}$	62 (88.6%)
	Na^+	$(C_{42}H_{69}O_{11})Na$	59 (85.5%)
Epi-deoxysalino-mycin	H^+	$C_{42}H_{70}O_{10}$	60 (85.7%)
Septamycin	H^+	$C_{48}H_{82}O_{16}$	76 (92.7%)
	Na^+	$(C_{48}H_{81}O_{16})Na$	79 (97.5%)
X-206	H^+	$C_{47}H_{82}O_{14}$	69 (84.1%)
	Na^+	$(C_{47}H_{81}O_{14})Na$	70 (86.4%)

n(+)	n(−)	$\overline{\text{ASIS(+)}}$	$\overline{\text{ASIS(−)}}$	f(+)	f(−)
47	34	29.25	19.12	0.67_9	0.32_1
26	10	20.1	19.0	0.73_4	0.26_6
20	14	20.4	28.0	0.51	0.49
50	27	16.5_2	19.5	0.61	0.39
46	30	25.1	27.0	0.59	0.41
46	22	16.9_4	19.8_6	0.64	0.36
42	33	21.2	20.4	0.57	0.43
28	17	17.2	10.2	0.73	0.27
19	18	18.8	8.2	0.71	0.29
37	30	28.1	20.7	0.62_5	0.37_5
44	25	18.4	16.7	0.66	0.34
50	19	29.2	18.1	0.81	0.19
25	32	41.1_5	21.6	0.59_8	0.40_2
23	34	14.8	12.5	0.44_5	0.55_5
31	25	21.9	14.8	0.64	0.36
30	32	16.7	15.0	0.51	0.49
33	26	19.3	18.6	0.57	0.43
45	15	15.0	14.5	0.76	0.24
44	32	19.7	19.3	0.58_5	0.41_5
38	41	31.6	18.9	0.61	0.39
40	29	15.9	13.0	0.63	0.37
53	17	26.2	12.0	0.87	0.13

2. Distribution of lipophilicity within the molecular architecture

Figures 5 to 11 show the distribution pattern for lipophilicity (ASIS effects) along the framework of some carboxylic ionophores. As expected, the most hydrophilic zone is concentrated around the head-to-tail hydrogen bond, especially in the ionized complexes. Highest lipophilicity occurs in a region situated near the midpoint. Nigericin and monensin (Figure 5) are typical representatives. This distribution may be more or less disturbed by the presence of extra (polar or polarizable) substituents. Thus in salinomycin and narasin the presence of the allylic alcohol function in ring C represents an uncharacteristic hydrophilic region at the center of the molecule (for stereorepresentation see Anteunis and Rodios, 1981).

The introduction of alkoxy substituents (methoxy, sugar fragments) and especially hydroxyl groups also serves to lessen the local lipophilic character. This is the case for ring A in lonomycin, carriomycin, septamycin (Figure 7), and especially in A204A (Figure 7) and etheromycin (Figure 8) [introduction of oxygenated functions O(5) and OH-4], and the same is observed for ring F in lonomycin, A204A, and etheromycin. In dianemycin (Figure 9) and lenoremycin (Figure 10) a long acyclic but relatively polar fragment attached to the carboxyl results in an analogous effect. A further illustration concerns the comparison between etheromycin and septamycin. Together with the epimeric state of C-2, etheromycin possesses an enantiomeric ring A. It contains an O(5)H instead of O(5)Me and an extra methoxy group in ring F, but lacks this group in ring C. As a consequence, hydrophilicity increases in ring A and F in etheromycin, but lipophilicity is gained in rings C and D. The reason why H-17 and H-18 behave more lipophilically in etheromycin than in septamycin is due to the fact that these protons in septamycin are close spatially to the hydrophilic O(10)Me. In spite of the presence of a free hydroxyl group in etheromycin and a more hydrophilic C ring, the overall fractional lipophilicity in etheromycin has *increased*, not decreased, in comparison to septamycin. The reason is related to a compensating increase in the lipophilic character in etheromycin of the sugar fragment G, especially for H-43 and H-45. An explanation for this is offered if one accepts the polar zone of ring G in etheromycin as being orientated toward O(5)H, which in turn is hydrogen bonded to O(15) by H bridging, e.g., O(5)H---O(15) $\{\tau[C(6)O(6)-C(42)C(43)] \approx 180°\}$. In this model O*H*-5 is screened off and the observed ASIS effects can be explained. Also, this solvent-screened character, as revealed by the spectral behavior of O*H*-5 (see Section III.E.7), corroborates the present hypothesis. It is clear, therefore, that lipophilicity has not to compensate for the presence of polar groups if the latter are buried within the complex. A comparison between lenoremycin and dianemycin reveals identical features. Dianemycin should display lowered fractional lipophilicity [presence of extra O(5)H]. It does not, however, because this hydroxyl oxygen is in the cavity, O(5) participating in cation coordination. In lenoremycin the extra coordination of the sugar ring oxygen, encapsulating the aqueous cavity, makes the lipophilic loop somewhat longer but less intense.

Ionophore X-206 and alborixin exhibit exceptional lipophilic distributions (Figure 11) and they represent, therefore, a quite different type of carboxylic ionophores. They are of the longest-chain species of the family and possess a remarkably high number of oxygenated functions, among which six are present as free hydroxyl groups. Not surprisingly, their fractional lipophilicity is low and especially so for the salts. It is possible that lipophilicity (Table 5) is somewhat underestimated, because most of the protons for which ASIS measurements were impossible may be lipophilic. Three hydroxyl groups [O(6)H, O(9)H, and O(11)H] are near the surface and solvent accessible, and two of these do not participate in complexation [O(9)H and O(11)]. The skeleton of these ionophores mimics the seam of a tennis ball [mutual O(6)H and O(11)H hydrogen bridging helps the anchoring of this form; see Section III.E.5]. In addition, the O(4) that participates in metal ion coordination is incompletely screened by aliphatic fragments. Only three zones with very localized lipophilicity are present, concentrated at Me(47) and at the regions C(4)Me−C(5)−C(6)H, C(18)Me−C(19), and C(29)−C(30)Me−C(31) together with the end-ethyl group. In the free acid, where lipophilicity typically increases, especially around the head-to-tail zone, the screening of Me(46) is substantial, the proton signal being found at an unusually high field position of δ 0.38 in C_6D_6. The atypical behavior of X-206 and alborixin is therefore due to the fact that the highest hydrophilic zone is *not* at the head-to-tail junction (note also the unique ASIS distribution pattern for ring F). The hydrophilic zone consists of a region where O(4)H, O(6)H, and O(11) are clustered together. The access for a cation is presumably best at that point, facing the C(7) to C(16) segment, as illustrated also later in Figure 29.

We will present in Section IV.C a proposal for the mechanism of ion trapping and release by membrane carriers as it follows from the recognition of general conformational features, e.g., whereby hinges can be defined as giving conformational mobility to certain segments. In most cases these hinges operate in order to give the molecule the ability to act as a "floodgate," giving access to the inner cavity. The entrance is constituted by a polar face as defined in the present discussion. The gate is almost invariably created by a rupture of the head-to-tail hydrogen bridge, but not, however, in X-206 and alborixin, where the ionophores remain most probably closed during the complexation-de-complexation process. Here, hinges are distributed in such a way that they provoke a rotation of only certain fragments together with their ligands, e.g., O(4), O(6), and O(11). The trajectory of the cation is such that this mechanism provides the most hydrophilic access during the entire process, so that some ligands escort this cation until they are exchanged for the solvent on decomplexation. It is clear that the recognition of regions of increased hydrophilicity, as disclosed by ASIS measurements, and the conceptualisms of lipophilicity and hinges strongly support each other in defining the mechanism of transport. But the observation of ASIS effects for localized regions at the boundary of the cyclic cation carrier must also allow a more detailed insight into the physical state of the ionophore near the water-membrane interface. As stated earlier, the distribution of the two kinds of zones along the surface not only helps one to determine the direction of approach of the vehicle (geometrical aspect), but I believe that the fractional lipophilicity must reflect the ease of carriage across the membrane, e.g., it helps to define the kinetic mode (energetic aspect).

3. ASIS and spectral assignments

The recognition of homogeneous zones of increased or decreased lipophilicity with attendant ASIS effects allows one to assign a posteriori some signals in the ^{1}H NMR spectrum, once the conformation of the ionophore has been revealed. This is also the only way to assign by ^{1}H NMR, e.g., methoxy protons and methyl groups on quaternary carbons. In carriomycin we were originally unable to distinguish between the CH−Me(31) and CH−Me(35) signals (Rodios and Anteunis, 1978a). According to the data obtained for septamycin (Rodios and Anteunis, 1978a) and with the expected ASIS effects for the corresponding regions in mind, Me(35) is at δ 1.10 and Me(31) at δ 0.97 in C_6D_6. Furthermore, this assignment of Me(35) corresponds to the observed $^3J(12,Me(35_{eq})) = 7.0$ Hz (congested Me) and $^3J(28,Me(31_{eq})) = 6.6$ Hz (normal equatorial Me). In Na$^+$-nigericin (Rodios and Anteunis, 1977) Rodios and I left the problem of assignment for CHMe(31) and CHMe(36) open. ASIS effects now allow an attribution in C_6D_6 (not in CDCl$_3$) that is the reverse of that reported in the original table. The original assignments of Me(34) and Me(35) are correct, however. This is also borne out by comparison with the ASIS effects on the structurally equivalent zonal positions in Na$^+$-monensin. Whereas now Et substitutes Me(34), the signal corresponding to Me(32) (being Me(35) in Na$^+$-nigericin) can be assigned unambiguously (as it is the only Me left that stays on a quaternary carbon).

   In etheromycin we tend to assign the values for Me(30), Me(33), Me(34), and Me(37) not in the order shown in Table 1 of the original publication (Anteunis and Rodios, 1978) but, rather, in the order Me(34), Me(37), Me(30), and Me(33). Solvent titration allows to corroborate the latter order. In order to avoid mistakes in the assignment of peaks to the correct groupings in different solvents (problem of "crossing-over" phenomena in relative peak locations), solvent titration can also be replaced by following the shifts in C_6D_6 (or toluene) with temperature. The ASIS effects decrease at higher temperature, as expected, and the tendency of the spectral displacements of the signals by raising the temperature discloses their ASIS capabilities.

IV. PRIMARY STRUCTURE AND PREDESTINATION TO CONFORMATIONAL BIAS

A. General Considerations: Definition of Hinges
   (Anteunis, 1981)

It is well known in peptide chemistry that the short-range interactions are of overwhelming importance, allowing the prediction of a more or less discrete number of energy minima in the conformational space. One may wonder if this can also be done for the polyether ionophores and if a predestination to a certain discrete number of favorable forms exists already by the mere succession of the different types of bonds, rings, and their substitution patterns along the backbone. Two facts seem to discount this possibility: (1) the stress upon the importance of head-to-tail bridging by hydrogen bonding as a prerequisite for the cyclization and (2) the degradation of the role of the several methyl, ethyl, and methoxy groupings to solely surrounding the polar cavity by a lipophilic surface. The importance of the hydrogen bonding in cyclization is overestimated, as illustrated by the facts that (1) often there is only one OH function available for doing the job (carriomycin, grisorixin, etc.), (2) the position of the hydroxyl is not critical (at the end or, alternatively, near-end of the backbone: X-206, etc.) and (3) some ionophores possess apparently strained polysubstituted tetrahydropyrane rings for which the H-bridge bonding alone would not suffice for compensation: grisorixin with one button shut, but ring A with one equatorial and two axial substituents believed to be the reason for bonding only weakly Na^+ (Chock et al., 1977); dianemycin, where ring A as well as ring C has three axial (plus syndiaxial strain!) next to two equatorial substituents, etc.

   A conclusive indication that other factors intervene in molding the polyether into its curled loop is laid open by the fact that the solid-state conformation of the salinomycin p-iodophenacyl *ester* possesses almost the entirely closed surface (Kinashi et al., 1973, 1975). One has only to detach the ester, perform two rotations (e.g., around C(24)-C(25) at the tail and C(2)-C(3) at the head), and the closure is achieved. All other rotors, including the long acyclic fragment C-7 to C-13, are in a predestined state to form the circle (Anteunis and Rodios, 1981). Also, the p-bromophenacyl ester of septamycin (Pretcher and Weber, 1974) can be closed after removal of the ester by simple rotation of only C(20)-C(21) (from ± to −) and C(24)-C(25) (from $\frac{+}{+}$ to +). The quasicyclic form was indeed already present in the ester in the fragments from C-1 to C-20 and C-21 to C-30! This is

not a mere fortuitous result of crystal packing, as convincingly demonstrated by the discovery that 17-epi-deoxy-(O-8)-salinomycin (epi-
salinomycin) free acid *in solution* is also a rigid structure, yet C-7 to
C-13 is acyclic (Anteunis and Rodios, 1981). But epi-salinomycin is
not cyclic, taking, rather the shape of a double sine wave with the
middle near C-17. It suffices to invert (eipmerize) C-17, however, in
order to obtain directly the original closed form of (deoxy)salinomycin.
Except for very minor relaxation changes, none of the other torsions
have to be varied.

When inspecting the tridimensional structures of most ionophores,
even those with apparent constraint fragments, one realizes that the
torsions, except here and there for one exception, are in their most
stable rotameric states, all concerted to result in a cyclic form. We
have recently discussed two cases (Ionomycin and salinomycin) where
a violation of predicted stabilization is observed (Anteunis, 1981). The
"floppy" fragments that can take several rotameric states will be called
the "hinge" rotors (symbol ⧄). They may be important during the
process of trapping or releasing the ion. Before I discuss some specific cases, I want first to enumerate the different rules that one can
apply in order to predict the secondary structures of the ionophores.
The principles behind these conformational rules are not new but well-
known in conformational analysis. Thus rule A-2 (see below) states
that instead of diaxial repulsion between two β-substituted oxygens in
six-membered rings, an appreciable stabilization may occur if one is
a hydroxylic group. This is especially so in entirely anhydrous me-
dium. One may presume that for ionophores, where water *in the cavity*
is totally excluded, the effect is important (Anteunis and Rodios, 1981),
as long as the hydrogen-bonding mechanism is not acting at the boundary.

B. Conformational Rules

The following principles (Figure 31) that may provoke conformational
rigidity seem to operate in polyether ionophores (the Dunitz-Prelog
nomenclature shall be followed: Dunitz and Prelog, 1960).

1. *Substituent constraints of tetrahydropyran and
   tetrahydrofuran fragments*

   A.1a A *quaternary* substituent (mimicking tert-butyl) stays always
        in the equatorial* position and a further vicinal substitution,
        either equatorial or axial, is disallowed.

---

*The terms equatorial and axial should be visualized as pseudoequa-
torial and pseudoaxial for tetrahydrofuran rings. A tetrahydrofuran
ring always possesses more mobility than the corresponding six-member
ring, however.

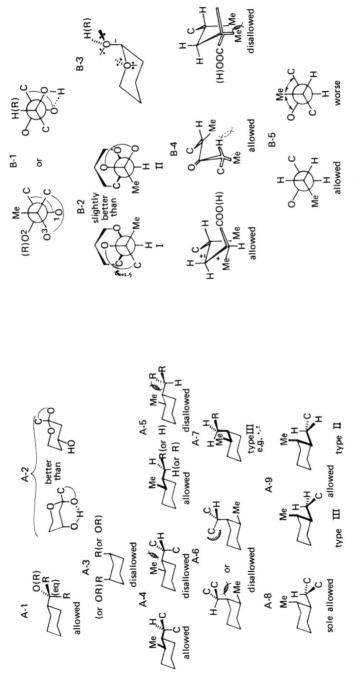

Figure 31 Illustration of conformational rules A and B. (From Anteunis, 1981.)

A.1b A tertiary substituent will act as a quaternary substituent if it does not point its C——H bond inward and over the ring. See, however, rule B.1.

A.2a An axial glycosidic function is preferred over an equatorial (anomeric effect: Lemieux, 1971), especially if stabilized by a syndiaxial OH group by forming a hydrogen-bridge (particularly in the cavity of the ionophore). See also rule B.3.

A.2b The anomeric effect may be annihilated if compensation by (poly)equatorial substitution is present or if rule A.1 applies.

A.3 Syndiaxial strain should be avoided (see rule B.4), except for O——H---O bridging (see rule A.2) and when screened from protic solvents.

A.4 An *equatorial tertiary* substituent can only be flanked by *one* equatorial (trans)vicinal R group if no type I sequence [(+,−) sequence] is present.

A.5a An *equatorial secondary* substituent has two allowed rotational states with respect to an equatorial (trans)vicinal R, i.e., in order of decreasing stability: (−, ±) or (+, ±) and (−, −) or (+, +) (type III and type II, respectively).

A.5b The type II sequence becomes disallowed when flanked by two equatorial (trans)vicinal R groups, unless the in-between substituent is Me.

A.6 An *axial tertiary* substituent is disallowed when flanked by one (and all the more so when flanked by two) equatorial (cis)vicinal R groups (R = Me, Et, OL, etc.).

A.7 Only a type III substitution pattern [either (+, ±) or (−, ±) sequence] is allowed when an *axial secondary* substituent is flanked by an equatorial (cis)vicinal R. When the axial secondary substituent is flanked on both sides by two equatorial R groups, much strain is created that only disappears when the axial substituent is Me.

A.8a An *equatorial tertiary* substituent has only one allowed rotational state with an adjacent (cis)axial R, e.g., the one avoiding a type I sequence.

A.8b An extra axial (cis)vicinal group will not destroy this preference, but an extra equatorial substituent is disallowed.

A.9a An *equatorial secondary* substituent may take two rotational states, one where a type II [(+, +) or (−, −)] sequence is realized, the other where a type III [(+, ±) or −, ±) sequence is realized.

A.9b An extra axial (cis)vicinal group will not compromise the foregoing situation, but an extra equatorial (trans) group will reduce the two possibilities to only one rotameric state for the secondary substituent.

2. Along acyclic rotors

B.1   Two adjacent *quaternary* centers are allowed if they are of
       a glyoxal acetal or glycolaldehyde acetal type [$-C(OR)R-$
       $C(OR)_2-$]. The preferred disposition is the one with max-
       imal gauche oxygen dispositions and with the minimum of
       parallel free-orbital orientations (anomeric effect), e.g., O(2)
       as the (pseudo) axial group. See also rule B.3 for the O(2)$-$R
       rotational state (Figure 31).

B.2a Rotors of the digol type [$-C(OR)R-C(OR)R-$] also prefer
       a gauche oxygen disposition.

B.2b If no other constraints are present (e.g., rule B.4), it is
       better to find an oxygen orientated over a ring than a car-
       bon, and the more so with respect to six-membered rings (see
       Figure 31: I moreover better than II; see rule B.2a).

B.3   Next to the anomeric effect itself (rule A.2), the exoanomeric
       effect further predicts that the best disposition is the one with
       a minimum of parallel orientations of unshared electron pairs
       [a (+, +) or (−, −) state] (Lemieux, 1971).

B.4   Among the three rotameric states along acyclic fragments,
       those possessing a minimum number of quasisyndiaxial dis-
       positions are the preferred ones. However, such a disposi-
       tion along a sp^2 carbon is allowed. In almost every case of
       the present ionophores this statement leads to the exclusion
       of two out of the three rotamers. In fact, this general prin-
       ciple has already been applied in rules A.1 to A.8. An ex-
       ception is found when a favorable hydrogen-bridge mechanism
       can operate (see rules A.2 and A.3).

B.5   One "sandwich" position is worse than two independent gauche
       dispositions.

C. Practical Applications of Conformational Rules:
    Static and Dynamic Features

The following discussions are based on an analysis of conformational
constraints that are initiated when changes in the "native" spatial
structures are considered. Although this rationale converges to a
consistent picture of proposals for geometric happenings during ionophoric action, alternative approaches may be worked out. Thus,
by deliberately imposing a change of one specific rotor, even when
"disallowed," it is possible that by virtue of a cascade of coupled
phenomena (i.e., while adopting neighbor torsions to the new situation) an alternative operational picture for action may emerge. These
second-order mechanisms may, by virtue of their gearing or wobble
character, become very effective.

Table 6 Indication of Conformational Strain Induced Along the Framework of Lenoremycin and Dianemycin When Altering the Native State

Rotor or ring	Strain in alternative states[a]	
	Rotor 2	Rotor 3
C(2)−C(3)	s.d. Me(39):C(1)−C(2)	s.d. Me(40):Me(39)
C(3)−C(4)	s.d. Me(40):C(1)−C(2)	s.d. C(4)−C(5):C(1)−C(2)
C(4)−C(5)	s.d. C(6)−C(7):C(3)−C(4)	s.d. C(6)−C(7):Me(40)
C(5)−C(6)		
C(6)−C(7)		
C(7)−C(8)	s.d. C(6)−C(7):Me(37)	s.d. C(6)−C(7):C(8)−C(9)
C(8)−C(9)	sa.·C(9)−O(4):Me(37):C(9)−C(10)	sa. C(9)−O(4):C(7)−C(8):C(9)−C(10)
Ring A		
Spiro ring B C(16)−C(17)	B.2b II allowed	Oxygens anti
Ring C		
Spiro ring D C(24)−C(25)	s.d. Me(32):C(23)−C(24)	s.d. Me(32):C(24)−O

[a]s.d. = (quasi)syndiaxial strain, with indication of opponents (e.g., Me(39):C(1)−C(2) quasisyndiaxial opposition of Me(39) with C(1)−C(2) bond); sa. = sandwich position with indication of situation [e.g., Me(37) guache between both C(9)−O(4) and C(9)−C(10) indicated as C(9)−O(4):Me(37):C(9)−C(10).

1. Lenoremycin and dianemycin

The native torsional states along the rotors C(2) to C(9) are stable ones. Table 6 recapitulates, with reference to the rules, the strains that are introduced for each of the corresponding two other rotameric alternatives. Most of the rotor are typically predestined to occur only in one conformational state as present in their native states. There might be two rotational states for C(5)−C(6) (partial double-

Inversed ring or other state	Conformational rule or remark
	B.4
	B.4
	B.4
Cisoid (C=O eclipses C(6)−H Transoid (C=O eclipses C(6)−Me(38)	Transoid is the native situation. Eclipsing with C=O occurs best with the most voluminous group (sic). Hinge rotor.
	Frozen double bond.
	See correct stereoview, Figures 9 and 10 or solid state.
	B.5 Even more restricted in dianemycin by axial Me(36); A.8
Antianomeric, syndiaxial	Note the application of rule A.2a in the native configuration (see also Section III.E-5)
Restricted flexibility allowed	
	Native of type B.2bI Hinge rotor.
Tert-butyl	A.1a
Restricted flexibility allowed	
	B.4

bond character), and this is certainly so for C(16)−C(17) together with a librational flexibility of the five-membered rings. Rotation along these fragments seems to be the most economical way to give access to the interior cavity. The conformational floppiness around the transoid bond allows dianemycin to expand and to incorporate an extra water molecule in the head-to-tail button-shut mechanism. This would, in principle, also be possible for lenoremycin, but the participation of the deoxy sugar fragment in coordination makes this superfluous.

In other rotors rotational freedom is especially allowed in the junctions between the furanoses, certainly if the latter are unsubstituted. It is clear that many of the aliphatic or methoxy groupings serve dual roles. Rules A.4 to A.9 typically illustrate the controlling effect on folding by syndiaxial strain caused during rotational changes. If, e.g., the equatorial C(26)—Me group on the last right is lacking, as in X-206 or (methyl)salinomycin, conformational restriction is lifted, rendering C(24)—C(25) a multistate rotor [and a two-state rotor if C(24)—Me(Et) is present]. Hinge rotors are not immediately at the head or tail of the molecule. They are much more efficient for opening and closing if they are somewhat removed from the extremities.

2. Dynamic aspects: Alborixin, X-206, and a proposal for a mechanism of trapping

Also in X-206 the rotor C(2)—C(3) is restricted by the presence of C(4)—Me(eq). Rotors C(7)—C(8) and C(8)—C(9) would be free, were it not that O(4)H---O(3) (directed toward the cavity in the salt!) serves as a "clip" (see rule A.2a).

When one inspects the location of mobile rotors, one comes to the consistent picture that C(10)—C(11) together with C(16)—C(17) and C(22)—C(23) together with C(30)—C(31) are two-state rotors that may control the cants of ring B [so that it may direct its ring oxygen O(5) toward the outside] and that of ring C [bridging O(7) toward the cavity and O(8)—H toward the exterior] and finally also that of the fragment C(23)—C(30), consisting of the two furanoses so that they too may direct their ring oxygens outward. One further notices that in counterpoising ring C, the oxygen O(7) comes in a syndiaxial disposition toward O(6)H, fixing the rotation by hydrogen-bond bridging. By these two cants a trapped ion can be displaced by mediation of four to five coordinators that move together [O(4),O(6)H, O(8), and O(12)] toward that ionophoric boundary which is also the most accessible and polar region of the ionophore (see Figure 29, Section III.E.4). The movement is not necessarily concerted, so that the solvation shell of the cation can be stripped off consecutively (Burgermeister and Winkler-Oswatitsch, 1977). This "crocodile" mechanism may be especially pronounced for those ionophores having a tennisball seam conformation. It is my feeling that where rigidity is abandoned, there might be a good reason for it: these multistate rotors define the hinges for action.

3. Etheromycin, A204A, carriomycin, lonomycin, and septamycin

Hinge rotors in common are C(8)—C(9) and C(20)—C(21), the latter being smoother in carriomycin and septamycin. In lonomycin the situation, even the native one, is bad for C(8)—C(9). The fragments C(1)—C(7) and C(21)—C(30) may open as a diptych, concomitantly

with the disconnection of the end-to-end H-bridge bond. The
C(11)−OMe, participating in complexation, is rotated from the inner
cavity toward the surroundings and may therefore play the role of a
handle. The flexibility of carriomycin is additionally increased at
C(7)−C(8) and in etheromycin and lonomycin by an even more effective
two-state rotor C(16)−C(17). Of all the ionophores out of the present
group, etheromycin seems to be the most flexible one, and this might
partly explain why it is also the least discriminating member against
several cations (Mitani and Ōtake, 1978) and prefers even directional,
asymmetric ions (NH_4^+). Flexibility has not only to deal with selectivity, however, but also with the rate of dissociation or recombination.
Because, in addition, etheromycin has a rather large lipophilicity number, it is possible especially for the recombination rate to be large.
Experimental kinetic data are, however, not available in that respect.

4. Nigericin and monensin

These two ionophores have two common two-state rotors (but differently numbered): C(16)−C(17) (Nigericin) or C(12)−C(13) (Monensin)
and C(20)−C(21) (Nigericin) or C(16)−C(17) (Monensin). [The first
rotor is even somewhat strained in the native state, the alternative
(+) disposition (as realized in lonomycin along C(20)−C(21) being
slightly better through avoiding a supplementary sandwich situation.]
The dynamic aspects are similar to the behavior of the foregoing ionophores. It is attractive to imagine that by rotations along these bonds
the fore-penultimate ring is tilted, consecutively followed by that of
the two last rings (more or less in concert).

This process would especially be assisted in monensin, because this
polyether possesses an extra hydroxylic group O(6)H that fixes the
rotation through H bridging with O(10)H and O(11)H as the latter
approach. In contrast, nigericin carries a methoxy grouping instead
[although a hydrogen bond with O(10)H and/or O(11)H as the donor(s)
is not excluded] and possesses additional flexibility along C(7)−C(8)
and C(8)−C(9). The following consequences may perhaps be visualized:
(1) the carboxylate group in nigericin participates in coordination,
while in monensin, being too far removed, it does not; and (2) nigericin
is, by its greater flexibility, capable of catching large cations (Lutz
et al., 1970), which might be the result of a recombination rate that
is higher than the dissociation rate. (The rate of formation of the Na^+
complex is reported to be almost diffusion controlled, e.g., $>1 \times 10^{10}$
mol^{-1} sec^{-1}; Chock et al., 1977.)

5. Lysocellin

Lysocellin is a quite mobile molecule [the hinges here are: C(2)−C(3),
C(8)−C(9), C(10)−C(11), C(11)−C(12), C(12)−C(13), and C(16)−
C(17)], some rotors being under strain even in the native form [quasi-
syndiaxial conditions, e.g., C(16)−C(17)]. It is not surprising that

selectivity is low, and by virtue of the bad screening, lysocellin prefers to adopt a dimeric form with divalent cations, for which association is much better (Mitani et al., 1977).

V. CONCLUSION

With the rise of ^{13}C spectroscopy, it was once thought that ^{1}H work would become of less consequence. The latter, however, produces quite a lot of unique information regarding conformation. ^{1}H NMR spectroscopy, especially with the new techniques offered by high-field instrumentation in FT, allow more and more insight into the spatial architecture of complex biomolecules.

Data such as shifts, couplings, relaxations, solvent accessibility, and ASIS effects produce more information than one might guess. It is fortuituous that ionophores have a rather discrete number of molecular conformations, a fact that greatly alleviates the interpretation of the spectral phenomena and makes them excellent objects for study. They represent perhaps the smallest biostructures, governed by simple and well-known conformational rules. The major outcome one may expect is a better understanding of biophysical mechanisms, for which ionophores are one of the easiest targets. One may hope that in the near future the tackling of *dynamic* processes by NMR spectroscopy will give a new dimension to our knowledge about the interplay between biological entities, which, although based on generalized and common rules, are astonishingly selective, specific, and elegantly designed. Dynamic processes such as recombination/dissociation rates can now be monitored by pulse NMR techniques, either by observation of ^{1}H or by other nuclei (Degani, 1977, 1978b; Degani and Friedman, 1975; Degani and Elgavish, 1978; Degani et al., 1976).

REFERENCES

Abraham, R. J., and Bakke, J. M. (1978). The calculation of ^{2}J(H, H) couplings in benzyl groups. *Org. Magn. Reson. 11*:373-374.
Alléaume, M. (1975), as reported in Gachon, P., and Kergomard, A. (1975). Grisorixin, an ionophorous antibiotic of the nigericin group. *J. Antibiot. 28*:351-357.
Alléaume, M., and Hickel, D. (1970). Crystal structure of grisorixin silver salt. *Chem. Commun. 1970*:1421-1423.
Alléaume, M. and Hickel, D. (1972). Crystal structure of the thallium salt of the antibiotic grisorixin. *J. Chem. Soc. Chem. Commun. 1972*:175-176.
Alléaume, M., Busetta, B., Farges, C., Gachon, P., Kergomard, A., and Staron, T. (1975). X-ray structure of alborixin, a new antibiotic ionophore. *J. Chem. Soc. Chem. Commun. 1975*:411-412.
Altona, C., and Haasnoot, C. A. G. (1980). Prediction of anti and

gauche vicinal proton-proton coupling constants in carbohydrates: A simple additivity rule for pyranose rings. *Org. Magn. Reson.* 13:417-429.

Anderson, W. A., and Freeman R. (1962). Influence of a second radiofrequency field on high resolution nmr spectra. *J. Chem. Phys.* 37:85-103.

Anet, F. A. L. (1974). ^{13}C Nmr at high magnetic fields. In *Topics in Carbon-13 Nmr Spectroscopy*, Vol. 1. G. C. Levy (Ed.). John Wiley and Sons, New York, pp. 209-227.

Anteunis, M. (1966). The influence of spatial orientation of free orbitals in PMR spectroscopy. Influence of vicinal orbitals on ^{3}J and ^{2}J. *Bull. Soc. Chim. Belg.* 75:413-425.

Anteunis, M. (1971). Vicinal exocyclic couplings and constitutional problems. *Bull. Soc. Chim. Belg.* 80:3-7.

Anteunis, M. (1977a). Solution conformation of the antibiotic 3823A (monensin-A)-sodium salt. *Bull Soc. Chim. Belg.* 86:367-381.

Anteunis, M. (1977b). Solution conformation of the ionophore X-206 and its sodium salt. *Bull. Soc. Chim. Belg.* 86:931-947.

Anteunis, M. (1977c). Solution conformation of the ionophore A23187 and its magnesium salt. *Bioorg. Chem.* 6:1-11.

Anteunis, M. (1977d). Solution conformation of lysocellin-Na$^+$; more than a simple structural analog of lasalocid-Na$^+$. *Bull. Soc. Chim. Belg.* 86:187−198.

Anteunis, M. (1981). Application of simple rules for the prediction of the conformation of carboxylic acid ionophores. *Bull. Soc. Chim. Belg.* 90:449-470.

Anteunis, M. (1982). ASIS effect and lipophilicity of biomolecules. In preparation.

Anteunis, M., and Rodios, N. A. (1978). Solution conformation of monensin free acid, a typical representative of the polyetherin antibiotic. *Bioorg. Chem.* 7:47-55.

Anteunis, M. J., and Rodios, N. (1981). Solution conformation of 17-epi-deoxy-(O-8)-salinomycin disclosing the predestination for closure of carboxylic acid antibiotics. Triggered flexibility by a hinge mechanism. *Bull. Soc. Chim. Belg.* 90:471-480.

Anteunis, M., and Verhegge, G. (1977). Solution conformation of the ionophore A204A Na$^+$-salt. *Bull Soc. Chim. Belg.* 86:353-

Anteunis, M., Tavernier, D., and Borremans, F. (1966). Experiments on ketals. VI. PMR spectra of alkyl substituted 3-dioxanes with rigid or anancomeric structures. *Bull Soc. Chim. Belg.* 75:396-412.

Anteunis, M., Swaelens, G., Anteunis-De Ketelaere, F., and Dirinck, P. (1971a). NMR-experiments on acetals. Part 28. 1,3-Dioxanes with non-chair conformations and the ^{2}J(OCH$_2$O) criterium. *Bull. Soc. Chim. Belg.* 80:409-422.

Anteunis, M., Swaelens, G., and Gelan, J. (1971b). NMR-experiments on acetals. Part 32. Dependency of geminal coupling constants of methylene groups on electronegativity, bond length and free orbital overlap of adjacent lobes, an empirical relationship as a tool for conformational description. *Tetrahedron* 27:1917-1929.

Anteunis, M., Becu, Chr., and Anteunis-De Ketelaere, F. (1974). NMR experiments on acetals. 45. Conformational aspects of 7,7-dimethyl-2,4-dioxabicyclo[3.3.1]-nonane. *J. Acta. Cienc. Indica* 1:1-6.

Anteunis, M., Rodios, N. A., and Verhegge, G. (1977). Solution conformation of dianemycin, its sodium salt and of lenoremycin-Na$^+$ (Ro 21-6150 or A-130-A). *Bull. Soc. Chim. Belg.* 86:609-632.

Axenrod, T., and Webb, G. A. (Eds.) (1974). *NMR Spectroscopy of Nuclei Other than Protons.* John Wiley and Sons, New York.

Baker, E. B. (1962). Two synthesizer nuclear spin decouplings; INDOR spectra of $^{13}CF_3COOH$ and $CF_3{}^{13}COOH$, $^{14}NH_4{}^+$, and $(CH_3)_4{}^{29}Si$. *J. Chem. Phys.* 37:911-912.

Barfield, M., and Grant, D. M. (1963). The effect of hyperconjugation on the geminal spin-spin coupling constant. *J. Am. Chem. Soc.* 85:1899-1905.

Barfield, M., Hruby, V. J. and Méraldi, J. -P. (1976). The dependence of geminal H-H spin coupling constants on ϕ and ψ angles of peptides in solution. *J. Am. Chem. Soc.* 98:1308-1314.

Bell, R. A. (1973). The chemical application of the nuclear Overhauser effect. In *Topics in Stereochemistry*, Vol. 7, N. L. Allinger and E. L. Eliel (Eds.). John Wiley and Sons, New York, pp. 1-92.

Berg, D. H., and Hamill, R. L. (1978). The isolation and characterization of narasin, a new polyether antibiotic. *J. Antibiot.* 31:1-6.

Biellmann, J. -F., Hanna, R., Ourisson, G., Sandris, C., and Waegell, S. (1960). Etude d'interactions 1-3. *Bull. Soc. Chim. Fr.* 1429-1430.

Bissel, E. C., and Paul, I. C. (1972). Crystal and molecular structure of a derivative of the free acid of the antibiotic X 537A. *J. Chem. Soc. Chem. Commun.* 1972:967-968.

Blount, J. F., and Westley, J. W. (1971). X-ray crystal and molecular structure of antibiotic X 206. *J. Chem. Soc. Chem. Commun.* 1971:927-928.

Blount, J. F., and Westley, J. W. (1975). Crystal and molecular structure of the free acid form of antibiotic X-206 hydrate. *J. Chem. Soc. Chem. Commun.* 1975:533.

Borremans, F. and Anteunis, M. J. O. (1981). Predictability of proton chemical shifts in polyether carboxylic acid ionophores. *Bull. Soc. Chim. Belg.* 90:1045-1053.

Bradbury, J. H., Crompton, M. W., and Warren, B. (1974). Determination of the sequence of peptides by PMR spectroscopy. *Anal. Biochem.* 62:310-316.

Briggs, R. W., and Hinton, J. F. (1979). Thallium-205 and ^{1}H NMR studies on the complexes of Tl(1) with the antibiotics nonactin, monactin and dinactin. *J. Magn. Reson.* 33:363-377.

Bucourt, R. (1974). The torsion angle concept in conformational analysis. In *Topics in Stereochemistry*, Vol. VIII, E. L. Eliel and N. L. Allinger (Eds.). John Wiley and Sons, New York. pp. 160-219.

Burgermeister, W., and Winkler-Oswatitsch, R. (1977). Complex formation of monovalent cations with biofunctional ligands. In *Topics in Current Chemistry. 69. Inorganic Biochemistry. II.* Fr. L. Boschke, (Ed.). Springer-Verlag, Berlin, Heidelberg, New York, pp. 91-196.

Bystrov, V. F., Gavilov, Yu. D., Ivanov, V. T., and Ovchinnikov, Yu. A. (1977). Refinement of the solution conformation of valinomycin. *Eur. J. Biochem.* 78:63-82.

Campbell, I. D., Dobson, C. M., Williams, R. J. P., and Wright, P. E. (1975). Pulse methods for the simplification of protein NMR-spectra. *FEBS Lett.* 57:96-99.

Chaney, M. O., Demarco, P. V., Jones, N. D., and Occolowitz, J. L. (1974). The structure of A23187, a divalent cation ionophore. *J. Am. Chem. Soc.* 96:1932-1933.

Chalmers, A. A., Pachler, K. G. R., and Wessels, P. L. (1974). Difference selective population inversion spectra and their application to the study of ^{13}C-H coupling constants in 2,3-dibromothiophene. *J. Magn. Reson.* 15:415-419.

Chivers, P., and Crabb, T. (1970). The NMR spectra of syn and anti perhydro 7,11-methanopyrido 1,2-C (1,3) diazorine and the influence of the nitrogen lone pair on the geminal coupling constant of an adjacent methylene group. *Tetrahedron* 26:3389-3399 and references cited therein.

Chock, P. B., Egger, F., Eigen, M., and Winkler, R. (1977). Relaxation studies on complex formation of macrocyclic and open chain antibiotics with monovalent cations. *Biophys. Chem.* 6:239-251.

Cookson, R. C., and Crabb, T. A. (1972). Geminal coupling constants in methylene groups. *Tetrahedron* 28:2139-2143.

Cox, H. E. (1921). Influence of the solvent of the temperature coefficient of certain relations. A test of the radiation hypothesis. *J. Chem. Soc. London* 119:142-158.

Cramer III, R. D. (1977). Hydrophobic interaction and solvation energies. Discrepancies between theory and experimental data. *J. Am. Chem. Soc.* 99:5408-5411.

Czerwinski, E. W., and Steinrauf, L. K. (1971). Structure of the antibiotic dianemycin. *Biochem. Biophys. Res. Commun.* 45: 1224-1287.

Dadok, J., and Sprecher, R. F. (1974). Correlation NMR spectroscopy. *J. Magn. Reson.* 13:243-248.

Danneels, D., and Anteunis, M. (1974). Influence of methyl substituents on the chemical shift of the ring protons in mono-, di- and trimethylcyclohexanes. *Org. Magn. Reson.* 6:617-621.

Davies R. (1975). Relationship between the magnitude of J_{gem} and the spatial orientation of β-substituents. *J. Chem. Soc. Perkin Trans.* 2:1400-1411.

Davies, R., and Hudec, J. (1975). Relationship between the magnitude of J_{gem} and the spatial orientation of α-substituents. *J. Chem. Soc. Perkin Trans.* 2:1395-1400.

De Bruyn, A., and Anteunis, M. (1976). Experimental data for gauche couplings in carbohydrates. *Org. Magn. Reson.* 8:228 and references cited therein.

Degani, H. (1977). Kinetics of monensin complexation with sodium ions by ^{23}Na NMR spectroscopy. *Biophys. Chem.* 6:345-349.

Degani, H. (1978a). NMR kinetic studies of the ionophore X-537A- (lasalocid). Mediated transport of manganous ions across phospholipid bilayers. *Biochem. Biophys. Acta* 509:364-369.

Degani, H. (1978b). Ionic permeabilities of membranes. NMR kinetic studies. In *N.M.R. Spectroscopy in Molecular Biology*, B. Pullman, (Ed.). D. Reidel, Dordrecht, Holland, pp. 393-403.

Degani, H., and Elgavish, G. A. (1978). Ionic permeabilities of membranes. ^{23}Na and ^{7}Li NMR studies of ion transport across the membrane of phosphatidylcholine vesicles. *FEBS Lett.* 90:357-360.

Degani, H., and Friedman, H. L. (1975). Ion binding by X-537A. Rates of complexation of Na^{2+} and Mn^{2+} in methanol. *Biochemistry* 14:3755-3761.

Degani, H., Hamilton, R. M. D., and Friedman, H. L. (1976). Ion binding by X-537A. Equilibrium and rate of complexation of Ca^{2+} in methanol. *Biophys. Chem.* 4:363-366.

De Keukeleire, D., Vanheertum, R., and Verzele, M. (1971). On the hydroxyl group P.M.R.-signals in 2- and 4-acylresorcinols and the structure of humulone. *Bull. Soc. Chim. Belg.* 80:393-396.

Dunitz, J. D., and Prelog, V. (1960). Röntgenographisch bestimmte Konformationen und Reaktivität Mittlerer Ringe. *Angew. Chem.* 72:896-902.

Dwek, R. A. (1973). *NMR in Biochemistry. Applications to Enzyme Systems.* Clarendon Press, Oxford.

Engler, E. M., and Laszlo, P. (1971). A new description of nuclear magnetic resonance solvent shifts for polar solutes in weakly associating aromatic solvents. *J. Am. Chem. Soc.* 93:1317-1327.

Ernst, R. R., and Anderson, W. A. (1966). Application of Fourier transform spectroscopy to magnetic resonance. *Rev. Sci. Instrum.* 37:93-102.

Feeney, J., and Partington, P. (1973). Pseudo Indor NMR spectra using double resonance difference spectroscopy and the Fourier transform technique. *J. Chem. Soc. Chem. Commun.* 1973:611-612.

Freeman, R. (1980). Nuclear magnetic resonance spectroscopy in two frequency dimensions. *Proc. R. Soc. London A* 373:149-178.

Gachon, P., and Kergomard, A. (1975). Grisorixin, an ionophorous antibiotic of the nigericin group. II. Chemical and structural study of grisorixin and some derivatives. *J. Antibiot.* 28:351-357.

Gachon, P., Farges, Chr., and Kergomard, A. (1976). Alborixin, a new antibiotic ionophore: Isolation, structure, physical and chemical properties. *J. Antibiot.* 29:603-610.

Gagnaire, D., and Vincendon, M. (1977). Easy identification of hydroxy-bearing carbon atoms in ^{13}C nuclear magnetic resonance spectroscopy: A new method for signal assignment in carbohydrates. *J. Chem. Soc. Chem. Commun.*:509-510.

Gagnaire, D., Mancier, D., and Vincendon, M. (1978). Spectres RMN des polysaccharides et de leurs dérivés: influence des substituents sur le déplacement chimique ^{13}C. *Org. Magn. Reson.* 11:344-349.

Glickson, J. D., Gordon, S. L., Pitner, T. Ph., and Walter, R. (1976). Intramolecular ^{1}H NOE effect studies (valinomycin in DMSO-d_6). *Biochemistry* 15:5721-5729.

Grandjean, J., and Laszlo, P. (1979). ^{23}Na-NMR study of the competition of biogenic amines with sodium ion for binding to lasalocid (X-537A). *Angew. Chem. Int. Ed. Engl.* 18:153-154; *Angew. Chem.* 91:166.

Gupta, R. K., Faretti, J. A., and Becker, E. D. (1975). Rapid scan Fourier transform NMR spectroscopy. *J. Magn. Reson.* 13:275-290.

Haasnoot, C. A. G., de Leeuw, F. A. A. M., and Altona, C. (1980). The relationship between proton-proton NMR coupling constants and substituent electronegativities. I. An empirical generalization of the Karplus equation. *Tetrahedron* 36:2783-2792.

Haasnoot, C. A. G., de Leeuw, F. A. A. M., de Leeuw, H. P. H., and Altona, C. (1981). The relationship between proton-proton NMR coupling constants and substituent electronegativities. II. Conformational analysis of the sugar ring in nucleosides and nucleotides in solution using a generalized Karplus equation. *Org. Magn. Reson.* 15:43-52.

Haynes, D. H., Kowalsky, A., and Pressman, B. C. (1969). Application of nuclear magnetic resonance to the conformational changes in valinomycin during complexation. *J. Biol. Chem.* 244:502-505.

Haynes, D. H., Pressman, B. C., and Kowalsky, A. (1971). NMR study of ^{23}Na^{+} complexing by ionophores. *Biochemistry* 10:852-860.

Hofer, O. (1976). The lanthanide induced shift technique: Applications in conformational analysis. In *Topics in Stereochemistry*, Vol. 9, N. L. Allinger and E. L. Eliel (Eds.). John Wiley and Sons, New York. pp. 36-198.

Imada, A., Nozaki, Y., Hasegawa, T., Mizuta, E., Igarasi, S., and Yoneda, M. (1978). Carriomycin, a new polyether antibiotic produced by streptomyces hygroscopicus. *J. Antibiot.* 31:7-14.

James, Th. L. (1975). *Nuclear Magnetic Resonance in Biochemistry. Principles and Applications.* Academic Press, New York.

Kinashi, H., Ōtake, N., Yonehara, H., Sato, S., and Saito, Y. (1973). The structure of salinomycin, a new member of the polyether antibiotics. *Tetrahedron Lett. 1973*:4955-4958.

Kinashi, H., Ōtake, N., Yonehara, H., Sato, S., and Saito, Y. (1975). Studies on the ionophorous antibiotics. I. The crystal and molecular structure of salinomycin p-iodophenacyl ester. *Acta Crystallog. B31*:2411-2415.

Kitame, F., Utsushikawa, K., Kohama, T., Saito, T., Kikuchi, M., and Ishida, N. (1974). Laidlomycin, a new antimycoplasmal polyether antibiotic. *J. Antibiot. 27*:884-889.

Kopple, K. D., and Go, A. (1977). Cyclodimerization of a hexapeptide unit at high concentration. Rationalization in terms of the conformation of the cyclic dodecapeptide. *J. Am. Chem. Soc. 99*:7698-7704.

Kopple, K. D., and Schamper, T. J. (1972). Proton magnetic resonance line broadening produced by association with nitroxyde radical in studies of amide and peptide conformation. *J. Am. Chem. Soc. 94*:3644-3646.

Kopple, K. D., Ohnishi, M., and Go, A. (1969). Conformation of cyclic peptides. III. Cyclopentaglycyltyrosyl and related compounds. *J. Am. Chem. Soc. 91*:4264-4272.

Kowalewski, V. J. (1969). The INDOR technique in high-resolution NMR. In *Progress in NMR Spectroscopy*, Vol. 5, J. W. Emsley, J. Feeney, and L. H. Sutcliffe, (Eds.). Pergamon Press, New York, pp. 1-32.

Krasne, S., and Eisenman, G. (1976). Influence of molecular variations of ionophore and lipid on the selective ion permeability of membranes: I. Tetranactin and the methylation of nonactin-type. *J. Membr. Biol. 30*:1-44.

Lallemand, J. Y., and Michon, V. (1978). Carbon-13 nuclear magnetic resonance studies on X537A (lasalocid), an ionophore antibiotic: free acid, sodium and thallium salts, and behaviour in solution. *J. Chem. Res.(S).*, 162-163.

Laszlo, P., and Stang, P. (1971). *Organic Spectroscopy; Principles and Applications.* Harper and Row, New York, pp. 76, 250.

Ledaal, T. (1968). Solvent effects in NMR spectroscopy. The geometry of solute/solvent collision complexes. *Tetrahedron Lett. 1968*:1683-1688.

Lehmann, J. (1976). Chemie der Kohlenhydrate. Monosaccharide und Derivate. In *Thieme Taschenlehrbuch der Organische Chemie*, Serie 10/B, George Thieme Verlag, Stuttgart, p. 44.

Lehn, J. M., Sauvage, J. P., and Dietrich, B. (1970). Cryptates. Cation exchange rates. *J. Am. Chem. Soc. 92*:2916-2918.

Lemieux, R. U. (1971). Effects of unshared pairs of electrons and their solvation on conformational equilibria. *Pure Appl. Chem.* 25:526-548.

Levy, G. C., and Lichter R. L. (1979). *Nitrogen-15 NMR Spectroscopy.* John Wiley and Sons, New York.

Lindenbaum, S., Rytting, J. H., and Sternson, L. A. (1979). Ionophores, biological transport mediators. In *Progress in Macrocyclic Chemistry* Vol. I, R. M. Izatt and J. J. Christensen (Eds.). John Wiley and Sons, New York, pp. 220-250.

Llinás, M., and Klein, M. P. (1975). Charge relay at the peptide bond. A PMR study of solvation effects on the amide electron density distribution. *J. Am. Chem. Soc.* 99:5408-5411.

Lohman, J. A. B., and MacLean, C. (1978). Alignment effects on high resolution NMR spectra induced by the magnetic field. *Chem. Phys.* 35:269-274.

Lutz, W. K., Wipf, H. -K., and Simon, W. (1970). Alkalikationen-Spezifität und Träger-Eigenschaften der Antibiotica Nigericin und Monensin. *Helv. Chim. Acta* 53:1741-1746.

Lutz, W. K., Winkler, F. K., and Dunitz, J. D. (1971). Crystal structure of the antibiotic monensin. Similarities and differences between free acid and metal complex. *Helv. Chim. Acta* 54:1103-1108.

Martin, J. S., and Dayly, B. P. (1963). Proton chemical shifts in polysubstituted benzenes. *J. Chem. Phys.* 39:1722-1728.

Mitani, M., and Otake, N. (1978). Studies on the ionophorous antibiotics. XV. The monovalent cation selective ionophorous activities of carriomycin, lonomycin and etheromycin. *J. Antibiot.* 31:750-755.

Mitani, M., Yamanishi, T., Ebata, E., Otake, N., and Koenuma, M. (1977). Studies on ionophorous antibiotics. VII. A broad cation selective ionophore, lysocellin. *J. Antibiot.* 30:186-188.

Miyazaki, Y., Shibuya, M., Sugawara, H., Kawaguchi, O., Hirose, Ch., and Nagatsu, J. (1974). Salinomycin a new polyether antibiotic. *J. Antibiot.* 27:814-821.

Morishima, I., Endo, K., and Yonezawa, T. (1971). Studies on nuclear magnetic resonance contact shifts induced by hydrogen bonding with organic radicals. I. [1]H and [13]C Contact shifts of protic molecules in the presence of the nitroxyde radical. *J. Am. Chem. Soc.* 93:2048-2050.

Morishima, I., Endo, K., and Yonezawa, T. (1973). Interaction between closed- and open-shell molecules. VI. [1]H and ^{13}C contact shifts and molecular orbital studies on the hydrogen bond of nitroxyde radical. *J. Chem. Phys.* 58:3146-3154.

Morris, A. T., and Dwek, R. A. (1977). Some recent applications of the use of paramagnetic centres to probe biological systems using NMR. *Q. Rev. Biophys.* 10:421-484.

Nieboer, E., and Falter, H. (1977). Peptide sequence analysis by NMR spectroscopy. In *Molecular Biology, Biochemistry and Bio-*

physics, Vol. 25, Advanced Methods in protein sequence determination. S. B. Needleman (Ed.). Springer-Verlag, Berlin.

Noggle, J. H., and Schiemer, R. E. (1971). Nuclear Overhauser effect. Academic Press, New York.

Ohnishi, M., and Urry, D. W. (1969). Temperature dependence of amide proton chemical shifts. The Secondary structures of gramicidin S and valinomycin. *Biochem. Biophys. Acta 36*:194-202.

Otake, N., Koenuma, M., Miyamae, H., Sato, Sh., and Saito, Y. (1975). Studies on the ionophorous antibiotics. Part III. The structure of lonomycin, a polyether antibiotic. *Tetrahedron Lett. 1975*:4147-4150.

Otake, N., Koenuma, M., Miyamae, H., Sato, S., and Saito, Y. (1977). Studies on the ionophorous antibiotics. IV. Crystal and molecular structure of the thallium salt of lonomycin. *J. Chem. Soc. Perkin Trans. 2, 1979*:494-496.

Patel, D. J., and Shen, C. (1976). Structural and kinetic studies of lasalocid A (X537A) and its silver, sodium and barium salts in nonpolar solvents. *Proc. Nat. Acad. Sci. USA 73*:1786-1790.

Pfeiffer, D. R., and Deber, C. M. (1979). Isosteric metal complexes of ionophore A 23187. A basis for cation selectivity. *FEBS Lett. 105*:360-364.

Pitner, T. P., and Urry, D. W. (1972). PMR studies in trifluorethanol solvent mixtures as a mean of delineating peptide protons. *J. Am. Chem. Soc. 95*:1399-1400.

Pressman, B. C. (1976). Biological applications of ionophores. *Annu. Rev. Biochem. 45*:501-530.

Prestegard, J. H., and Chan, S. I. (1969). Studies of the cation-binding properties of nonactin. I. The K^+-nonactin complex. *Biochemistry 8*:3921-3927.

Prestegard, J. H., and Chan, S. I. (1970). Studies of the cation-binding properties of nonactin. II. Comparison of the sodium ion, potassium ion and cesium ion complexes. *J. Am. Chem. Soc. 92*:4440-4446.

Pretcher, T. J., and Weber, H. P. (1974). X-ray crystal structure and absolute configuration of p-bromophenylacyl-septamycin monohydrate. *J. Chem. Soc. Chem. Commun. 1974*:697-698.

Rodios, N. A., and Anteunis, M. (1977). Solution conformation of nigericin-free acid and nigericin-sodium salt. *Bull. Soc. Chim. Belg. 86*:917-929.

Rodios, N. A., and Anteunis, M. (1978a). Solution conformation of septamycin and its sodium salt. *J. Antibiot. 31*:294-301.

Rodios, N. A., and Anteunis, M. J. O. (1978b). Solution conformation of lonomycin-free acid and lonomycin-sodium salt. A ^{1}H NMR study. *Bull. Soc. Chim. Belg. 87*:447-457.

Rodios, N. A., and Anteunis, M. J. O. (1978c). High resolution ^{1}H NMR study of carriomycin free acid and its sodium salt. *Bull. Soc. Chim. Bdg. 87*:437-446.

Rodios, N., and Anteunis, M. J. O. (1979a). Lonomycin-Na⁺. A recall of its ¹H NMR spectrum. *Bull. Soc. Chim. Belg. 88*:37-41.

Rodios, N. A., and Anteunis, M. J. O. (1979b). ¹H NMR spectrum and solution conformation of alborixin free acid. *Bull. Soc. Chim. Belg. 88*:279-288.

Rodios, N. A., and Anteunis, M. J. O. (1980). Non-closed forms of monensin and nigericin-free acid in protic solvents. *Bull. Soc. Chim. Belg. 89*:537-550.

Samek, Z. (1971). Configurational assignment of secondary methyl groups based on the average coupling constant J(CH₃——CH). *Tetrahedron Lett. 1971*:1709-1712.

Sandrus, C., and Ourisson, G. (1958). Etude des cétones cycliques (V): Un effet conformationnel nouveau. *Bull. Soc. Chim. Fr.* :1524-1526.

Schmidt, P. G., Wang, A. H. -J. and Paul, I. C. (1974). A structural study on the sodium salt of the ionophore, X-537A (lasalocid), by X-ray and NMR analysis. *J. Am. Chem. Soc. 96*:6189-6191.

Schwetlick, K. (1971). In *Kinetische Methoden zur Untersuchung von Reaktionsmechanismen.* VEB Deutscher Verlag der Wissenschafften, p. 114 (1971).

Schwyzer, R., and Ludescher U. (1969). Untersuchungen über die Konformation des Cyclischen Hexapeptids Cyclo-Glycyl-L-Prolyl-Glycyl-Glycyl-L-Prolyl-Glycyl Mittels PMR und Parallelen zum Cyclodecapeptid Gramicidin S. *Helv. Chem. Acta 52*:2033-2040.

Shen, C., and Patel, D. J. (1976). Free acid, anion, alkali and alkaline earth complexes of lasalocid A (X537A) in methanol: Structural and kinetic studies at the monomer level. *Proc. Nat. Acad. Sci. USA 73*:4277-4281.

Shiro, M., and Koyama, H. (1970). Crystal structure of silver polyetherin A. *J. Chem. Soc. B*:243-253.

Sorenson, S., Hansen, R. S., and Jacobson, H. J. (1974). Assignments and relative signs of ¹³C-X coupling constants in ¹³C FT NMR from selective population transfer (SPT). *J. Magn. Reson. 14*:243-245.

Spoormaker, T., and de Bie, M. J. A. (1978). Long-range carbon-proton spin-spin coupling constants. A ¹³C NMR study of mono-halogen substituted ethanes and propanes. *Rec. Trav. Chim. Pays-Bas 97*:135-144.

Spoormaker, T., and de Bie, M. J. A. (1979). An additivity relation for vicinal carbon proton spin-spin coupling constants in aliphatic compounds. *Rec. Trav. Chim. Pays-Bas 98*:59-64.

Srivanavit, Ch., Zink, J. I., and Dechter, J. J. (1977). A thallium NMR determination of polyether cation selectivity sequences and their solvent dependences. *J. Am. Chem. Soc. 99*:5876-5881.

Steinrauf, L. K., Czerwinski, E. W., and Pinkerton, M. (1971). Comparison of the monovalent cation complexes, nigericin and dianemycin. *Biochem. Biophys. Res. Commun. 45*:1279-1287.

Urry, D. W., Mitchell, L. W., and Onishi, T. (1974). ^{13}C Magnetic resonance evaluation of polypeptide secondary structure and correlation with proton magnetic resonance studies. *Proc. Natl. Acad. Sci. USA 71*:3265.

Urry, D. W., Long, M. M., Jacobs, M., and Harris, R. D. (1975). Molecular mechanism of ion-ionophore complexation. Part V. Conformation and molecular mechanisms of carriers and channels. *Ann. N.Y. Acad. Sci. 264*:203-220.

Wen-Chih Liu, Slusarchyk, D. S., Astle, G., Trejo, W. H., Brown, W. E., and Meyers, E. (1978). Ionomycin, a new polyether antibiotic. *J. Antibiot. 31*:814-819.

Westley, J. W. (1976). A proposed numbering system for polyether antibiotics. *J. Antibiot. 29*:584-586.

Westley, J. W., Blount, J. F., Evans, R. H. Jr., and Chao-Min Liu (1977). C-17 Epimers of deoxy-(O-8)-salinomycin from streptomyces albus (ATCC 21838). *J. Antibiot. 30*:610-612.

White, R. J., Martinelli, E., Gallo, G. G., Lancini, G., and Beynon, P. (1973). Rifamycin biosynthesis studies with ^{13}C-enriched precursors and carbon magnetic resonance. *Nature 243*:273-277.

Witanowski, M., Stefaniak, L., and Webb, G. A. (1977). Nitrogen NMR spectroscopy. *In Annual Reports on NMR-Spectroscopy* Vol. 7, G. A. Webb, (Ed.). Academic Press, New York, pp. 117-244.

Wong, D. T., Horng, J. -S., and Hamill, R. L. (1971). Effect of a new monocarboxylic acid antibiotic A 204 on the monovalent cation permeability of rat liver mitochondria. *Biochem. Pharmacol. 20*:3169-3177.

Wüthrich, K. (1976). *NMR in Biological Research: Peptides and Proteins*. North-Holland/American Elsevier, New York.

chapter 6

13C NMR SPECTRA OF POLYETHER ANTIBIOTICS

Haruo Seto and *Noboru Ōtake*
Institute of Applied Microbiology, University of Tokyo, Tokyo, Japan

I. INTRODUCTION

The polyether antibiotics characterized as possessing several cyclic ether systems are mainly produced by the *Streptomyces* genus (Westley, 1977b). Due to structural complexity, easier preparation of heavy metal-containing derivatives, difficulty to obtain degradation products useful for structural studies, and extensively overlapping ^{1}H NMR spectra, x-ray analysis has been the only practical method for structural elucidation of these compounds (see Chapter 3). Until a few years ago, on the other hand, ^{13}C NMR spectroscopy, which has played an important role in natural product chemistry, was not a method of choice for structural studies of polyether antibiotics due apparently to the difficulty in analyzing very complicated ^{13}C NMR spectra. This obstacle has been overcome in recent years by the aid of the biosynthetic labeling method, as well as Anteunis' extensive ^{1}H NMR works (see Chapter 5) which enable unambiguous assignments of ^{13}C signals to be made through selective proton decoupling. As a result, enough ^{13}C NMR spectral data have accumulated to establish the relationships between specific structures and chemical shifts of relevant carbons in the ^{13}C NMR spectra of polyether antibiotics (Seto et al., 1979a).

Thus ^{13}C NMR spectroscopy, which allows one to observe almost all carbon resonances without overlapping, is now becoming a very attractive methodology for researchers working in the field of polyether antibiotics.

In this chapter assignments of almost all of the polyethers will be presented, together with their application to structural studies. These data will be useful for analyzing solution conformations of the polyether antibiotics, their interactions with metal cations, and structures of new polyether antibiotics to be isolated in the future.

II. TECHNIQUES USED FOR ^{13}C ASSIGNMENTS OF POLYETHER ANTIBIOTICS

One of the structural features of most polyether antibiotics is the repetition of similar partial structures in the molecules, which results in complicated ^{13}C NMR spectra with many methylene and methine signals crowded in a narrow region. Therefore, in addition to commonly employed techniques such as single-frequency off-resonance decoupling (sford) and selective proton-carbon decoupling, partially relaxed Fourier transform (PRFT) NMR techniques and biosynthetic methods are required to obtain total assignments of ^{13}C NMR spectra of polyether antibiotics. Some explanations of these methods will be given in the following.

A. Differentiation of Methyl, Methylene, Methine, and
   Quaternary Carbon Signals

The first step in analyzing ^{13}C NMR spectra is to discriminate methyl,
methylene, methine, and quaternary carbons. This can be accomplished
mostly by sford or sometimes by weak-noise off-resonance decoupling,
which enables to detect nonprotonated carbons (Roth, 1977). In case
of the polyether antibiotics, however, sford is not necessarily a useful
technique for identifying methylenes and methines (and occasionally
tert-methyls) in the region of about 25-40 ppm, due to extensive signal
overlap under the sford conditions (see Figure 1e). Higher-order
couplings as well as unequivalent chemical shifts of some methylene
protons make the situation even worse (Roth, 1977).

The first step in analyzing this problem can be solved by the PRFT NMR technique (Nakanishi
et al., 1974; Smith, 1978). In this method a 90° monitor pulse is applied to the sample under investigation after some time interval following a 180° pulse which is utilized to invert ^{13}C signals. This pulse
sequence is repeated until satisfactory signal/noise ratio is obtained.
During the waiting time between the two pulses ^{13}C signals begin to
recover to the original state according to their longitudinal relaxation
times (T_1) (Lyerla and Levy, 1974). Since the relaxation time usually
increases in the order of CH_2 < CH ⩽ CH_3 < $-C-$, these signals
can be distinguished from each other by setting an appropriate waiting
time.*

For example, in the PRFT spectrum of nigericin sodium salt (Figure
1b; waiting time 0.20 sec) methylene resonances appear as positive
signals while the methine and methyl peaks remain negative. It should
be noted that the distinction of these signals can be hardly made by
sford (Figure 1e). Although time-consuming, one can obtain more
precise information by measuring the relaxation time, which further
enables the distinction of carbon resonances due to the deoxy sugar
showing longer T_1 values, from those of the aglycone, with much
shorter T_1 values in glycosidic polyether antibiotics (groups 2 and 3b,
see later). A detailed explanation was given by Wehrli (1976) of the use
of ^{13}C spin relaxation data in organic structure assignments.

In special cases observation of the sford spectra under a PRFT condition (Figure 1d) or selective excitation condition (Martin, et al.,
1979) may be necessary to analyze overlapping signals. The latter
technique facilitates the selective observation of signals in a very

---

*T_1 is dependent on several factors, such as molecular weight, molec-
ular shape, sample concentration, temperature, solvent, and strength
of the magnetic field of NMR spectrometers. The author's experiences,
however, show that the suitable waiting time for this purpose falls in
the relatively narrow range of 0.1-0.2 sec for 0.2-0.5 mol solutions of
most polyethers at 25 MHz.

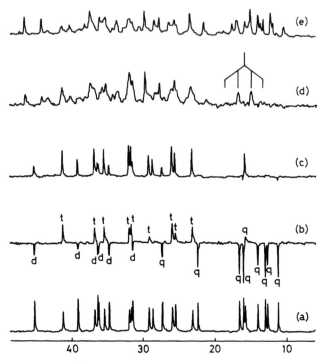

Figure 1 ^{13}C NMR spectra of nigericin sodium salt in CDCl$_3$. (a) Proton noise decoupled. (b) PRFT spectrum (waiting time 0.2 sec; q,t, and d represent methyl, methylene, and methine, respectively). (c) PRFT spectrum (waiting time 0.35 sec). (d) Off-resonance decoupled under PRFT conditions (waiting time 0.35 sec). (e) Off-resonance decoupled.

narrow range, thus preventing the undesirable overlapping of un-necessary peaks.

B. Selective Proton Decoupling

This method is widely utilized in the assignments of ^{13}C NMR spectra. The prerequisites for successful selective proton decoupling are good separation and detailed assignments of ^{1}H signals to be irradiated in the ^{1}H NMR spectra. As explained later, most ^{13}C NMR works were made (and still will be made in future) by using spectrometers operating at 25 MHz (100 MHz with regard to ^{1}H resonance frequency). Under such experimental conditions, these requirements can be hardly satisfied due to overlapping of ^{1}H signals (see Figure 2).

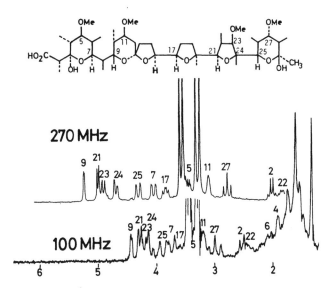

Figure 2 ^{1}H NMR spectra of Ionomycin A sodium salt taken at 100 and 270 MHz in CDCl$_3$. Note the good separation of oxymethine signals in the upper trace.

On the other hand, by taking advantage of better separation obtained by NMR instruments operating at a higher magnetic field, Anteunis et al. made an almost complete analysis of ^{1}H signals, excepting for some methylenes, of the following antibiotics: dianemycin and lenoremycin (Anteunis et al. 1977), X-206 (Anteunis, 1977a), carriomycin (Rodios and Anteunis, 1978a), etheromycin (Anteunis and Rodios, 1978), lonomycin (Rodios and Anteunis, 1978b and 1979), septamycin (Rodios and Anteunis, 1978c), nigericin (Rodios and Anteunis, 1977), monensin (Anteunis, 1977b), lasalocid (Anteunis, 1976), and lysocellin (Anteunis, 1977c). For details of ^{1}H NMR spectra of polyether antibiotics, see chapter 5.

Thus the assignments of ^{13}C resonances of these antibiotics were made possible by selective proton decoupling. For example, based on their work with lonomycin A, signals due to H-2, H-5, H-7, H-9, H-11, H-17, H-22, H-25 and H-27 could be assigned as shown in Figure 2, and the carbons appended to them were unambiguously identified by selective proton-decoupling experiments. Although the protons combining to C-21, C-23, and C-24 are not well separated from each other, it can be seen from Figure 2 that these carbons could be distinguished as a set from the remaining carbons by this technique. Rigorous assignments of C-21, C-23, and C-24 were obtained by the use of other methods such as comparison to structurally related compounds or the biosynthetic method (see Section II.C). Useful explanation on selective proton-decoupling experiments are given in detail by Johnson (1979).

C. Biosynthetic Labeling Method

It has been well recognized that ^{13}C NMR spectroscopy in combination with the use of ^{13}C-labeled precursors is a very useful tool to investigate the biosynthesis of natural products (Tanabe, 1974, 1975, 1976). Utilization of ^{13}C-^{13}C couplings has made this technique more attractive not only for studying reaction mechanisms such as the rearrangement involved in the biosynthetic process, but also for its power in making assignments of ^{13}C signals of complex molecules (Seto et al., 1973).

Biosynthetic studies reported for lasalocid (Westley et al., 1974), narasin (Dorman et al., 1976), salinomycin (Seto et al., 1977a), and lysocellin (Ōtake et al., 1978b) by ^{13}C NMR spectroscopy have revealed that these metabolites are derived from lower fatty acids such as acetic acid, propionic acid, and butyric acid. The polyketide origin of monensin was also confirmed by ^{14}C tracers (Day et al., 1973).

Taking account of structural similarities between the polyether antibiotics, it can be reasonably assumed that all the remaining members of this group would also be built up from the same biosynthetic precursors. This hypothesis enables one to choose a proper precursor to selectively increase signal intensities of desired carbons, thereby enabling one to make easier and more reliable ^{13}C assignments. An application of this technique for analyzing ^{13}C chemical shifts of lonomycin A is explained in the following (Mizoue et al., 1978).

Based on this hypothesis, lonomycin A is expected to derive from 5 acetate and 10 propionate units, as shown in Figure 3. Therefore use of $CH_3{}^{13}COOH$ will enable one to distinguish three oxymethines C-11, C-17, and C-23, and two (hemi)ketals, C-13 and C-29, from the remaining carbons. Furthermore, the carbons adjacent to these functional groups can also be identified by $^{13}CH_3{}^{13}COOH$, which causes $^{13}C-^{13}C$ couplings to occur between C(11)−C(12), C(13)−C(14), C(17)−C(18), C(23)−C(24), and C(29)−C(30). It should be noticed in this case that the partial structures of O−C(O)−CH_2, O−CH−CH−O, and O−C(O)−CH_3 are only found at C(13)−C(14), C(23)−C(24), and C(29)−C(30) to give conclusive evidences for the unambiguous assignments of these carbons.

Distinction of the two combinations between an oxymethine and a methylene, i.e., C(11)−C(12) and C(17)−C(18) can be made with ease by selective proton-decoupling experiments irradiating at the H-11 or H-17 proton. Although the H-11 and H-17 signals are overlapped by other signals in the 100-MHz ^{1}H NMR spectrum, as shown in Figure 2, separation of these two signals is large enough for selective proton decoupling to be successfully carried out at 25 MHz.

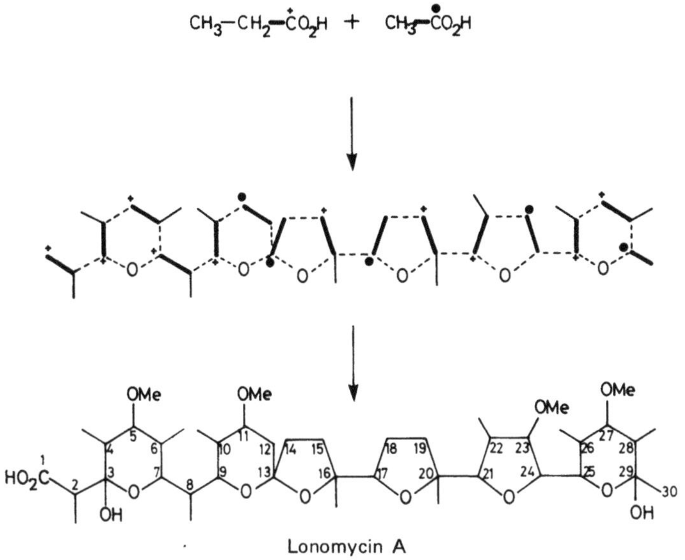

$$CH_3-CH_2-\overset{*}{C}O_2H \; + \; CH_3-\overset{\bullet}{C}O_2H$$

Lonomycin A

Figure 3   Biosynthetic pathway of lonomycin A.

By analogy, it will be easily understood from Figure 3 that $CH_3CH_2{}^{13}COOH$ and $CH_3{}^{13}CH_2{}^{13}COOH$ can be a great help for signal assignments of the remaining carbons, C(1)−C(2), C(3)−C(4), C(5)− C(6), C(7)−C(8), C(9)−C(10), C(15)−C(16), C(19)−C(20), C(21)− C(22), C(25)−C(26), and C(27)−C(28).

As mentioned earlier, the assignments of methylene carbon signals by selective proton decoupling are frequently complicated by severe overlapping and unequivalent chemical shifts of the methylene protons to be irradiated. Biosynthetic labeling, on the other hand, will supply a reliable method to obtain unambiguous assignments of methylene carbons.

In addition to the antibiotics mentioned earlier, this technique has been also used for analyzing ^{13}C NMR spectra of X-206, dianemycin, antibiotic 6016, and nigericin (see later), and the results are contained in Tables 1, 2, 4, 5, 7, 9, and 10.

III. CLASSIFICATION OF POLYETHER ANTIBIOTICS

In Chapter 1, Vol. 1, of this book, Westley has classified the polyether antibiotics according to their affinity for mono or divalent cations. His classification can be accepted for better understanding of the structure-biological activity relationships of the antibiotics under consideration.

However, since the ^{13}C NMR spectral characteristics of the poly-ether antibiotics are determined by their structural features but not by their selectivity against metal cations, in this chapter a different classification system is employed which would be more appropriate to analyze the ^{13}C NMR spectra of the polyether antibiotics.

They are divided into five major groups depending on the characteristic partial structures which are reflected in the chemical shifts of ^{13}C NMR spectra. Representatives of each group are shown in Figure 4. In this chapter explanation will be given to compounds whose ^{13}C NMR data were analyzed in detail.

1. Group 1

An isolated ketone resonance appearing at about 210-220 ppm specifies the members of this group, which are further separated into the following four subgroups.

    1a.   Lasalocid with a 6-substituted 2-hydroxy-3-methyl benzoic acid moiety. Seven signals due to the chromophoric part are observed between 115-175 ppm.

    1b.   Salinomycin, 20-deoxysalinomycin, and narasin (4-methyl-salinomycin) with a tricyclic spiroketal system. Two ketal carbon signals appear at about 99 and 105-107 ppm, together with two olefinic resonances at about 122 and 125-132 ppm.

    1c.   Noboritomycins A and B and CP-44,161. The ^{13}C-spectral features common to 1a and 1b are observed with these metabolites, which can be regarded as hybrids of both the groups.

    1d.   Lysocellin with no olefinic or aromatic carbons.

2. Group 2

Dianemycin, lenoremycin, and leuseramycin are in group 2. The members of this group are characterized by the resonances due to an α-substituted α,β-unsaturated ketone system appearing at about 206-207, 134, and 145-146 ppm.

3. Group 3

There exists the following carbon skeleton common to all the members of this group, with the exception of monensin (Figure 5). The antibiotics of this group possess methoxy carbons appearing at 50-62 ppm, more frequently at 55-60 ppm. The number of the methoxy function ranges from 1 (mutalomycin) to 5 (K-41A and K-41B). This group is further divided into the following subgroups. The members of 3a and 3b contain three (hemi)ketal carbons, whereas those of 3c and 3d possess two (hemi)ketal functions.

    3a.   Lonomycin and mutalomycin without a deoxy sugar.

    3b.   Carriomycin, A204A, etheromycin, septamycin, 6016, K-41A, and K-41B with one or two deoxy sugars. The resonance of

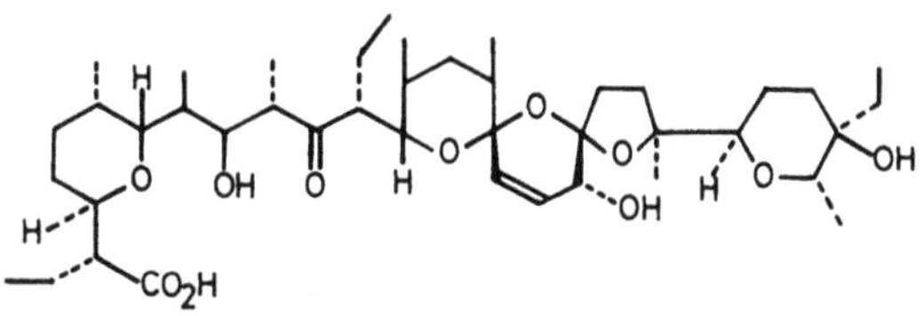

group 1   Salinomycin

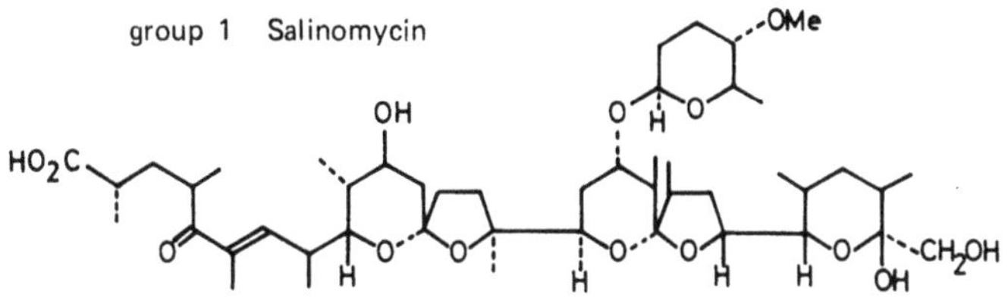

group 2   Dianemycin

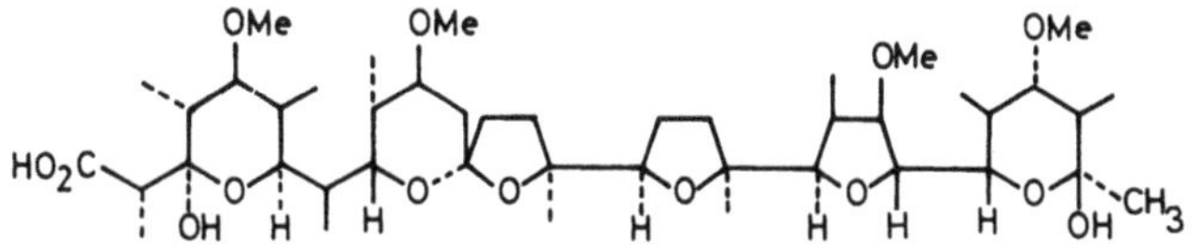

group 3   Lonomycin A

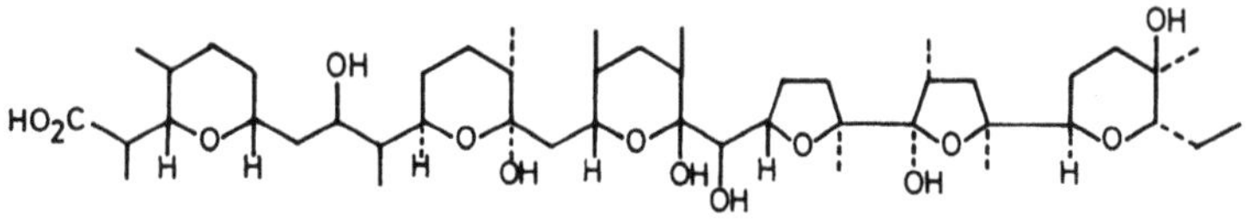

group 4   X - 206

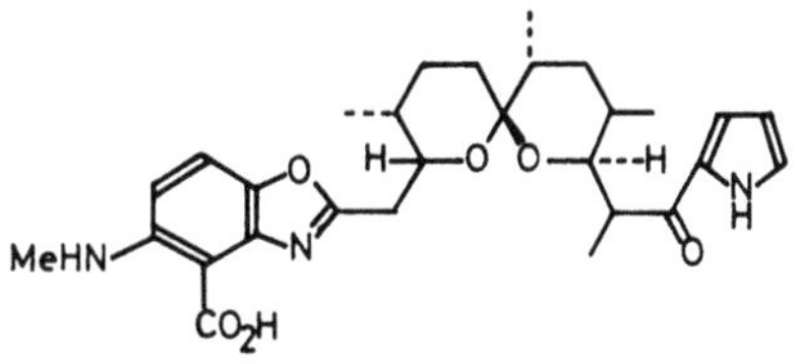

group 5   A 23187

Figure 4   Representative members of the five major groups of polyether antibiotics.

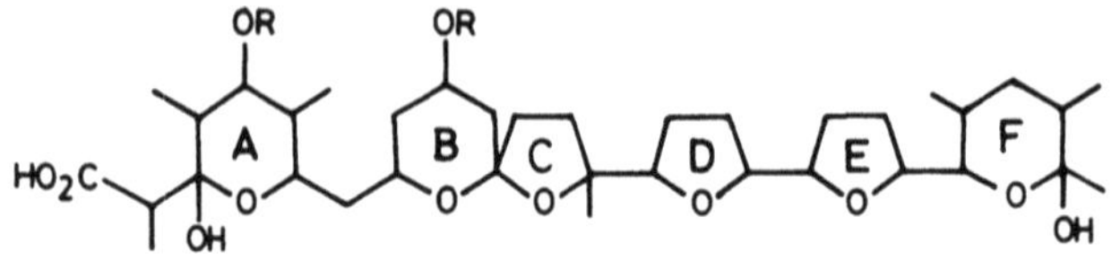

Figure 5 The basic carbon skeleton common to the members of group 3.

an acetal signal (95-103 ppm) due to O-methylamicetose is found only in this group and group 2.

3c. Nigericin and grisorixin lacking a hemiketal function at $C-3$ appearing at 99-100 ppm.

3d. Monensin without the A ring common to the other members of groups 3a to 3c.

4. Group 4

X-206 and alborixin are in group 4. The ^{13}C NMR spectra of these antibiotics are not so characteristic as compared to those of the other groups. The three hemiketal signals together with the lack of any methoxy signals between 50 and 60 ppm specify X-206 and alborixin.

5. Group 5 (miscellaneous)

Ionomycin and A23187 are in group 5.

IV. ^{13}C NMR SPECTRA OF POLYETHER ANTIBIOTICS

Explanation of the ^{13}C NMR spectra of polyether antibiotics are given in the following. For convenient comparison the numbering systems proposed by Westley (1977a) and Westley et al. (1979) are employed in this chapter, with the modification that alkyl or methoxy substituents are referred to the numbers of the carbons to which they attach themselves. This makes it easier to correlate the chemical shifts of methyl, ethyl, or methoxy carbons in similar environments, but with different numbers by the proposed systems.

Most ^{13}C NMR works described in this chapter were made at 25 MHz in CDCl$_3$ or C$_6$D$_6$ solution, using tetramethylsilane as the internal standard. It should be kept in mind that ^{13}C chemical shifts are somewhat dependent on sample concentration, temperature, and solvents. Dorman et al., (1976) described that even a small amount of water contained in CDCl$_3$ affected the ^{13}C chemical shift of narasin. Therefore care must be taken when one compared experimental data with literature values.

A. Group 1

1. Group 1a: lasalocid

Partial assignments of the ^{13}C NMR spectrum of lasalocid (Westley
et al., 1970) appeared in 1974 for the first time based on the incorporation patterns of ^{13}C-enriched precursors (Westley et al., 1974).
Later on, Seto et al., (1978a) completed the assignments of all the
carbon resonances of lasalocid free acid and sodium salt by comparing
their ^{13}C NMR data with those of 2-hydroxy-3-methyl benzoic acid and
the retroaldol ketone obtained by alkaline treatment of lasalocid (Figure 6) (Westley et al., 1970). The ketone, which is an epimeric mixture
of the C-14 center, gave double peaks for 10 of the 12 carbons adjacent
or close to C-14, whereas the 8 carbons associated with the terminal
tetrahydropyran all gave single peaks. The paired signals were assigned by partially relaxed Fourier transform (PRFT) spectra, assum-

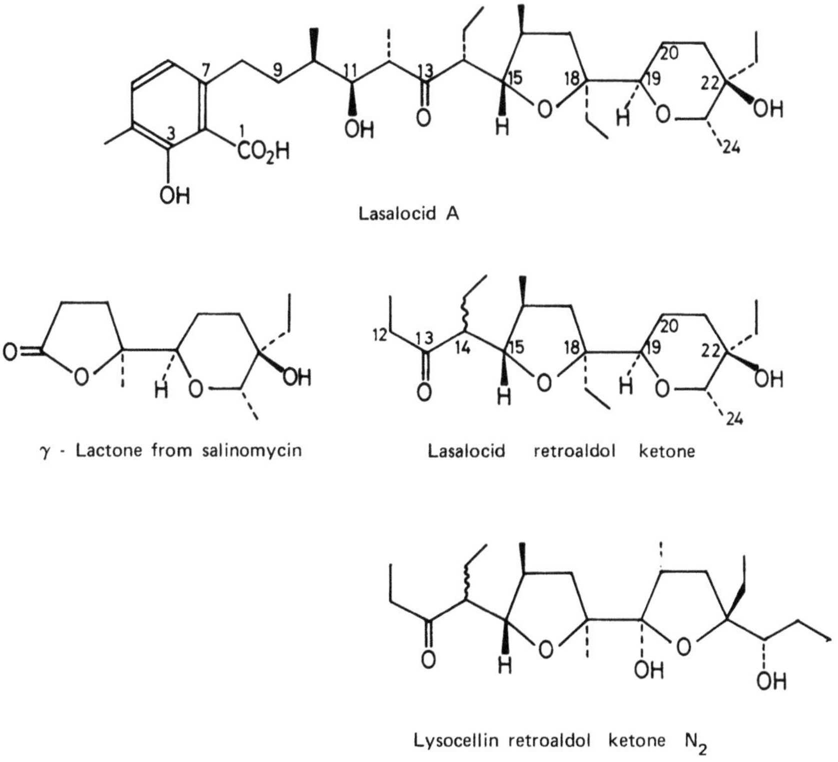

Lasalocid A

γ - Lactone from salinomycin   Lasalocid retroaldol ketone

Lysocellin retroaldol ketone N_2

Figure 6 The structures of lasalocid A, its retroaldol ketone, lysocellin
retroaldol ketone N_2, and γ-lactone from salinomycin.

Table 1 ^{13}C Chemical Shifts of Lasalocid A and Its Retroaldol Ketone

Carbon	Functionality	Lasalocid A free acid (in CD_2Cl_2)	Enriched by[b]	Lasalocid A sodium salt (in CD_2Cl_2)	Retroaldol ketone[a] (in $CDCl_3$)	2-hydroxy-3-methyl benzoic acid ($CDCl_3$)
1	COOH	173.6	1A	176.4		173.4
2	C=	111.2		118.2		112.6
3	HO—C=	161.6	1P	161.3		160.8
4	C=	124.1		131.5		126.7
5	CH=	135.1	1A	131.5		136.8
6	CH=	121.6		119.6		118.9
7	C=	144.4	1A	143.5		128.6[c]
8	CH_2	34.8		33.4		
9	CH_2	37.0	1P	38.1		
10	CH	34.9		34.5		
11	CH—OH	72.8	1P	71.0	37.1(36.4)[c,d]	
12	CH	48.9		49.0	212.6	
13	C=O	214.1	1B	219.9	58.9(57.2)	
14	CH	55.4		55.9	86.5(85.7)	
15	CH—O	84.2	1P	83.1	38.3(36.9)	
16	CH	34.8		34.1	41.0(40.7)	
17	CH_2	38.7	1B	37.9	84.4(84.3)	
18	C—O	86.7		87.6	72.9	
19	CH—O	70.9	1A	68.6		

Carbon	Group					
20	CH_2	20.0		19.5	21.3	
21	CH_2	30.2	1B	29.2	29.5	
22	$C{-}O$	72.4		71.5	70.5	
23	$CH{-}O$	76.6	1A	77.2	76.6	
24	CH_3	14.0		13.6	14.2	15.5
4-Me		15.7		15.3		
10-Me		13.4		13.3		
12-Me		13.2		12.6	7.4[c]	
14-Me		12.9		12.4	12.5(12.2)	
16-Me		15.9		16.0	17.6(16.7)	
18-Me		9.2		9.5	8.1	
22-Me		6.6		6.7	6.4	
14-CH_2		16.7		16.2	21.3(21.0)	
18-CH_2		30.6		29.8	28.7(28.4)	
22-CH_2		30.7		31.1	30.6	

[a] Mixture of epimers at C-14.

[b] 1A, 1P, and 1B represent $CH_3{}^{13}COOH$, $CH_3CH_2{}^{13}COOH$, and $CH_3CH_2CH_2{}^{13}COOH$, respectively.

[c] The functionalities or chemical environments of these carbons are different from those of the corresponding carbons in lasalocid A.

[d] Where two peaks were observed for a single carbon, the one appearing at higher field is arbitrarily expressed in parentheses. Therefore chemical shift values in parentheses do not necessarily correspond to one epimer.

Source: Seto et al., 1978a.

ing that the relaxation times of similar carbons in both the epimers are roughly equal.

The assignments of the ^{13}C signals [C(19)−CH(24), C-22(CH$_2$), and C-22(CH$_3$)] of this ketone were assigned by the γ-lactone obtained from salinomycin (Seto et al., 1977a). The remaining part of the ketone is identical to the corresponding part of the lysocellin retroaldol ketone N$_2$($\overline{O}$take and Koenuma, 1977), and signals common to both the compounds were ascribed to C(12)−C(18), CH$_3$(C-12), CH$_2$(C-14), CH$_3$(C-14), and CH$_3$(C-16). The results are summarized in Table 1.

Independently, Lallemand and Michon (1978) made the ^{13}C NMR assignment of lasalocid by a unique method which utilized coupling between ^{13}C and thallium cation in lasalocid thallium salt. Although most assignments of carbon resonances made by the two groups were identical, discrepancies were observed, especially with C-20 and CH$_2$(C-22). Assuming the involvement of the hydroxy group at C-22 in thallium complex formation, Lallemand and Michon (1978) claimed that the carbon signal at 19.9 ppm showing strong ^{13}C-Tl coupling must be ascribed to CH$_2$(C-22), whereas the other group attributed this resonance to C-20, based on the chemical shift of the corresponding carbon in the γ-lactone (see salinomycin). Selective proton-decoupling experiments based on the work by Anteunis (1976) have proved that the signal in question must be ascribed to C-20 (J. Y. Lallemand, private communication).

2. Group 1b: salinomycin, 20–deoxysalinomycin, and narasin (4–methylsalinomycin)

The structure of narasin (4–methylsalinomycin)
The structural determination of narasin was carried out by comparing its mass-spectral data with those of salinomycin (Figure 7) (Occolowitz et al., 1976). This work, however, only established that narasin is a 4-methyl derivative of salinomycin, and no experimental evidence could be obtained with regard to the stereochemical disposition of the new methyl group. This problem has been solved by ^{13}C NMR investigation (Seto et al., 1977b), which may be taken as evidence showing the advantage of ^{13}C NMR over mass spectroscopy for stereochemical studies of polyether antibiotics.

Comparison of the ^{13}C NMR spectra of narasin and salinomycin revealed the following spectral differences between them (see Figure 8): (1) A new methyl signal appeared at 18.9 ppm in narasin; (2) C-4 methylene (20.1 ppm) in salinomycin changed to a methine (28.9 ppm) in narasin, shifting downfield by 8.8 ppm; and (3) C-5 methylene (26.4 ppm) in salinomycin shifted downfield by 9.1 ppm in narasin. These spectral changes supported the structure of narasin (4-methyl-salinomycin) established by mass spectroscopy.

The equatorial orientation of CH$_3$(C-4) was determined by the small downfield shift (+0.9 ppm) of CH$_3$(C-6). This value can be explained

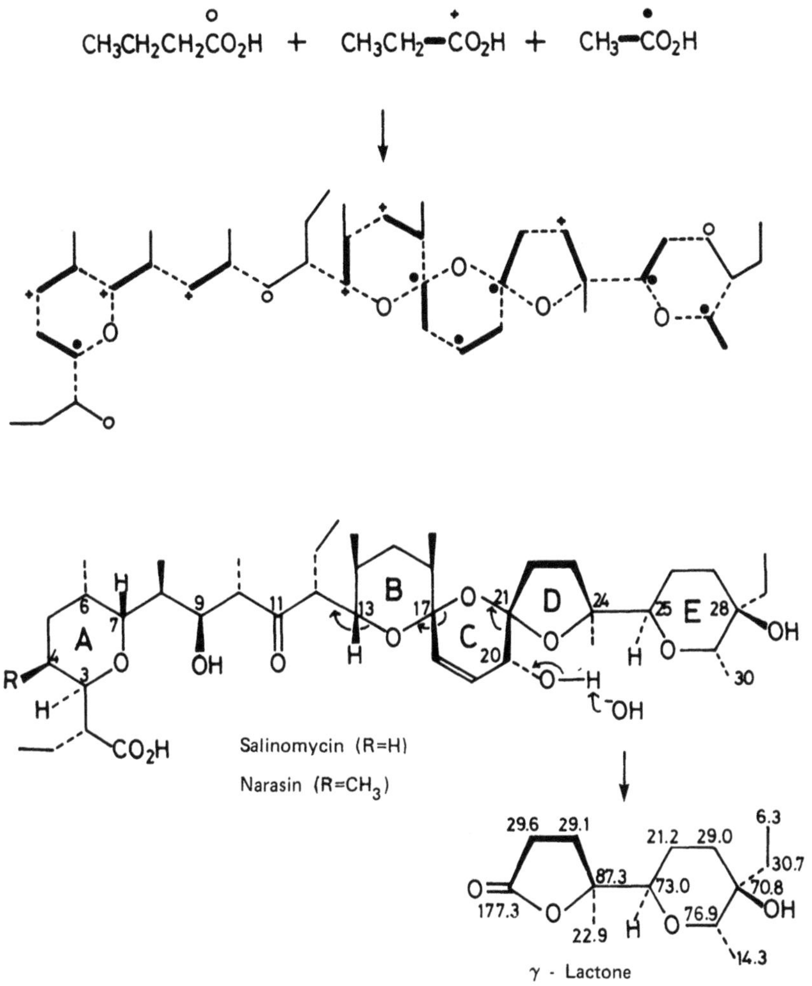

$$CH_3CH_2CH_2CO_2H \quad + \quad CH_3CH_2\overset{+}{-}CO_2H \quad + \quad CH_3\overset{\bullet}{-}CO_2H$$

Salinomycin (R=H)

Narasin (R=CH$_3$)

γ - Lactone

Figure 7 The structures of salinomycin, its γ-lactone and narasin (4-methylsalinomycin), and the biosynthetic pathway of salinomycin.

by the δ effect reported for gauche-trans orientation [CH$_3$(C-6) against equatorial CH$_3$(C-4)] (Grover et al., 1973). This conclusion was further corroborated by measurements of T_1 of narasin. The relaxation time of the new methyl group [CH$_3$(C-4), T_1 0.09 sec] can be compared with those of methylenes (T_1 0.05-0.12 sec) in length and is in marked contrast to those of the remaining methyl groups [T_1 CH$_3$(C-24) 0.22 sec, CH$_3$(C-6) 0.58 sec, other methyls 0.31-0.65 sec].

Table 2 ^{13}C Chemical Shifts of Salinomycin, 20-Deoxysalinomycin, and Narasin (4-Methylsalinomycin) in $CDCl_3$

Carbon	Functionality	Salinomycin free acid	Enriched by[a]	Salinomycin sodium salt	20-Deoxy salinomycin free acid	Narasin free acid	Enriched by[a]
1	COOH	177.2	1B	184.8	177.1	178.4	2B
2	CH	48.9	1A	51.1	48.2	49.3	
3	CH–O	74.9	2A	75.8	74.7	78.4b	2P
4	CH₂ or CH	20.1	1P	19.7	20.1	29.0b	2P
5	CH₂	26.4	2P	26.8	26.6	35.5b	
6	CH	28.0	1P	28.0	28.1	28.0b	2P
7	CH–O	71.7	2P	71.3	71.6	72.0b	
8	CH	36.5	1P	35.9	36.2	36.6b	2P
9	CH–O	68.7	2P	67.8	68.5	68.5b	
10	CH	49.2	1B	49.6	49.6	49.9	2P
11	C=O	214.5		217.6	213.8	216.5	2B
12	CH	56.5	1P	55.5	56.3	56.1	
13	CH–O	75.2	2P	75.6	75.6	75.1b	2P
14	CH	32.6	1P	32.5	32.7	32.9	
15	CH₂	38.6	2P	38.6	38.8	38.7b	2P
16	CH	40.7	1A	40.6	41.0	41.1b	
17	O–C–O	99.2	2A	99.1	99.0	99.6	
18	CH=	121.6	1A	122.1	121.8	122.0	
19	CH=	132.4	2A	130.8	125.6	132.0	
20	CH–O or CH₂	67.2	1A	66.6	33.1	67.6	
21	O–C–O	106.4	2A	107.1	105.0	106.5	
22	CH₂	36.2	2A	36.1	40.0	36.2b	

Carbon						
23 CH$_2$	30.2	1P	32.5	30.0	30.5	
24 C–O	88.5	2P	88.3	88.5	88.5	2P
25 CH–O	73.7	1A	74.6	74.1	73.9[b]	
26 CH$_2$	21.9	2A	19.9	22.2	21.8	
27 CH$_2$	29.3	1B	29.1	29.7	29.4	
28 C–O	70.9		70.5	71.3	70.8	2B
29 CH–O	77.2	1A	76.5	76.4	77.1	
30 CH$_3$	14.5	2A	14.7	14.4	14.3	
2-Me	13.2		13.2	13.4	13.2	4B
4-Me	—		—	—	19.0	3P
6-Me	11.2		10.7	11.2	12.1[b]	3P
8-Me	7.0		6.8	7.0	7.0[b]	3P
10-Me	12.8		12.1	13.2	13.0[b]	3P
12-Me	11.9		12.4	11.9	12.1	4B
14-Me	15.6		15.7	15.7	15.7[b]	3P
16-Me	17.9		17.6	17.9	18.0[b]	3P
24-Me	25.8		27.7	25.8	26.1	3P
28-Me	6.3		6.5	6.5	6.3	4B
2-CH$_2$	16.6		15.7	16.6	16.4[b]	3B
12-CH$_2$	22.7		23.7	22.7	24.0[b]	3B
28-CH$_2$	30.6		32.1	31.9	30.9	3B

[a] 1A, 2A, 1P, 2P, 3P, 1B, 2B, 3B, and 4B represent $CH_3{}^{13}COOH$, $^{13}CH_3COOH$, $CH_3CH_2{}^{13}COOH$, $CH_3{}^{13}CH_2COOH$, $^{13}CH_3CH_2COOH$, $CH_3CH_2CH_2{}^{13}COOH$, $CH_3CH_2{}^{13}CH_2COOH$, $CH_3{}^{13}CH_2CH_2COOH$, and $^{13}CH_3CH_2CH_2COOH$, respectively.

[b] Assignments in the original report of Dorman et al. (1976) have been revised.

Source: Seto et al., 1977a, for salinomycin and 20-deoxysalinomycin; and Dorman et al., 1976, for narasin (4-methylsalinomycin).

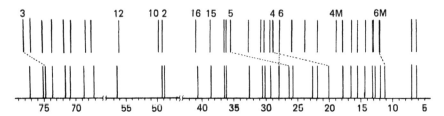

Figure 8 ^{13}C NMR spectra of narasin (upper) and salinomycin (lower) in CDCl$_3$. (Source: Seto et al., 1977b.)

This unusually short relaxation time of CH$_3$(C-4) is compatible with the energetically preferred conformation shown in Figure 9, in which free rotation of CH$_3$(C-4) is prevented by a proton of CH$_2$(C-2). Such spatial relationship is possible only when the methyl is equatorially oriented at C-4. It should be emphasized that due to the extensive overlapping of ^1H signals and equatorial orientation of the proton at C-3, ^1H NMR was useless for this stereochemical investigation.

Assignments of the ^{13}C NMR spectra of salinomycin, 20-deoxysalinomycin and narasin

By selectively increasing signal intensities through the incorporation of ^{13}C-labeled sodium butyrate and sodium propionate, Dorman et al., (1976) reported the total assignments of the ^{13}C chemical shifts of narasin. However, about half of their assignments were not made on a one-to-one-basis.

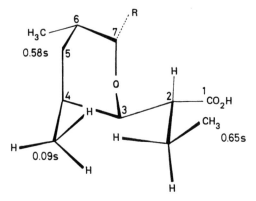

Figure 9   The stereochemical relationship of ring A of narasin and its substituents. Values given are the relaxation times T$_1$ in second. (Source: Seto et al., 1977b.)

Seto et al. (1977a) made the complete assignments of salinomycin free acid and sodium salt utilizing ^{13}C-^{13}C couplings. As shown in Figure 7, labeling experiments with $^{13}CH_3^{13}COOH$ enabled one to establish the relationships C(3)−C(4), C(17)−C(18), C(19)−C(20), C(21)−C(22), C(25)−C(26), and C(29)−C(30). In addition, the couplings were also observed between C(1)−C(2), CH_2(C-2)−CH_3(C-2), C(11)−C(12), CH_2(C-12)−CH_3(C-12), C(27)−C(28), and CH_2(C-28)−CH_3(C-28). Since C-1, C-11, and C-27 were specifically enriched by $CH_3CH_2CH_2^{13}CO_2H$, acetic acid was incorporated into these positions after its conversion to butyric acid. It should be noticed that two ketal carbon signals C-17 and C-21 were firmly and straightforwardly distinguished by this double labeling method, since the former was coupled to an olefinic signal and the latter to a methylene resonance. On the other hand, use of $CH_3^{13}CH_2^{13}COOH$ revealed the following sets of carbon signals: C(5)−C(6), C(7)−C(8), C(9)−C(10), C(13)−C(14), C(15)−C(16), and C(23)−C(24).

In addition to this biosynthetic technique, comparison of salinomycin with 20-deoxysalinomycin (Miyazaki et al., 1978) and the γ-lactone obtained via the mechanism shown in Figure 7 (Seto et al., 1977a) played an important role for the total assignment of salinomycin. The reported assignments of C-7 and C-13 including their counterparts of ^{13}C-^{13}C coupling (C-8 and C-14) have been recently interchanged (H. Seto, unpublished data) based on the comparisons with noboritomycin A (Keller-Juslén, et al., 1978) and CP-44,161 (Tone et al., 1978).

The established assignments of salinomycin free acid, its sodium salt, and 20-deoxysalinomycin free acid are summarized in Table 2, which also contains the reassigned ^{13}C NMR data of narasin (via comparison to salinomycin).

3. Group 1c: noboritomycins A and B, and CP-44,161

The structural elucidation of noboritomycin A by x-ray analysis was reported together with tentative assignments of the ^{13}C NMR spectra of noboritomycins A and B (Keller-Juslén et al., 1978). Based on the ^{13}C NMR spectral differences, noboritomycin B was determined as a derivative of noboritomycin A with an ethyl substituent at C-4. Since noboritomycin A can be regarded as a hybrid of lasalocid A (Westley et al., 1970) and salinomycin (Kinashi et al., 1975), its ^{13}C assignment could be made with ease by making reference to these antibiotics.

During reinvestigation of the ^{13}C NMR spectral data it was found that the configuration of the ketal carbon C-23 of noboritomycins A and B was incorrectly represented in the original report and their structures have been revised as shown in Figure 10 (Fehr et al., 1979). Detailed comparison of noboritomycin A with salinomycin and selective proton decoupling showed some original assignments of the antibiotics to be corrected as shown in Table 3 (H. Seto, K. Furihata, and N. Otake, unpublished data). The results, however, do not affect the

Table 3 ^{13}C Chemical Shifts of Sodium Salts of Noboritomycins A and B and CP-44,161 in CDCl$_3$

Carbon	Functionality	Noboritomycin A	Noboritomycin B	CP-44,161
1	COOH	173.9	173.9	175.3
2	C=	119.6	119.7	117.2
3	HO–C=	156.4	155.9	161.5
4	C=	121.4	127.5	123.2
5	CH=	130.7	129.0	131.6
6	CH=	115.0	115.0	119.3
7	C=	146.0	145.8	143.1
8	CH or CH$_2$	29.6	29.6	33.3
9	CH$_2$	43.8	43.8	37.3b
10	CH	30.4	30.3	33.3
11	CH–O	68.7a	68.7a	71.6
12	CH	48.5	48.4	48.3
13	C=O	216.7	216.6	218.7
14	CH	46.7	46.7	55.8
15	CH–O	75.9a	75.9a	76.6
16	CH	32.0	32.0	32.4
17	CH$_2$	38.6	38.6	38.3b
18	CH	40.5	40.5	40.3
19	O–C–O	98.9	98.9	99.0
20	CH=	122.5	122.5	121.8
21	CH=	131.2	131.2	125.9
22	CH–O or CH$_2$	64.1a	64.1a	30.8
23	O–C–O	104.7	104.7	104.6
24	CH	45.0	44.9	43.7
25	CH–O or CH$_2$	95.0	94.9	39.4b
26	C–O	85.4	85.4	88.1b

Position	Type			
27	CH–O	82.0[a]	81.9[a]	78.2
28	CH$_2$	35.1	35.0	32.6[b]
29	CH–O or CH$_2$	71.5[a]	71.4[a]	25.7[b]
30	CH–O or C–O	81.4[a]	81.4[a]	86.2[b]
31	COOR or CH–O	170.5[a]	170.4[a]	71.6
32	CH$_3$	—	—	19.3
4-Me		15.9	13.9	16.2
8-Me		18.9[a]	18.9[a]	—
10-Me		13.1[a]	13.1[a]	12.5[b]
12-Me		12.7	12.6	12.9[b]
14-Me		7.6[a]	7.5[a]	13.2[b]
16-Me		17.4[a]	17.4[a]	17.8
18-Me		15.6[a]	15.6[a]	15.8
24-Me		12.7[a]	12.6[a]	13.5[b]
26-Me		28.7[a]	28.7[a]	9.3
30-Me		—	—	23.6
31-Me		13.8[a]	13.7[a]	—
4-CH$_2$		—	23.0	—
14-CH$_2$		—	—	15.4
26-CH$_2$		—	—	29.5[b]
31-OCH$_2$		61.4	61.4	—
25-OCH$_3$		59.6	59.6	—

[a] Assignments in the original report of Keller-Juslén et al. (1978) have been revised.
[b] Assignments may be interchanged.

Source: Keller-Juslén et al., 1978, for noboritomycins A and B; and H. Seto, K. Furihata, and N. Ōtake (unpublished data) for CP-44,161.

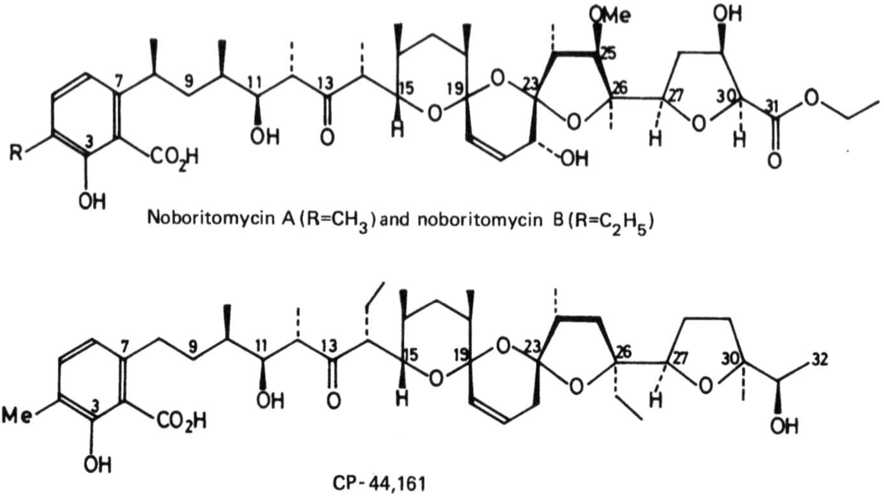

Noboritomycin A (R=CH₃) and noboritomycin B (R=C₂H₅)

CP-44,161

Figure 10   The structures of noboritomycins A and B and CP-44,161.

structure of noboritomycin B. It should be noted that the C-25 signal appears at an unusually low field (95.2 ppm). This value can be compared with those of C-15 in carriomycin, septamycin, and A204A (see later).

CP-44,161 is the first ionophore antibiotic produced by a microorganism other than *Streptomyces*, i.e., *Dactilosporangium salmoneum* (Tone et al., 1978). Its ^{13}C NMR assignment has been made by selective proton decoupling as well as by comparison with noboritomycin A, salinomycin, and lasalocid and is summarized in Table 3 (H. Seto, K. Furihata, and N. Ōtake, unpublished data).

4. Group 1d: lysocellin

On alkaline treatment, lysocellin (Ōtake et al., 1975) gave the retro-aldol ketone N₂ (Ōtake and Koenuma, 1977), which is a mixture of two epimers at the C-12 center. ^{13}C NMR data of this ketone were analyzed by utilization of chemical shift differences between the two epimers as well as by comparison to the lasalocid retroaldol ketone as explained previously. The results summarized in Table 4 gave a reliable basis for the assignments of carbon resonances due to the right half of the lysocellin structure.

Total ^{13}C NMR assignment of lysocellin sodium salt (see Table 4) has been completed with the aid of the biosynthetic labeling method using CH₃[13]CH₂[13]COOH (Ōtake et al. 1978b). In agreement with the biosynthetic hypothesis, seven propionic acid molecules were incorpor-

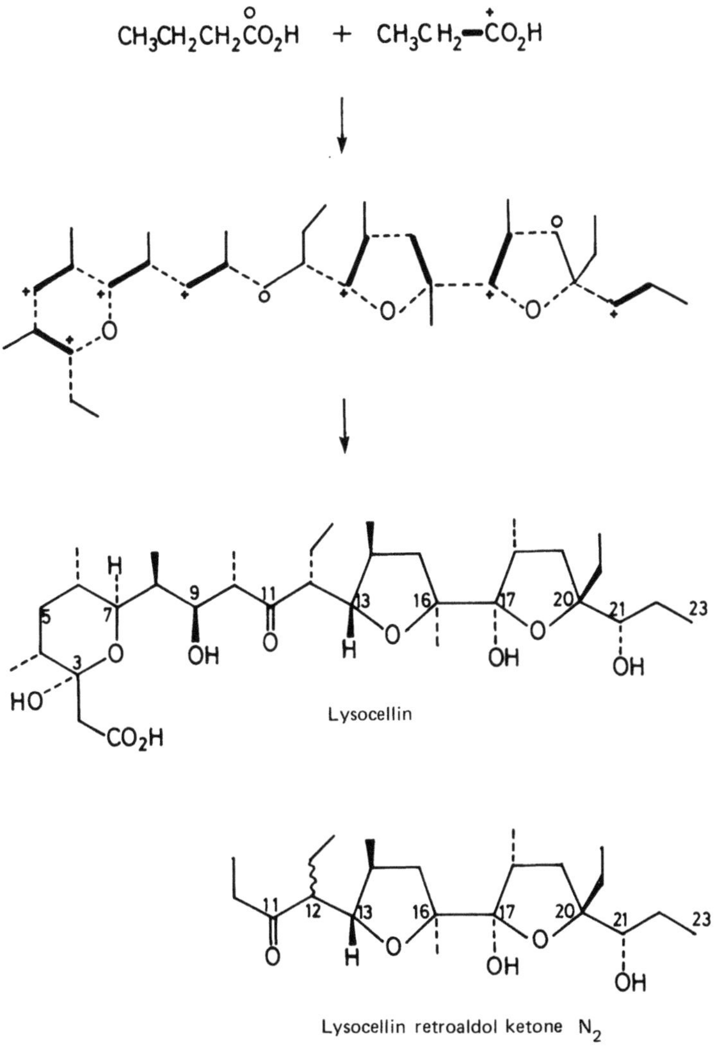

$$CH_3CH_2CH_2\overset{O}{\overset{\|}{C}}O_2H \quad + \quad CH_3C\overset{\cdot}{H}_2\!-\!\overset{+}{C}O_2H$$

Lysocellin

Lysocellin retroaldol ketone N_2

Figure 11   The structure of lysocellin and its biosynthetic pathway.

ated to lysocellin, giving ^{13}C-^{13}C couplings which confirmed the relationships between C(3)−C(4), C(5)−C(6), C(7)−C(8), C(9)−C(10),
C(13)−C(14), C(15)−C(16), C(17)−C(18), and C(21)−C(22). Selective proton decoupling was also utilized to distinguish some methine
carbons based on the ^1H NMR analysis by Anteunis (1977c).

Table 4 ^{13}C Chemical Shifts of Lysocellin Sodium Salt and Its Retroaldol Ketone in CDCl$_3$

Carbon	Functionality	Lysocellin	Enriched by[a]	Retroaldol ketone[b]
1	COOH	177.7		
2	CH$_2$	45.9	1P	
3	O–C–O	98.1	2P	
4	CH	39.3	1P	
5	CH$_2$	36.6	2P	
6	CH	32.3	1P	
7	CH–O	79.3	2P	
8	CH	32.3	2P	
9	CH–O	75.7	1P	
10	CH	47.5	2P	37.3(37.1)[c,d]
11	C=O	214.6	1B	213.6
12	CH	55.0		59.3(57.2)
13	CH–O	83.5	1P	87.3(86.7)
14	CH	34.6	2P	36.9(36.4)
15	CH$_2$	42.7	1P	42.5
16	C–O	86.0	2P	85.2(84.9)
17	O–C–O	108.1	1P	107.6
18	CH	38.3	2P	37.9(37.7)
19	CH$_2$	37.6	1B	37.0

Position	Group		1P / 2P	
20	C—O	87.1		88.0(87.9)
21	CH—OH	71.6	1P	73.1
22	CH$_2$	25.4	2P	24.7
23	CH$_3$	11.3		11.0
4-Me		15.5		
6-Me		16.6		
8-Me		5.4		
10-Me		12.8		7.3[d]
12-Me		12.6		12.5(12.2)
14-Me		16.6		16.8(16.2)
16-Me		23.8		24.5
18-Me		14.7		14.1(13.9)
20-Me		7.5		7.5
12-CH$_2$		14.9		21.5(21.0)
20-CH$_2$		31.4		30.4(29.7)

[a] 1P, 2P, and 1B represent $CH_3CH_2{}^{13}COOH$, $CH_3{}^{13}CH_2COOH$, and $CH_3CH_2CH_2{}^{13}COOH$, respectively.

[b] Mixture of epimers at C-12.

[c] Where two peaks were observed for a single carbon, the one appearing at higher field is arbitrarily expressed in parentheses. Therefore, chemical shift values in parentheses do not necessarily correspond to one epimer.

[d] Functionalities or chemical environments of these carbons are different from those of the corresponding carbons in lysocellin.

Source: Otake et al., 1978.

B. Group 2

The ^{13}C NMR spectrum of dianemycin sodium salt was analyzed by the aid of the biosynthetic labeling method and selective proton decoupling to give its complete assignments as shown in Table 5 (Mizoue et al., 1980). The resonances due to C-11, C-13, C-17, C-23, and C-29 were separated from the remaining signals by being enriched with $CH_3^{13}COOH$, and C-1, C-3, C-5, C-7, C-9, C-15, C-19, C-21, C-25, and C-27 with $CH_3CH_2^{13}COOH$. The distinction of these signals within each group was accomplished by use of chemical shift trends and selective proton decoupling based on the work by Anteunis et al. (1977). Table 5 also contains the ^{13}C NMR assignments of dianemycin free acid made by comparison to its sodium salt.

The established assignment of dianemycin free acid enabled one to determine the structure of leuseramycin, a new antibiotic produced by *Streptomyces hygroscopicus* (Mizutani et al., 1980). Most of the ^{13}C chemical shifts of dianemycin free acid and leuseramycin free acid agree very well within experimental error, as shown in Table 5. However, the hydroxymethyl carbon (C-30, 65.9 ppm) in dianemycin has been replaced by a new methyl carbon resonance at 28.3 ppm in leuseramycin. Downfield shifts of C-25, C-27, and C-28 by 0.6, 0.8, and 4.2 ppm, respectively, were also observed in the ^{13}C NMR spectrum of leuseramycin free acid. These spectral features of the new antibiotic are in accord with the structure with a methyl carbon (C-30) at the right terminal of the main framework, as shown in Figure 12.

The structural relationship between dianemycin and leuseramycin can be compared with that between nigericin (Steinrauf et al., 1968) and grisorixin (Gachon et al., 1970).

The assignments of the ^{13}C NMR data of lenoremycin sodium salt were also made by comparison with dianemycin as well as by selective proton decoupling based on the ^{1}H NMR study on lenoremycin (Anteunis et al., 1977).

The structures of A-130B and A-130C

Tsuji (1980) independently reported the ^{13}C NMR analysis of antibiotic A-130A (identical with lenoremycin) in C_6D_6 solution. The differences of the ^{13}C chemical shifts of A-130A in $CDCl_3$ and C_6D_6 (see Table 5 and 6) do not exceed 0.7 ppm for most carbon signals. The larger differences observed with some carbons, such as C-10, C-12, C-20, and C-23, may be attributed to the misassignment of these carbons to one of the two groups.

Based on the assignment of A-130A made by selective proton decoupling aided by the ^{1}H NMR analysis of lenoremycin (Anteunis et al., 1977) and comparison to related compounds, Tsuji et al. determined the structures of its congeners, A-130B and A-130C. As shown in Table 6, A-130B is composed of 54 carbons, while A-130A, as well as A-130C, has 47 carbons. The precise comparison of these three antibiotics led to the conclusion that A-130B has an additional deoxy-sugar

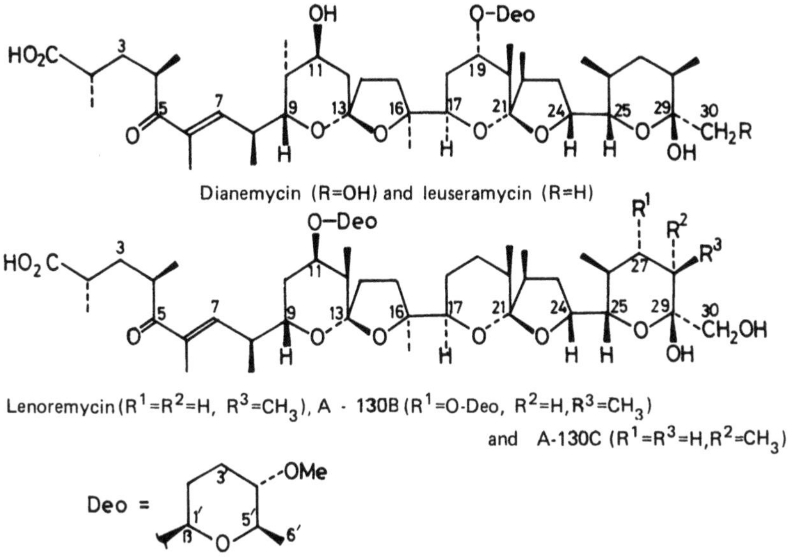

Dianemycin (R=OH) and leuseramycin (R=H)

Lenoremycin (R^1=R^2=H, R^3=CH$_3$), A - 130B (R^1=O-Deo, R^2=H,R^3=CH$_3$)

and A-130C (R^1=R^3=H,R^2=CH$_3$)

Deo =

Figure 12 The structures of dianemycin, leuseramycin, lenoremycin, A-130B, and A-130C.

moiety at C-27. Marked and slight changes (footnotes c and d, respectively, in Table 6) in the ^{13}C chemical shifts were exhibited from A-130A to A-130B as CH$_2 \rightarrow$CH−O (37.2→82.6 ppm), upfield shifts of two methyl signals (17.5 and 17.9→12.9 and 14.0 ppm, respectively), downfield shifts of two methine signals (36.9 and 33.3→45.4 and 40.0 ppm, respectively), and slight signal shifts of CH−O (73.5→72.8 ppm) and O−CH−O (99.1→100.3 ppm). Taking account of the structure of A-130A, these spectral changes can be explained only by locating the sugar at C-27 in ring E (see Figure 12).

The comparison between the ^{13}C spectra of A-130A and A-130C revealed chemical shift changes of seven carbons which are assigned to those on the E ring. The changes including a remarkable upfield shift of the C-26 signal are compatible with the structure in which CH$_3$(C-28) is epimeric (α axial conformation) to that of A-130A. Thus A-130C has been assigned to the structure as shown in Figure 12.

Even allowing for the influence of the different solvents, i.e., CDCl$_3$ and C$_6$D$_6$, disagreements remain in the ^{13}C chemical shifts of some signals (C-10, C-12, C-23, and C-2') reported by the two groups. These discrepancies, however, do not affect the structural determination of leuseramycin, A-130B, and A-130C.

Table 5 ^{13}C Chemical Shifts of Lenoremycin, Dianemycin, and Leuseramycin in CDCl$_3$

Carbon	Functionality	Lenoremycin Na⁺ salt	Dianemycin Na⁺ salt	Enriched by[a]	Dianemycin free acid	Leuseramycin free acid
1	COO	181.3	183.8	1P	179.3	179.2
2	CH	39.5	40.2	1P	37.5	37.1
3	CH₂	41.2	41.5		40.4	40.1
4	CH	37.3	37.5		36.6	36.8
5	C=O	207.4	206.2	1P	204.8	204.4
6	C=	134.0	133.6		134.2	134.2
7	CH=	146.2	144.9	1P	144.9	144.9
8	CH	41.2	37.8		37.8	38.1
9	CH-O	68.0	69.6	1P	69.8	69.6
10	CH₂ or CH	28.1	35.9		36.6	36.8
11	CH-O	73.1	70.4	1A	70.6	70.6
12	CH or CH₂	36.4	34.0		33.7	33.9
13	O-C-O	108.9	106.9	1A	107.1	107.0
14	CH₂	35.6	39.7		39.5	39.7
15	CH₂	32.2	32.2	1P	32.7	32.8
16	C-O	85.8	86.6		86.9	87.0
17	CH-O	80.9	75.7	1A	75.7	75.4
18	CH₂	17.5	25.4		25.2	25.2
19	CH₂ or CH-O	26.1	79.2	1P	80.1	80.1
20	CH	39.6	34.6		34.0	34.4
21	O-C-O	111.1	109.8	1P	109.6	109.0
22	CH	35.1	35.9		36.1	35.8
23	CH₂	29.8	29.9	1A	29.9	29.4
24	CH-O	79.4	77.9		77.2	76.9
25	CH-O	73.1	73.2	1P	73.9	74.5

Position	Group	C-11	C-19	G-19	C-19
26	CH	33.0		32.9	32.5
27	CH_2	36.3		37.3	38.1
28	CH	36.4		34.8	39.0
29	O–C–OH	98.5	1P	98.2	98.7
30	CH_2OH or CH_3	64.1	1A	65.9	28.3
2-Me		20.3		18.4	18.6
4-Me		17.1		16.3	16.5
6-Me		11.2		11.3	11.3
8-Me		14.6		14.7	14.5
10-Me		—		10.4	10.4
12-Me		13.9		—	—
16-Me		27.0		27.0	27.1
20-Me		13.9		13.4	13.6
22-Me		15.3		16.3	16.5
26-Me		17.8		17.8	17.8
28-Me		17.0		17.3	17.2
Deoxy sugar at:		C-11	C-19	G-19	C-19
1'	O–CH–O	102.6	102.4	102.2	101.9
2'	CH_2	30.0	30.6	30.8	30.7
3'	CH_2	27.5	27.0	27.1	27.7
4'	CH–O	79.4	79.9	80.2	80.1
5'	CH–O	76.1	74.5	74.5	74.6
6'	CH_3	18.3	18.5	18.4	18.4
4'-OMe		56.7	56.7	56.8	56.8

[a] 1P and 1A represent $CH_3CH_2{}^{13}COOH$ and $CH_3{}^{13}COOH$, respectively.

Source: Mizoue et al., 1980, for lenoremycin and dianemycin; and Mizutani et al., 1980, for leuseramycin.

Table 6 ^{13}C Chemical Shifts of Sodium Salts of A-130A, A-130B, and A-130C in C_6D_6

Carbon	Functionality	A-130A	A-130B	A-130C
1	COOH	181.3	181.6	181.9
2	CH	39.8	39.8	39.8[b]
3	CH$_2$	41.9	41.8	41.9
4	CH	38.4	38.3	38.4
5	C=O	205.8	205.8	206.0
6	C=	134.5	134.5	134.8
7	CH=	146.0	145.9	145.8
8	CH	41.9	41.8	41.9
9	CH−O	68.5	68.5	68.4
10[a]	CH$_2$	29.8	29.7	29.6
11	CH−O	73.5	73.5	73.7
12	CH	39.8	39.8	39.9
13	O−C−O	109.3	109.0	109.1
14	CH$_2$	36.0	36.0	36.1
15	CH$_2$	32.5	32.4	32.5
16	C−O	85.8	85.9	85.9
17	CH−O	80.9	80.9	81.0
18	CH2	17.7	17.7	17.7
19[a]	CH$_2$	27.6	27.4	27.6
20	CH	30.4	30.3	30.4
21	O−C−O	111.1	111.3	111.1
22	CH	35.4	35.4	35.8
23	CH$_2$	36.7	36.7	36.8
24	CH−O	79.6	79.8	79.6
25	CH−O	73.5	72.8[c]	74.2[c]
26	CH	33.3	40.0[b]	26.3[b]
27	CH$_2$ or CH−O	37.2	82.6[b]	36.1[c]
28	CH	36.9	45.4[b]	36.4[c]
29	O−C−OH	99.1	100.3[c]	98.0[c]
30	CH$_2$−OH	64.7	64.6	65.0
2-Me[a]		20.9	20.8	20.9
4-Me[a]		17.7	17.7	17.7
6-Me		11.7	11.7	11.8
8-Me[a]		14.3	14.2	14.3
12-Me		13.9	13.9	13.9
16-Me		27.3	27.4	27.6
20-Me[a]		15.0	15.1	15.1
22-Me[a]		15.3	15.2	15.3
26-Me		17.9	14.0[b]	18.3[c]
28-Me		17.5	12.9[b]	15.5[b]

Table 6 (Continued)

Sugar at C-11				
1'	O−CH−O	103.3	103.2	103.5
2'[a]	CH$_2$	28.7	28.6	28.8
3'[a]	CH$_2$	26.6	26.5	26.7
4'	CH−O	79.5	79.5	79.6
5'	CH−O	76.8	76.7	76.8
6'	CH$_3$	18.6	18.7	18.7
4'-OMe		56.3	56.3	56.4

Sugar at C-27		
1'	O−CH−O	103.2
2'	CH2	30.9
3'	CH$_2$	27.4
4'	CH−O	80.6
5'	CH−O	74.5
6'	CH$_3$	18.7
4'-OMe		56.2

[a]Assignments may be interchanged.
[b]As compared to A-130A, marked change in the ^{15}C chemical shifts was observed in A-130B and A-130C.
[c]As compared to A-130A, slight change in the ^{13}C chemical shifts was observed in A-130B and A-130C.
Source: Tsuji et al., 1980.

C. Group 3

1. *Group 3a: Ionomycin and mutalomycin*

The complete assignment of Ionomycin A sodium salt was obtained by biosynthetic labeling as described previously (Mizoue et al., 1978). The results (Table 7) were exploited to establish "some empirical rules for the structural elucidation of polyether antibiotics" (Seto et al., 1979a), which will be explained later.

Precise selective proton decoupling and comparison to mutalomycin also facilitated the assignment of methyl and methine resonances which were not labeled by ^{13}C-labeled precursors. The ^1H NMR study of Ionomycin had been reported by Rodios and Anteunis (1978b, 1979).

Lallemand et al. (1979) carried out selective proton decoupling of emericid (identical with Ionomycin A), using a spectrometer operating at 62.9 MHz, to obtain the almost identical results more easily. Some methylene and methoxy signals, however, remain unassigned.

Table 7 ^{13}C Chemical Shifts of Sodium Salts of Lonomycin, Mutalomycin, Etheromycin, A204A, Carriomycin, Septamycin, and 6016 in CDCl$_3$

Carbon	Functionality	Lonomycin	Mutalomycin	Etheromycin	A204A	Carriomycin	Septamycin	6016
1	COOH	181.5[a]	181.2	180.7	180.3	180.4	180.2	178.4[b]
2	CH	46.0	47.1	45.1	45.5	46.0	45.3	72.1
3	O–C–OH	100.4[a]	99.6	99.5	99.3	100.1	99.4	99.2[a]
4	CH	35.4	35.0	40.2[c]	41.1	35.2[c]	39.5	34.0[c]
5	CH–O	82.2[a]	82.0	76.6	79.5	77.6	88.5	82.3[a]
6	CH or C–O	31.1	31.1	82.7	77.3	34.6[c]	80.0	33.4[c]
7	CH–O	70.8[a]	71.5	71.4	64.1	64.0	67.3	64.8[b]
8	CH or CH$_2$	37.7	36.6	39.7[c]	32.7	37.3	32.4	36.9
9	CH–O	63.3[a]	64.1	63.0	61.2	61.2	61.4	60.9[b]
10	CH or CH$_2$	33.7	40.2	32.5[c]	31.2[c]	31.3[c]	31.1[c]	31.2[c]
11	CH–O	82.0[b]	70.3	79.9	79.3	79.4	79.5	79.6[b]
12	CH$_2$ or CH	34.1[d]	33.4[c]	39.0[c]	36.8	36.7	36.7	36.7
13	O–C–O	107.1[b]	106.8	109.2	106.5	106.4	106.4	107.9[b]
14	CH$_2$ or CH	39.4[d]	39.0	36.9	46.0[c]	45.9	46.0	39.3
15	CH$_2$ or CH–O	30.4[a]	30.7	30.5	94.4	94.4	94.5	38.9[b]
16	C–O	84.2	84.3	85.2	83.1	82.9	83.0	82.6
17	CH–O	81.4[b]	81.6	83.0	83.2	83.2	83.2	89.9[b]
18	CH$_2$	25.9[c]	26.9	24.4	22.9	23.0	23.0	79.0
19	CH$_2$	33.5[a]	33.3[c]	32.9	25.5	25.6	25.6	30.5[b]
20	C–O or CH–O	85.8	83.8	86.1	78.7	78.9	78.9	73.9
21	CH–O	84.3[a]	86.4	84.0	79.1	79.0	79.1	78.6[b]
22	CH or CH$_2$	36.1	34.3	29.8[c]	29.1[c]	29.1[c]	29.1[c]	29.1[c]

Position	Type	1	2	3	4	5	6	7
23	CH₂ or CH–O	80.5b	32.3	24.4	24.1	24.1	24.1	24.3b
24	CH–O	79.8d	78.8	80.7	80.0	80.3	80.2	80.7
25	CH–O	73.8a	73.4	73.6	73.7	75.3	75.2	74.5a
26	CH	37.7	33.1	39.3	39.2	32.7	32.7	32.7
27	CH₂ or CH–O	84.0a	36.4	84.6	84.4	36.8	36.8	36.5a
28	CH	46.6	40.2	46.3	46.2c	39.6	40.6	39.4
29	O–C–OH	98.8b	96.5	98.4	98.1	96.6	96.6	96.6b
30	CH₃	26.5c	25.7	26.6	26.5	26.4	26.4	26.5
2-Me		11.5	11.7	11.0	11.5	11.5	11.5	—
4-Me		11.1	11.1	11.8	13.1	11.7	11.9	11.7
6-Me		4.1	4.1	8.1	12.6	5.5	9.9	5.0
8-Me		10.2	10.0	11.8	—	—	—	—
10-Me		12.0	10.6	—	—	—	—	—
12-Me		—	—	13.2	12.5	12.6	12.6	12.5
14-Me		—	—	—	11.5	11.6	11.5	13.0
16-Me		29.2	29.0	29.2	28.4	28.4	28.4	28.0
20-Me		22.3	23.2	22.6	—	—	—	—
22-Me		9.0	16.2	—	—	—	—	—
26-Me		13.8	17.6	13.6	13.5	17.3	17.3	17.3
28-Me		12.5	17.0	12.4	12.5	16.9	16.9	16.8
5-OMe		56.0	55.8	—	49.5	—	61.5	55.8
6-OMe		—	—	58.8	58.8	—	—	—
11-OMe		58.6	—	—	60.0	58.8	58.7	58.8
15-OMe		—	—	—	—	60.0	60.0	—
23-OMe		57.3	—	—	59.7	—	—	—
27-OMe		59.9	—	59.6	—	—	—	—

Table 7 (Continued)

		Deoxy sugar at				
		C-6	C-5	C-5	C-6	C-18
1'	O-CH-O	95.2	98.3	97.6	96.3	98.9
2'	CH_2	28.7	29.8	30.8	31.8	30.6
3'	CH_2	27.3	23.3	27.2	27.6	26.9
4'	CH-O	79.9	81.2	80.3	80.0	79.9
5'	CH-O	74.7	68.2	74.4	74.1	74.4
6'	CH_3	18.2	18.5	18.3	18.5	18.2
4'-OMe		56.9	56.2	56.7	56.6	56.7

[a] Enriched by $CH_3CH_2{}^{13}COOH$.
[b] Enriched by $CH_3{}^{13}COOH$.
[c] Assignments may be interchanged.
[d] Enriched by $^{13}CH_3COOH$.

Source: Mizoue et al., 1978, and Seto et al., 1979a, for lonomycin and mutalomycin; Seto et al. 1979a, and H. Seto, H. Nakayama, and N. Ōtake (unpublished data) for etheromycin, A204A, carriomycin, and septamycin; and Seto et al., 1979c, for 6016.

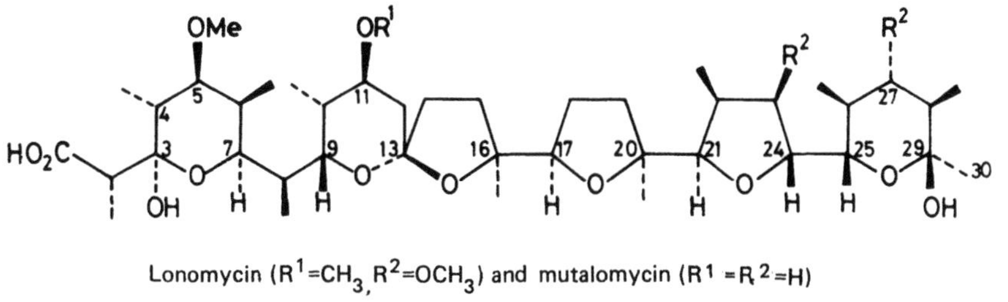

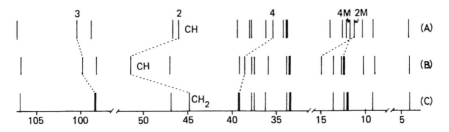

Lonomycin (R^1=CH$_3$, R^2=OCH$_3$) and mutalomycin (R^1 = R^2 =H)

Figure 13   The structures of lonomycin A and mutalomycin.

^{13}C NMR spectral analysis of mutalomycin was accomplished based on the established chemical shifts of lonomycin carbon signals (Seto et al., 1979a, H. Seto, K. Mizoue, and N. Ōtake, unpublished work). During this study it was found that the configuration of C-4 of mutalomycin reported earlier (Fehr et al., 1977) must be revised as shown in Figure 13 (Fehr et al., 1979).

The structures of lonomycins B and C

Lonomycins B (B) and C (C) were isolated from the fermentation broth of *Streptomyces ribosidificus* as minor components of lonomycin A (A) (Mizoue et al., 1978). B was easily converted to A in organic solvents such as acetone and ethyl acetate at room temperature, whereas the reverse reaction under the same condition was almost negligible. This phenomenon together with the identical mass spectra of both compounds implies that these two antibiotics are interconvertible through inversion at a ketal or hemiketal function.

Seto et al. (1978b) determined the position in question by ^{13}C NMR spectroscopy. As shown in Figure 14, the ^{13}C NMR spectra of A and B are very similar, suggesting for the most part that the two antibiotics are identical. However, the following remarkable differences between them were observed around the C-3 hemiketal carbon.

Figure 14   Pertinent region of the ^{13}C NMR spectra of lonomycins A, B, and C in CDCl$_3$. (Source: Seto et al., 1978b.)

Lonomycin A   Lonomycin B

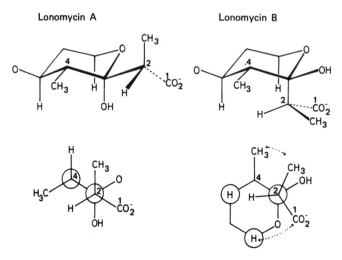

Figure 15   The stereochemical relationship around C-3 in lonomycins A and B.   (Source: Seto et al., 1978b.)

1. The C-2 signal at 46.0 ppm in A was shifted downfield by 6.0 ppm.
2. The absorption of C-4 at 35.4 ppm also suffered a downfield shift by 3.0 ppm in B.
3. The methyl resonance CH_3(C-2) at 11.1 ppm in A was replaced by a methyl peak at 14.9 ppm in B.
4. A methyl signal due to CH_3(C-4) at 11.6 ppm moved to 12.7 ppm in B.
5. A slight shift was observed with the carboxyl (C-1) and hemiketal (C-3) signals.

The structure of A given by an x-ray analysis (Ōtake et al., 1977) shows that the relationship of H-2 and CH_3(C-4) and that of H-4 and CH_3(C-2) are *syn* axial, as shown in Figure 15. Therefore it is reasonable to assume that the γ effect (Stothers, 1972; Levy and Nelson, 1972) acted strongly on C-2, C-4, CH_3(C-2), and CH_3(C-4) in A. The downfield shift of these carbons in B can be reconciled only by the configurational change at C-3 as shown in Figure 15. Thus C-2 and its substituents in B are oriented so as not to interfere sterically with H-4 and CH_3(C-4), resulting in the absence of the γ effect. The similarity of the chemical shifts of the carbons adjacent to the ketal (C-13) and hemiketal (C-29) functions in both the compounds indicated the structural identities of the remaining parts of A and B.

  C is similar to A in its physicochemical properties; however, it contains one less carbon and two less hydrogen atoms than A. The

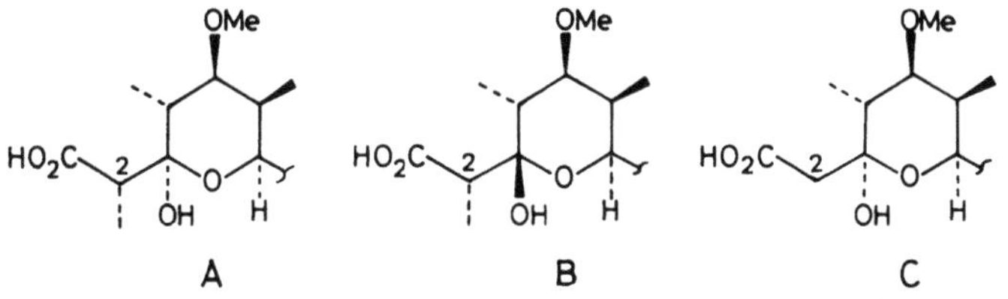

Figure 16 The partial structures of lonomycins A, B, and C. The remaining parts of lonomycins B and C are identical to that of lonomycin A.

^{13}C NMR spectrum of C showed close similarity to that of A, except for (1) the disappearance of the methyl resonance $CH_3(C-2)$ present in A, (2) the downfield shift by 3.0 ppm of the C-4 signal, and (3) the upfield shift of the C-3 peak by 2.0 ppm. In addition, the signal at 46.5 ppm corresponding to C-2 in A was shown to be a methylene by the sford spectrum of C. These chemical shift changes are reasonably accounted for by the disappearance of the β or γ effect (Stothers, 1972; Levy and Nelson, 1972) on C-3 and C-4 exerted by the methyl substituent $CH_3(C-2)$ in A. Thus the structures of B and C are illustrated as shown in Figure 16.

2. *Group 3b: etheromycin, A204A, carriomycin, septamycin, 6016, K-41A, and K-41B*

This subgroup contains the largest number of polyether antibiotics, which are very close to each other in their structures. Carriomycin (Nakayama et al., 1979), septamycin (Petcher and Weber, 1974), A204A (Jones et al., 1973), 6016 (Otake et al., 1978a), K-41A, and K-41B (Tsuji, 1979) can be distinguished by the positions of methoxy and/or deoxy sugar substituents. Furthermore, the latter three compounds are characterized by the presence of a hydroxy function at C-2. These structural similarities made the comparison of the ^{13}C chemical shift data within the group a very useful method to achieve total assignments of ^{13}C NMR spectra.

In addition, selective proton decoupling was also effective to achieve ^{13}C assignments of etheromycin, A204A, carriomycin, and septamycin, as summarized in Table 7 (Seto et al., 1979a; H. Seto, H. Nakayama, and N. Otake, unpublished data). Again, extensive ^1H NMR analytical works by the Anteunis group on etheromycin (Anteunis and Rodios, 1978), A204A (Anteunis and Verhegge, 1977), carriomycin (Rodios and Anteunis, 1978a), and septamycin (Rodios and Anteunis, 1978c) were the basis for the selective proton-decoupling experiments.

Table 8 ^{13}C Chemical Shifts of Sodium Salts of K-41A and K-41B in C_6D_6

Carbon	Functionality	K-41A	K-41B
1	COOH	179.8	179.7
2	CH−OH	72.5	72.4
3	O−C−OH	99.8	99.7
4	CH	39.4	39.3
5	CH−O	86.9	86.9
6	C−O	78.8	78.8
7	CH−O	67.6	67.6
8[a]	CH$_2$	33.3	33.3
9	CH−O	61.9	62.0
10[a]	CH$_2$	31.3	31.4
11[a]	CH−O	79.9	79.9
12	CH	37.0	37.2
13	O−C−O	107.2	106.6[b]
14	CH	46.4	46.5
15	CH−O	94.9	93.3[b]
16	C−O	83.7	84.3[b]
17	CH−O	83.8	84.3
18[a]	CH$_2$	25.9	25.8
19[a]	CH$_2$	23.3	23.4
20[a]	CH−O	79.6	79.6
21[a]	CH−O	79.4	79.3
22[a]	CH$_2$	29.2	29.2
23[a]	CH$_2$	24.3	24.3
24[a]	CH−O	81.1	81.1
25	CH−O	74.6	74.6
26	CH	39.8	39.8
27	CH−O	82.9	83.0
28	CH	48.2	48.2
29	O−C−OH	98.9	98.8
30	CH$_3$	27.2	27.1
4-Me[a]		12.5	12.5
6-Me[a]		11.0	10.9
12-Me		12.6	12.6
14-Me		11.7	11.1
16-Me		28.7	26.3[b]
26-Me[a]		13.8	13.8
28-Me[a]		13.2	13.2
5-OMe		60.8	60.8
6-OMe		50.9	50.9
11-OMe		59.4	59.5
15-OMe		59.9	—

Table 8 (Continued)

Carbon	Functionality	K-41A	K-41B
	Sugar at C-27		
1'	O–CH–O	103.0	103.0
2'	CH_2	31.0	31.0
3'	CH_2	27.4	27.4
4'	CH–O	80.6	80.6
5'	CH–O	74.7	74.7
6'	CH_3	18.8	18.8
4'-OMe		56.2	56.2
	Sugar at C-15		
1'	O–CH–O		103.8[c]
2'	CH_2		31.0[c]
3'	CH_2		27.1[c]
4'	CH–O		80.2[c]
5'	CH–O		74.9[c]
6'	CH_3		18.5[c]
4'-OMe			56.4[c]

[a]Tentatively assigned and may be changed.
[b]These slightly shifted signals supported the structure of K-41B.
[c]Signals observed only in K-41B.
Source: Tsuji et al., 1979.

As explained later, the structural determination of 6016 was made by using "empirical rules" (Seto et al., 1979c). During this process about half of the signals of 6016 were analyzed. Its total assignment has been obtained by selective proton decoupling and the biosynthetic method, the results of which are also contained in Table 7 (H. Seto, H. Nakayama, and N. Otake, unpublished data).

The ^{13}C signals of K-41A sodium salt obtained in C_6D_6 were assigned by making reference to the ^{13}C spectra of septamycin sodium salt, A204A sodium salt, K-41A potassium salt, and three derivatives (A, B and C in Figure 17) of K-41A (Tsuji et al., 1979). The spectrum of A confirmed the C(1)—C(4) and C-7 signal assignments in K-41A sodium salt, and the spectrum of C sodium salt verified the C-29

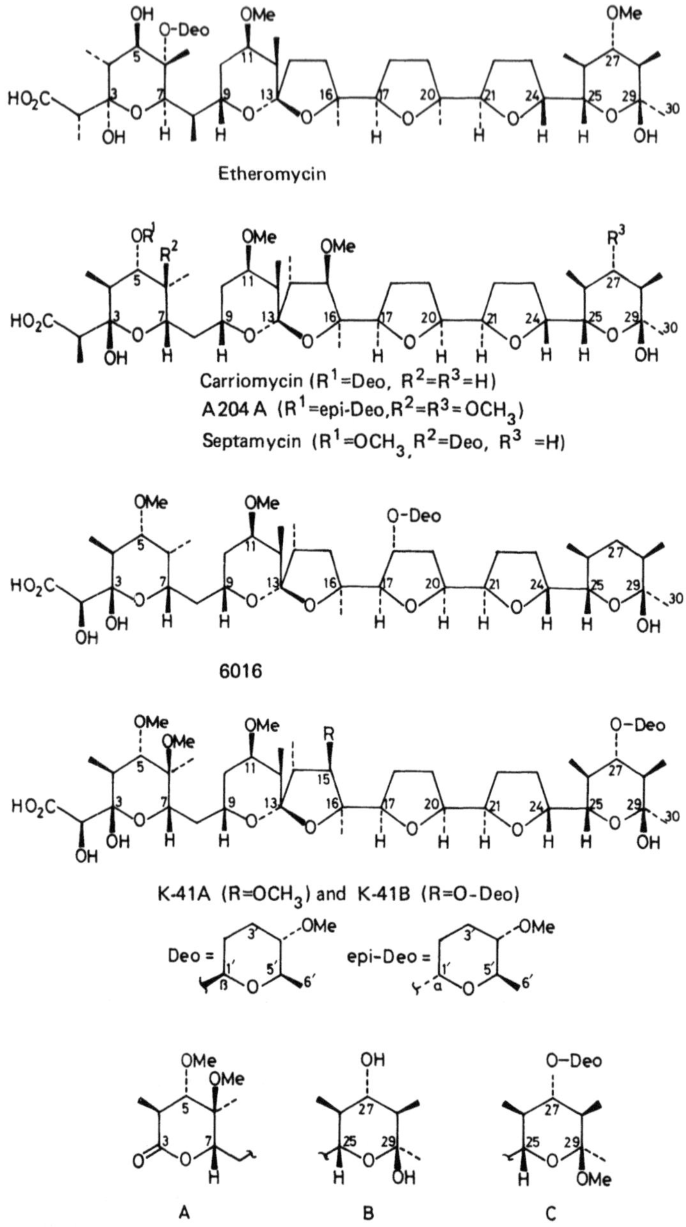

Figure 17 The structures of etheromycin, carriomycin, A204A, septamycin, 6016, K-41A, K-41B, and derivatives of K-41A, (A), (B), and (C). The remaining parts of (A), (B), and (C) are identical to K-41A.

and C-30 signal assignments. The signals due to the deoxy sugar moiety as well as C(25)—C(28), and CH$_3$(C-26), and CH$_3$(C-28) in K-41A were easily assigned by comparison with those of septamycin and B sodium salt, in which signals due to the deoxy sugar at C-27 disappeared. The total assignments of K-41A together with its minor component, K-41B, produced by *Streptomyces hygroscopicus* are summarized in Table 8.

The structural determination of K-41B was accomplished by comparison to K-41A. As seen from Table 8, the ^{13}C signals of K-41B correspond well with those of K-41A, but K-41B has seven additional signals (footnote f in Table 8) assignable to the second deoxy sugar moiety. Since K-41B lacks the CH$_3$O(C-15) signal, the second deoxy sugar was situated at C-15, as shown in Figure 17 (Tsuji et al., 1979).

3. Group 3c: nigericin and grisorixin

Nigericin (Steinrauf, et al., 1968) and grisorixin (Gachon et al., 1970; Alléaume and Hickel, 1970) are closely related to mutalomycin (Fehr et al., 1979) in the right-half side structure and to 6016 (Seto et al., 1979c; Otake et al., 1978a) in the substitution patterns of B and C rings (see Figure 17). However, these two antibiotics can be discriminated from the subgroups 3a and 3b by the disappearance of hemiketal signals at 99-100 ppm in the ^{13}C NMR spectra. The ^{13}C chemical shifts of nigericin sodium salt (see Table 9) were assigned by selective proton decoupling based on ^1H NMR analysis by Rodios and Anteunis (1977). Ambiguities with regard to the chemical shifts of some methylene carbons were eliminated by the aid of the biosynthetic method using CH$_3$^{13}COOH, ^{13}CH$_3$^{13}COOH, and CH$_3$CH$_2$^{13}COOH (H. Seto, K. Mizoue, and N. Otake, unpublished data).

Based on comparison to nigericin, the assignments of the ^{13}C signals of grisorixin were also accomplished, as shown in Table 9 (H. Seto, K. Mizoue, and N. Otake, unpublished data).

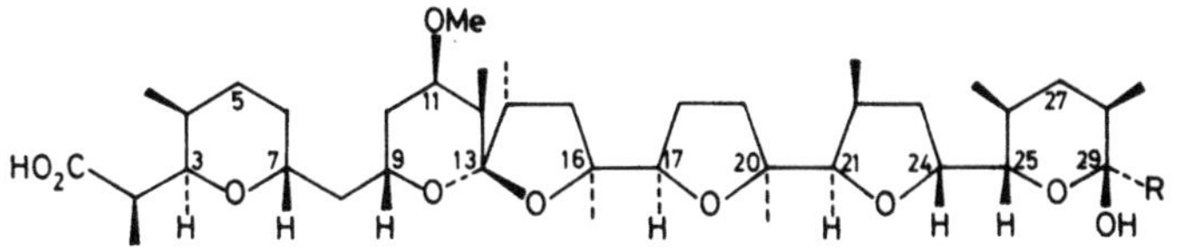

Nigericin (R=CH$_2$OH)
Grisorixin (R = CH$_3$)

Figure 18 The structures of nigericin and grisorixin.

Table 9 ^{13}C Chemical Shifts of the Sodium Salts of Nigericin, Grisorixin, and Monensin in CDCl$_3$

Carbon	Functionality	Nigericin	Enriched by[a]	Grisorixin	Monensin
1	COOH	183.9	1P	180.9	181.2
2	CH	45.9		45.8	45.0
3	CH–O	73.2	1P	73.4	83.0
4	CH	29.0		28.9	37.5
5	CH$_2$	26.4	1A	26.4	–
6	CH$_2$	23.4	2A	23.4	–
7	CH–O	68.4	1A	68.0	–
8	CH$_2$	35.8	2A	35.5	–
9	CH–O	60.4	1A	60.3	68.3
10	CH$_2$ or CH	32.3	2A	32.5^b	34.3
11	CH–O	79.5	1P	79.3	70.4
12	CH or CH$_2$	36.6^c		36.7	33.5
13	O–C–O	107.7	1P	107.4	107.0
14	CH or CH$_2$	39.6		39.5	39.2
15	CH$_2$	41.7	1P	41.8	33.2
16	C–O	82.4^e		82.2^d	85.8^f
17	CH–O	81.5	1A	81.7	82.5
18	CH$_2$	25.9	2A	25.6	27.3
19	CH$_2$	29.6	1P	29.7	29.8
20	C–O	84.8^e		85.0^d	85.2^f
21	CH–O	85.3	1P	85.8	84.9

Position	Type		value 1	value 2	value 3
22	CH		35.2	35.1	34.8
23	CH$_2$		32.1	32.6^b	33.3
24	CH–O	1A	76.5	75.9	76.4
25	CH–O	2A	76.9	77.8	74.5
26	CH	1P	31.9	31.9	31.8
27	CH$_2$		37.2	36.9	35.7
28	CH	1P	36.8^c	40.3	36.5
29	O–C–OH	1A	97.2	96.6	98.3
30	CH$_3$ or CH$_2$OH	2A	67.2	25.7	64.9
2-Me			14.4^g	14.1^h	16.8^i
4-Me			11.6	11.9	11.0^i
10-Me			—	—	10.5
12-Me			13.0	12.8	—
14-Me			13.4	13.3	—
16-Me			27.7	27.9	27.4
20-Me			22.8	22.4	8.1
22-Me			16.2^g	16.5^h	14.5
26-Me			17.0	17.0	16.8^i
28-Me			16.4^g	17.5^h	16.0
16-CH$_2$					30.6
3-OMe					
11-OMe			59.5	59.3	57.8

^{a}1A, 2A, and 1P represent CH$_3$^{13}COOH, ^{13}CH$_3$COOH, and CH$_3$CH$_2$^{13}COOH, respectively.
$^{b-i}$Assignments may be interchanged.
Source: H. Seto, K. Mizoue, and N. Ōtake (unpublished data).

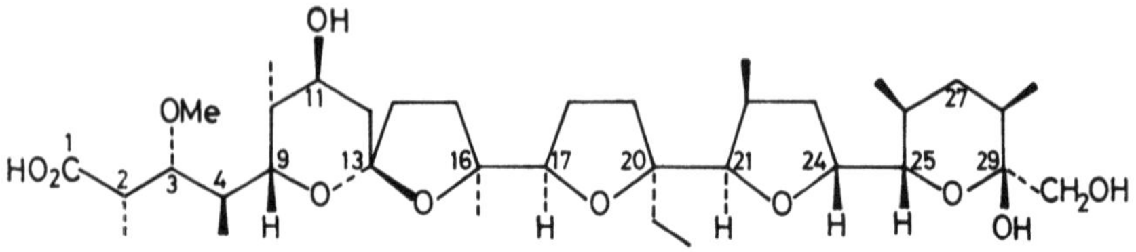

Figure 19 The structure of monensin.

4. Group 3d: monensin

The ^{13}C NMR spectrum of monensin (Pinkerton and Steinrauf, 1970) was analyzed partly by selective proton decoupling. Its structural similarities to mutalomycin (with regard to B and C rings) and nigericin (with regard to E and F rings) were utilized to advance further assignments of the remaining resonances, as shown in Table 9 (H. Seto and N. Ōtake, unpublished work). However, the partial structures specific to monensin, i.e., the presence of an ethyl group at C-20 and a linear structure (C-1 to C-4) left some ambiguity in the assignments of relevant carbon signals. The ^{1}H NMR spectral analysis of monensin had been made by Anteunis (1977b).

D. Group 4

Structural revision of alborixin

Alborixin (Gachon et al., 1976) and X-206 (Blount and Westley, 1975) are characterized as having six cyclic ether systems, three ketal carbons, and no methoxy substituent. Structures [I] and [II] in Figure 20, both determined by x-ray analysis, have been reported for alborixin and X-206, respectively, the difference being the presence of a methyl at C-6 in alborixin and the configuration at C-22. In an attempt to make complete assignments of these antibiotics the ^{13}C spectral data of both the antibiotics were compared. Taking account of the structural differences, a close similarity between the two spectra (Figure 21) was more than expected. In particular, the chemical shifts of three hemiketal carbon signals (C-27, 108.4 ppm; C-21, 99.6 ppm; and C-15, 97.9 ppm in alborixin; and C-27, 108.3 ppm; C-15, 97.7 ppm, and C-21, 99.5 ppm in X-206) were completely identical, within experimental errors.

Since it is well known that the chemical shift of a given carbon is affected by the stereochemical modification of an adjacent carbon (Stothers, 1972; Levy and Nelson, 1972), this result strongly implied that the configuration at C-22 must be identical in both the compounds. Reexamination of the x-ray analysis data of alborixin and X-206 revealed that the stereochemistry of C-22 in the former must be amended

Table 10 ^{13}C Chemical Shifts of X-206 and Alborixin Free Acids in CDCl$_3$

Carbon	Functionality	X-206	Enriched by[a]	Alborixin
1	COOH	176.2	1P	176.4
2	CH	40.6	2P	40.5
3	CH−O	84.2	1P	84.0
4	CH	31.2	2P	29.7[b]
5	CH$_2$	32.4	1A	36.1[b]
6	CH$_2$ or CH	32.6	2A	38.3[b]
7	CH−O	81.0	1A	86.8[b]
8	CH$_2$	41.3	2A	41.7
9	CH−OH	70.0	1P	70.0
10	CH	46.1	2P	46.4
11	CH−O	68.8	1A	68.9
12	CH$_2$	31.2	2A	31.8
13	CH$_2$	27.2	1P	27.2
14	CH	39.2	2P	39.2
15	O−C−OH	97.7	1A	97.9
16	CH2	40.0	2A	39.9
17	CH−O	72.4	1P	72.5
18	CH	34.9	2P	35.0
19	CH$_2$	36.0	1P	36.1
20	CH	33.4	2P	33.4
21	O−C−OH	99.5	1A	99.6
22	CH−OH	70.4	2A	70.4
23	CH−O	77.1	1A	77.1
24	CH$_2$	29.1	2A	29.1
25	CH2	32.8	1P	32.9
26	C−O	89.4	2P	89.4
27	O−C−OH	108.3	1P	108.4
28	CH	38.9	2P	38.9
29	CH2	42.3	1P	42.4
30	C−O	82.8	2P	82.9
31	CH−O	71.8	1A	71.9
32	CH2	21.5	2A	21.5
33	CH$_2$	31.2	1P	31.3
34	C−O	69.5	2P	69.6
35	CH−O	83.8	1P	83.8
36	CH2	20.0	2P	20.0
37	CH$_3$	10.5		10.5
2-Me		8.5		8.6
4-Me		16.9		16.9
6-Me		—		17.7[b]

Table 10   (Continued)

Carbon	Functionality	X-206	Enriched by	Alborixin
10-Me		8.9		9.0
14-Me[c]		16.7		16.7
18-Me		18.3		18.3
20-Me		14.8		14.8
26-Me[c]		25.5		25.5
28-Me[c]		16.3		16.3
30-Me[c]		25.0		25.0
34-Me[c]		24.2		24.3

[a] 1P, 2P, 1A, and 2A represent $CH_3CH_2{}^{13}COOH$, $CH_3{}^{13}CH_2COOH$, $CH_3{}^{13}COOH$, and $^{13}CH_3COOH$, respectively.
[b] Changes observed in the ^{13}C NMR spectrum of alborixin.
[c] Assignments may be interchanged.
Source: H. Seto, K. Mizoue, and N. Ōtake, unpublished data.

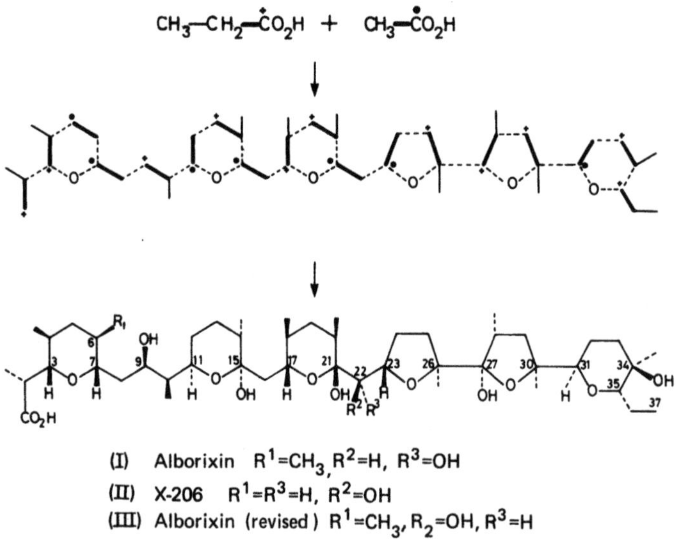

(I)   Alborixin $R^1=CH_3$, $R^2=H$, $R^3=OH$
(II)   X-206 $R^1=R^3=H$, $R^2=OH$
(III)   Alborixin (revised) $R^1=CH_3$, $R_2=OH$, $R^3=H$

Figure 20   The structures of X-206 and alborixin and biosynthetic pathway of X-206.

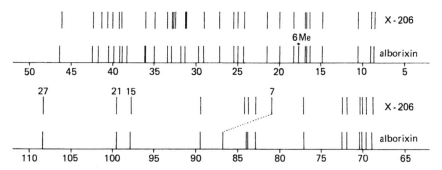

Figure 21 ^{13}C NMR spectra of X-206 and alborixin free acids in CDCl₃. (Source: Seto et al., 1979b.)

so as to be identical to that of the latter. Thus the correct structure of alborixin is represented by structure [III] in Figure 20 (Seto et al., 1979b).

Assignments of the ^{13}C NMR spectra of X-206 and alborixin

Since X-206 seemed to be the most difficult target to accomplish in complete ^{13}C NMR assignments, extensive use was made of biosynthetic labeling with $CH_3{}^{13}COOH$, $^{13}CH_3{}^{13}COOH$, $CH_3CH_2{}^{13}COOH$, and $CH_3{}^{13}CH_2{}^{13}COOH$ (K. Mizoue, H. Seto, and N. Ōtake, unpublished data). As expected from the biosynthetic assumption illustrated in Figure 20, 7 molecules of $CH_3{}^{13}COOH$ were incorporated into X-206 to enhance the signal intensities of C-5, C-7, C-11, C-15, C-21, C-23 and C-31, while 11 molecules of $CH_3CH_2{}^{13}COOH$ specified the resonances due to C-1, C-3, C-9, C-13, C-17, C-19, C-25, C-27, C-29, C-33, and C-35. When $^{13}CH_3{}^{13}COOH$ and $CH_3{}^{13}CH_2{}^{13}COOH$ were used as precursors, 7 and 11 ^{13}C-^{13}C couplings were observed, respectively. The incorporation pattern of these precursors (see Table 10), selective proton decoupling based on ^{1}H NMR analysis by Anteunis (1977a), as well as comparison to the Jone's oxidation product containing C1-C9 of X-206 (Blount and Westley, 1975) established the sequence from C-1 to C-37 of X-206 free acid. Methyl carbon resonances which were not labeled by the above precursors were mainly discriminated by selective proton decoupling. The results are summarized in Table 10.

The assignment of the ^{13}C NMR spectrum of alborixin has been easily obtained by taking account of the substitution effects by a methyl group (Stothers, 1972; Levy and Nelson, 1972) introduced to C-6 of X-206. The result is contained in Table 10 (K. Mizoue, H. Seto, and N. Ōtake, unpublished data).

E. Group 5

1. Ionomycin

Ionomycin is a metabolite of *Streptomyces conglobatus* sp. nov. Trejo isolated very recently (Toeplitz et al., 1979). The structure of iono-mycin determined by x-ray analysis, as shown in Figure 22, is novel among the polyether antibiotics in that it contains no (hemi)ketal func-tions, a minimum number of cyclic ether systems, and an enolizable β-diketone structure. Toeplitz et al. (1979) also reported the ^{13}C NMR spectral data of ionomycin calcium salt measured in $CDCl_3$ solution. Based simply on the calculated chemical shifts, they made tentative assignments of some carbon signals of the antibiotic as shown in Table 11, which also contains the advanced assignments of C-26, C-30, C-31, C-32, CH_3(C-26), and CH_3(C-30) made by comparison with CP-44,161 and X-206.

Table 11 ^{13}C Chemical Shifts of Ionomycin Calcium Salt in $CDCl_3$

Carbon	Functionality	Chemical shifts
20-Me	CH_3	12.5
32	CH_3	19.6
30-Me	CH_3	24.0
26-Me	CH_3	26.7
4-Me, 6-Me, 8-Me, 12-Me, 14-Me, 18-Me	CH_3	18.8, 19.6, 20.2, 21.4, 21.4, 22.2
4, 6, 14	CH	27.0, 28.2, 29.0
2, 3, 5, 7, 8, 12, 13, 15, 18, 20, 22	CH and/or CH_2	29.6, 33.1, 33.2, 34.1, 36.8, 34.8, 40.1, 40.3, 40.9, 42.2, 42.4, 42.6, 43.6, 47.8
31	CH−OH	71.0
19, 21, 23, 27	CH−O	78.1, 82.6, 84.1, 84.5
30	C−O	86.1
26	C−O	89.0
10	CH=	102.5
16, 17	CH=	133.4, 134.2
1	COO$^-$	186.1
9, 11	C=O and O−C=	197.5, 198.7

Source: Toeplitz et al., 1979.

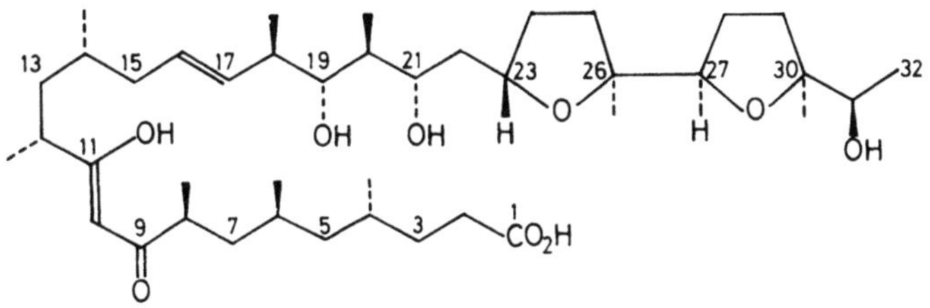

Figure 22   The structure of ionomycin.

The α-carbon signal (C-10) of the enolizable β-diketone system appears in the acetal carbon region (102.5 ppm). Therefore it should be noticed that without knowledge of the structure of ionomycin this resonance may be easily misinterpreted as evidence supporting the presence of a sugar in the molecule.

2. A23187

This compound contains two nitrogen atoms and is structurally very unique among the polyether antibiotics. Since about half of the ^{13}C signals appear in the sp^2 carbon region, A23187 can be easily distinguished from the remaining polyether antibiotics by ^{13}C NMR spectroscopy.

Deber and Pfeiffer (1976) reported the ^1H and ^{13}C NMR spectral data of A23187. Based on chemical shift trends and comparison to 2-methylbenzoxazole and pyrrole-2-carboxaldehyde, they made partial assignments of ^{13}C signals of the free acid and calcium complex of the antibiotic (see Table 12). Chemical shifts of some carbon signals were not given in their work.

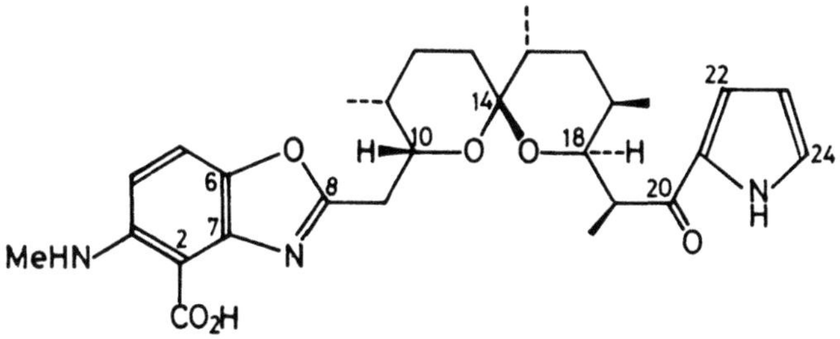

Figure 23   The structure of A23187.

Table 12 ^{13}C Chemical Shifts of A23187 Free Acid and Calcium Salt in CDCl$_3$

Carbon	Functionality	Free acid	Calcium salt
1	COOH	168.1	171.8
2	C=	97.8	105.8
3	N−C=	141.6[a]	141.6[a]
4	CH=	110.1[a]	110.6[a]
5	CH=	108.2[a]	108.4[a]
6	O−C=	150.7[a]	151.0[a]
7	N−C=	140.7[a]	140.7[a]
8	O−C=N	166.0	168.3
9	CH$_2$	b	b
10	CH−O	68.2[a]	70.8[a]
11	CH	b	b
12	CH$_2$	b	b
13	CH$_2$	b	b
14	O−C−O	97.5	98.0
15	CH	b	b
16	CH$_2$	b	b
17	CH	b	b
18	CH−O	72.7[a]	74.9[a]
19	CH	b	b
20	C=O	186.3	182.1
21	N−C=	133.0[a]	134.1[a]
22	CH=	116.3[a]	121.0[a]
23	CH=	116.8[a]	113.2[a]
24	N−CH=	124.4[a]	129.9[a]
3-NMe, 11-Me, 15-Me, 17-Me, 19-Me		10.7-16.1 (b)	10.7-15.9 (b)

[a] Assignments of these carbons are tentative and may be exchanged within each group.
[b] These signals were observed in the region 25.3-42.4 ppm in free acid and 24.9-42.6 ppm in calcium salt.
Source: Deber and Pfeiffer, 1976.

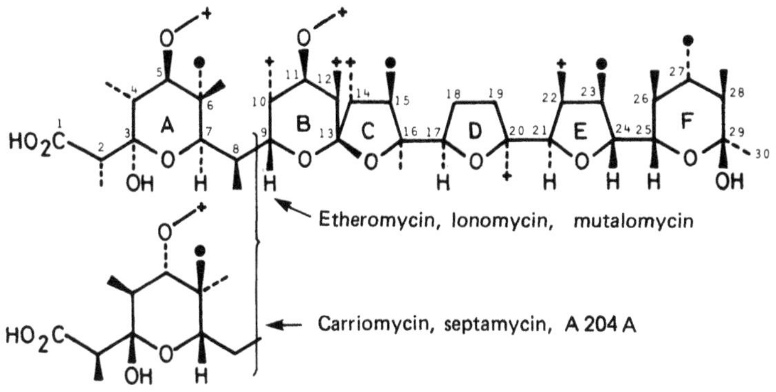

Figure 24 Basic carbon skeleton common to etheromycin, lonomycin, mutalomycin, carriomycin, septamycin, A204A, and nigericin. (Source: Seto et al., 1979a.)

V. ^{13}C CHEMICAL SHIFT TRENDS OF POLYETHER ANTIBIOTICS

A. Some Empirical Rules for the Structural Elucidation of Polyether Antibiotics by ^{13}C NMR Spectroscopy

As a result of extensive studies on the assignments of the ^{13}C NMR spectra of polyether antibiotics of group 3 (see before), Seto et al., (1979a) established some empirical rules that are useful for structural elucidation of antibiotics possessing the basic carbon skeleton common to groups 3a to 3c. (Figure 24). The rules can also be applied to compounds with similar partial structures, such as dianemycin and lenoremycin.

As shown in the following, in extracting the empirical rules from the established assignments, only those signals appearing in the characteristic regions or that were easily distinguishable from other signals by several ^{13}C NMR techniques were utilized.

1. A ring

The absolute configuration of the A ring of carriomycin, septamycin, and A204A is opposite to that of lonomycin, mutalomycin, and etheromycin, as shown. Its stereochemistry is related to the presence of a methyl at C-8. This methyl causes a downfield shift of the C-7 signal (carriomycin, septamycin, and A204A).

The presence of a substituent other than the methyl at C-6 can be detected by the characteristic chemical shifts of the axial methyl at C-6. A methoxy or sugar substituent at C-6 causes a large downfield shift of this methyl carbon (4.1-5.5 ppm for mutalomycin, lonomycin, and carriomycin, compared with 8.1-12.6 ppm for etheromycin, septa-

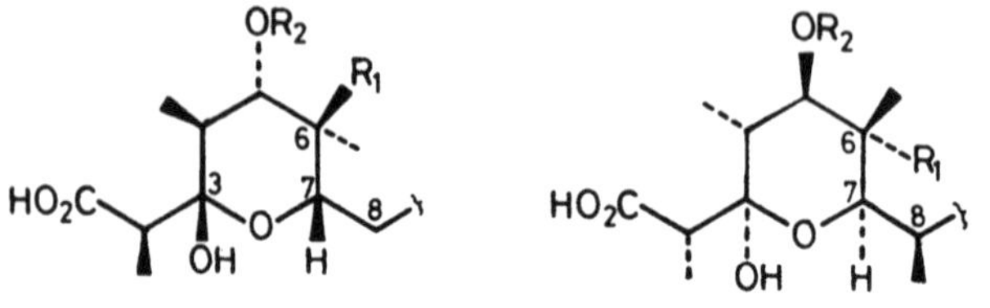

Carriomycin (R₁=H, R₂=sugar)

Septamycin (R₁=sugar, R₂=CH₃)

A 204 A (R₁= OCH₃, R₂= sugar)

C-7: 64.0 ~ 68.4

Etheromycin (R₁=sugar, R₂=H)

Lonomycin and

Mutalomycin (R₁=H, R₂= CH₃)

C-7: 70.8 ~ 71.5

Figure 25   The structures of the A ring present in the members of group 3.

mycin, and A204A. The signal due to the hemiketal carbon C-3 appearing at 99.2-100.4 ppm in the members 3a and 3b is absent in nigericin and grisorixin, which have no hydroxy function at C-3.

2. B and C rings

Three structures have been reported for the B-ring. The differences are due to the presence of a methyl at C-8 and the position of a methyl at C-10 or C-12. As shown in Figure 26, a methyl at C-8 causes a downfield shift of C-9 by about 3 ppm. Among the members with a methyl at C-8, etheromycin can be distinguished from lonomycin and mutalomycin by the chemical shift of C-13.

Two kinds of structures exist for the C ring. One has a methyl substituent at C-14 and the other has not. This difference can be detected by the chemical shift of C-16. In compounds with a methyl at C-14, C-16 is observed at a rather higher field than in those compounds lacking the substituent at C-14. The methoxy group at C-15 in carriomycin, septamycin, and A204A can be detected by the very characteristic oxymethine signal at 94.5 ppm due to C-15. The value can be compared with that of C-25 in noboritomycin (see above).

3. D and E rings

There are two kinds of structures for the D ring. One has a methyl at C-20 and the other has not. The latter group includes carriomycin, septamycin, and A204A. Since the methyl at C-20 resonates at a characteristic region (22.3 to 23.3 ppm), its presence can be revealed very easily.

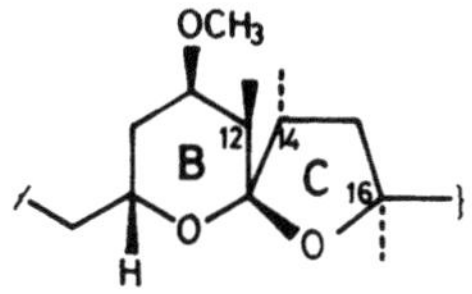

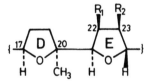

Nigericin

C-9: 60.4
C-13: 107.7
C-16: 82.4
CH₃(16): 27.7

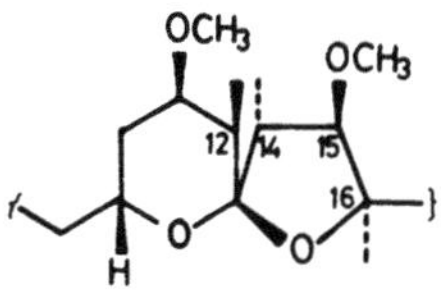

Carriomycin, septamycin, A 204 A

C-9: 61.2-61.4
C-13: 106.4-106.5
C-16: 82.9-83.1
CH₃(16): 28.4

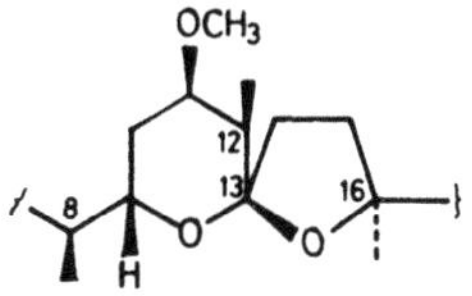

Etheromycin

C-9: 63.0
C-13: 109.2
C-16: 85.2
CH₃(16): 29.2

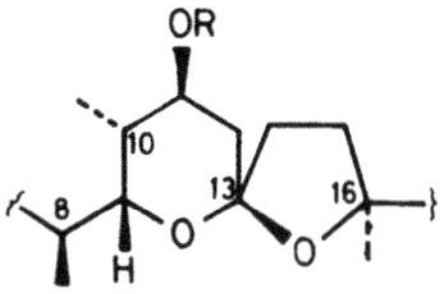

Lonomycin (R=CH₃) mutalomycin (R=H)

C-9: 63.3-64.1
C-13: 106.8-107.0
C-16: 84.2-84.3
CH₃(16): 29.0-29.2

Figure 26 The structures of the B and C rings present in the members of group 3.

Etheromycin (R₁, R₂ =H)

Lonomycin (R₁=CH₃, R₂= OCH₃)

Mutalomycin (R₁=CH₃, R₂=H)

C-20: 83.8 – 86.1

CH₃(20): 22.3 – 23.3

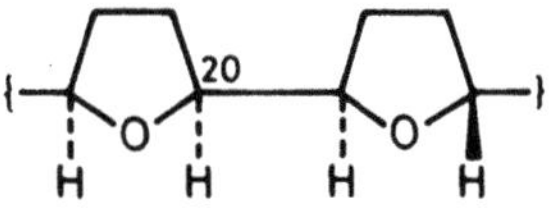

Carriomycin

Septamycin

A 204 A

C-20: 78.8 – 78.9

Figure 27 The structures of the D and E rings present in the members of group 3.

The structure of the E ring can be conveniently established by the characteristic resonances of a methyl at C-22 (16.2 ppm for mutalomycin, and 9.0 ppm for lonomycin) and a methoxy at C-23 (57.3 ppm for lonomycin). There exists no substituent on the E ring for compounds without a methyl at C-20, such as for carriomycin and septamycin.

4. F ring

Three kinds of structures are known for the F ring, the differences being due to the presence of a methoxy at C-27 and a hydroxy at C-30. Two methyls at C-26 and C-28 move to higher field due to the γ effect of the methoxy at C-27. Since the chemical shift values of these methyls unsubstituted at C-27, such as for carriomycin, mutalomycin, and septamycin, are characteristic among the methyl resonances, distinction of the nigericin and carriomycin types from the etheromycin type is very straightforward. The chemical shifts of the hemiketal carbon C-29 are also useful for detecting the methoxy at C-27.

Distinction of the nigericin type with a hydroxy substituent at C-30 from the other types can be made by the characteristic hydroxy methyl signal at 65-67 ppm.

5. 4'-O-Methylamicetose

The sugar found in polyether antibiotics is always 4'-O-methylamicetose. Advantageously, the oxymethine carbons in the sugar moiety can be detected by taking PRFT spectra. Since the chemical shift of an anomeric

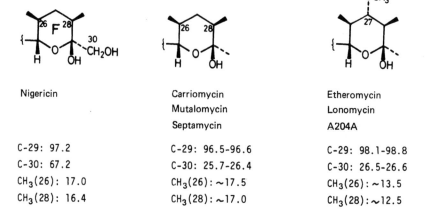

Nigericin	Carriomycin Mutalomycin Septamycin	Etheromycin Lonomycin A204A
C-29: 97.2	C-29: 96.5-96.6	C-29: 98.1-98.8
C-30: 67.2	C-30: 25.7-26.4	C-30: 26.5-26.6
$CH_3(26)$: 17.0	$CH_3(26)$: ~17.5	$CH_3(26)$: ~13.5
$CH_3(28)$: 16.4	$CH_3(28)$: ~17.0	$CH_3(28)$: ~12.5

Figure 28 The structures of the F ring present in the members of group 3.

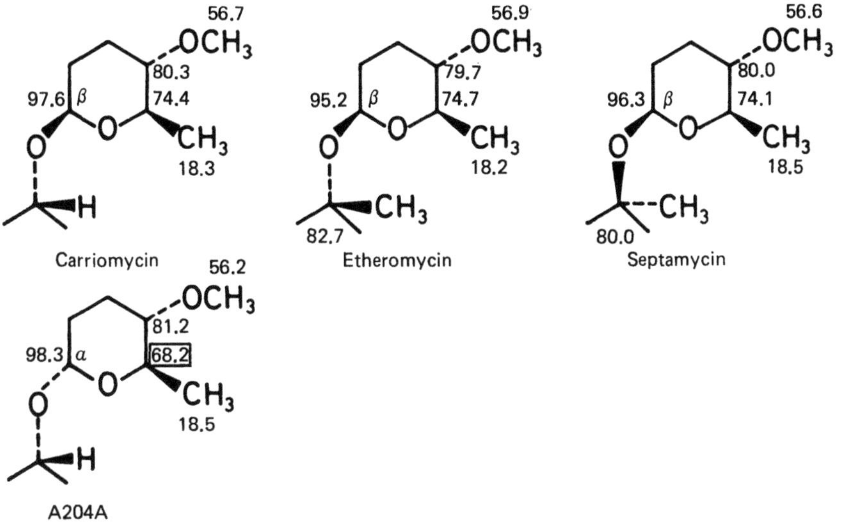

Figure 29   4'-O-Methylamicetose in carriomycin, etheromycin, septamycin, and A204A.

carbon is affected by the anomeric configuration as well as by the environment of the carbon to which the sugar is attached (Seo et al., 1978), it is much better to utilize the chemical shift of C-5' for obtaining information about the anomeric configuration. The chemical shift of C-5' in A204A clearly shows the anomeric configuration to be α. The upfield shift of this carbon is due to the γ effect of the axial oxygen at C-1'. Anomeric carbons attached to a quaternary carbon appear at a considerably higher field than those combined to a methine carbon.

6. *Methoxy signals*

The most characteristic signal in the region is the methoxy signal (49.5 ppm) linked to the quaternary carbon C-6 in A204A. Another signal showing discernible chemical shift (61.5 ppm) in septamycin is assigned to a methoxy carbon at C-5, which is connected to the quaternary oxycarbon C-6. Thus the chemical shifts of these methoxy carbons are very useful to know when seeking the substitution pattern at C-6.

The chemical shifts of the methoxy carbons at C-15 and C-27 are very close. However, as previosuly explained, the methoxy at C-15 is always accompanied by a very characteristic signal at 94.5 ppm.

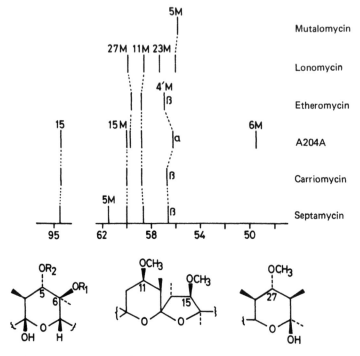

Figure 30   Characteristic carbon signals appearing at 50 to 62 and 95 ppm.

A204A (R₁=CH₃, R₂=sugar)

Septamycin (R₁=sugar, R₂=CH₃)

7. Signals appearing at 45–47 ppm

This region is usually specific to the methine carbon (C-2) adjacent to the terminal carboxylic acid. In addition, two different methine signals may sometimes be observed. One of them is ascribed to the C-28 methine with a methoxy substituent at C-27. In this case, two methyls at C-26 and C-28 do not resonate at ~17 ppm and the C-29 hemiketal carbon appears at a much lower field (98-99 ppm). The other signal is due to the methine signal of C-14, which is accompanied by a characteristic oxymethine signal at 94.5 ppm assignable to C-15.

The aforementioned rules have been extracted from the chemical shifts of group 3 antibiotics. The following additional rules are established by comparing all the polyether antibiotics described in this chapter.

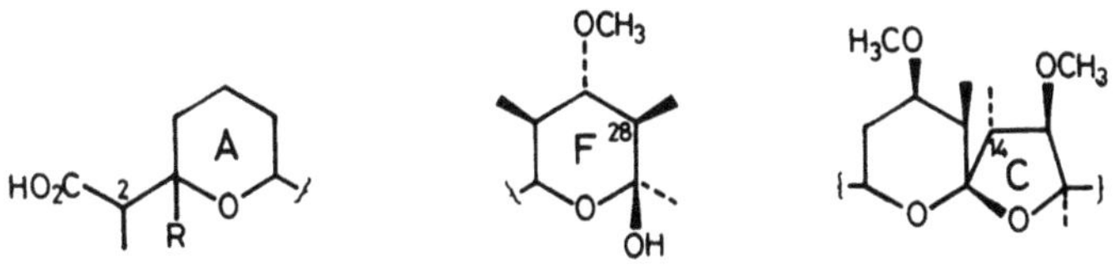

OCH₃ → OCH_3

A

F 28

O

OH

HO₂C → HO_2C ... 2 ... R

H₃CO → H_3CO ... OCH₃ → OCH_3

14

C

O   O

| Most polyethers (R=H or OH) | Etheromycin Lonomycin A204A C-29:98-99 | Carriomycin Septamycin A204A C-15:94.5 |

Figure 31 Carbons appearing at 45 to 47 ppm (C-2, C-14, and C-28).

8. Chemical shifts of (hemi)ketal carbons

The (hemi)ketal carbons of polyether antibiotics are all involved in ring formation. The chemical shifts of these carbons in a six-membered ring range from 96.5 (C-29 of mutalomycin) to 100.4 ppm (C-3 of lonomycin), whereas those in a five-membered ring cover 104.6 (C-23 of CP-44,161) to 111.3 ppm (C-21 of A-130B). Since the differences between the two groups are large enough, it is concluded that the number of six- and five-membered (hemi)ketal rings can be determined by the chemical shifts of quaternary carbons appearing at 96-112 ppm. In this case spiroketal carbons connecting five- and six-membered rings are regarded as part of the former ring. No systematic differences are observed in the chemical shifts between hemiketal and ketal carbons.

Signals other than (hemi)ketal in this characteristic region are due to the anomeric carbon of 4-O-methylamicetose (95.2-103.8 ppm), the α-carbon in an enolizable β-diketone system in ionomycin (102.5 ppm), and the oxymethine C-15 in carriomycin, A204A, septamycin, K-41A, and K-41B (93.3-94.5 ppm). However, these methine carbons can be easily differentiated by sford experiments.

9. Chemical shifts of tert-methyl carbons

All tert-methyl carbons in the polyether antibiotics are linked to quaternary oxycarbons. Except for signals due to CH_3(C-6) in etheromycin (8.1 ppm), A204A (12.6 ppm), septamycin (9.9 ppm), K-41A (11.0 ppm), and K-41B (10.9 ppm), which are strongly shielded by the γ effect due to their axial orientation, these methyl carbons resonate at between 22.3 [CH_3(C-20) of lonomycin] and 29.2 ppm [CH_3(C-16) of lonomycin and etheromycin].

Since the chemical shift of the sec-methyl carbon appearing at the lowest field is 20.3 ppm [CH_3(C-2) of lenoremycin], tert-methyl carbons in the polyether antibiotics may be identified simply by their chemical shifts. However, the distinction can be made more firmly by selective proton decoupling of singlet methyl resonance in the ^{1}H NMR spectra.

The exception for these chemical shift trends may be found in the four methyl signals appearing at 20.4-22.2 ppm for ionomycin (see Table 11), which has only two tert-methyls. The downfield shifts of the sec-methyl signals in this case are probably caused by the weaker γ effect associated with the noncyclic structure of ionomycin.

B. Application of the "Empirical Rules" for the Structural
    Elucidation of Antibiotic 6016

The usefulness of the "empirical rules" has been exemplified by their application to the structural determination of the new antibiotic 6016 (Seto et al., 1979c). Antibiotic 6016, $C_{46}H_{77}O_{16}Na$, is produced by *Streptomyces* sp. and active against gram-positive bacteria, mycobacteria, fungi, and yeast.

Its ^{13}C NMR spectrum (Figure 32) shows the presence of a carboxylate (178.4 ppm), three (hemi)ketals (107.9, 99.2, and 96.6 ppm), three methoxys (58.8, 56.7, and 55.8 ppm), and an anomeric carbon (98.9 ppm). These spectral data indicate that the antibiotic possesses the same basic carbon skeleton common to carriomycin, septamycin, and A204A, and, in fact, the structural determination of the antibiotic could be accomplished by application of the empirical rules, as shown in Figure 33. [13]C Chemical shift data supporting the structures of the A, B, C, and F rings are given in Figure 33 and are connected by dotted lines to the relevant carbons. It should be noted that only carbon signals numbered in Figure 32 were utilized for the structural determination of 6016. Readers are advised to confirm the structure by using the "empirical rules" themselves.

Some comments may be necessary for the carbinol carbon C-2 and the position of the 4'-O-methylamicetose.

Carbinol carbon C-2

The most striking feature of the ^{13}C NMR spectrum of 6016 is the absence of signals between 40 and 55 ppm, the region being specific to the C-2 methine carbons as explained previously. Since removal of the methyl from the C-2 methine does not considerably affect its chemical shift (cf. C-2 methylene in lysocellin 45.9 ppm, see Table 4), the only reasonable explanation for this spectral feature can be given by placing a hydroxy function on C-2.

The position of the deoxy sugar on the main framework

Since the structures (and ^{13}C assignments) of A, B, C, and F rings have been established without doubt by the empirical rules (for ^{13}C assignments of these rings see Table 7), the sugar must be placed on either the D or the E ring (see Figure 33). Its position was determined by ^{1}H NMR spectroscopy as follows. A sharp doublet at 3.61 ppm in

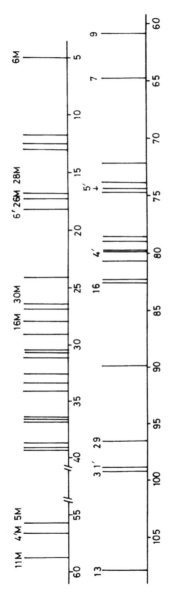

Figure 32 ^{13}C NMR spectrum of 6016 sodium salt in CDCl₃. The suffix M represents either a methyl or methoxy group on the numbered carbon. The carboxylic acid (C-1) at 178.4 ppm is not shown in this figure. (Source: Seto et al., 1979c.)

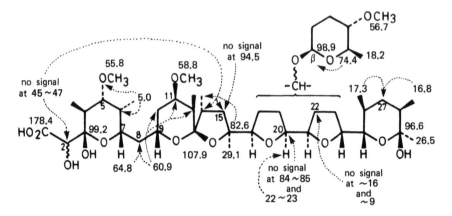

Figure 33 The structure of 6016 obtained by analysis of its ^{13}C NMR spectral data. The chemical shift values are bases of the partial structures connected by dotted lines. (Source: Seto et al., 1979c.)

the ^{1}H NMR spectrum of the antibiotic was proved by selective proton decoupling to be on the carbon at 89.9 ppm, which is not contained in A, B, C, or F ring. Moreover, this proton was coupled to an oxymethine at ~4.4 ppm. This spectral feature can only be accommodated by a D ring with the sugar at C-18. This structure resulted in a large upfield shift of C-20 (78.9 in carriomycin → 73.9 ppm in 6016), which may be rationalized by the stereochemistry with the sugar substituent and the hydrogen at C-20 on the same plane of the D ring (due to the strong γ effect). Thus the structure of 6016 has been determined as shown in Figure 17. The stereochemistry of C-2 has been proved to be R by x-ray analysis (Ōtake et al., 1978a).

    The rules can be also applied to other polyether antibiotics belonging to groups 3a to 3c. Therefore it may be again of interest for the readers to attempt the structural determination of K-41A using the ^{13}C NMR data given in Table 8.

VI. CONCLUSION

^{13}C NMR spectroscopy is well known to be a very useful tool for the structural elucidation of natural products. This is also true with the polyether antibiotics, especially when good crystals suitable for x-ray analysis are not obtainable, as evidenced in case of narasin. The structures of 6016 and K-41B could be also determined by the aid of ^{13}C NMR spectroscopy.

In addition to structural investigation, this methodology will further enable one to study important problems associated with the mechanisms of action of the polyether antibiotics, such as interaction with metal cations in solution. Subtle conformational changes of the antibiotics caused by complex formation will be amply reflected in their ^{13}C NMR spectra. Therefore detailed analysis of the spectral change will give valuable information which can hardly be obtained by other techniques.

The basic requirement for ^{13}C NMR spectroscopy to be fully powerful in such kinds of works, i.e., complete assignment of the ^{13}C NMR spectra of the polyether antibiotics, has almost been satisfied by extensive works, as explained in this chapter, and accumulated ^{13}C chemical shift data will become vital to physical, chemical, and biochemical studies of the polyether antibiotics in future.

REFERENCES

Alléaume, M., and Hickel, D. (1970). The crystal structure of grisorixin silver salt. *J. Chem. Soc. Chem. Commun. 1970*:1422-1423.

Anteunis, M. J. O. (1976). Solution conformation of lasalocid and lasalocid-Na$^+$. *Bioorg. Chem. 5*:327-337.

Anteunis, M. J. O. (1977a). Solution conformation of the ionophore X-206 and its sodium salt. *Bull. Soc. Chim. Belg. 86*:931-947.

Anteunis, M. J. O. (1977b). Solution conformation of the antibiotic 3823A (monensin A) sodium salt. *Bull. Soc. Chim. Belg. 86*:367-381.

Anteunis, M. J. O. (1977c). Solution conformation of lysocellin-Na$^+$. More than a simple structural analog of lasalocid-Na$^+$. *Bull. Soc. Chim. Belg. 86*:187-198.

Anteunis, M. J. O., and Verhegge, G. (1977). Solution conformation of the ionophore A204A Na$^+$-salt. *Bull. Soc. Chim. Belg. 86*:353-366.

Anteunis, M. J. O., and Rodios, N. A. (1978). A proton nmr study of the polyether antibiotic etheromycin monosodium salt (CP-38 295-Na$^+$). *Bull. Soc. Chim. Belg. 87*:753-764.

Anteunis, M. J. O., Rodios, N. A., and Verhegge, G. (1977). Solution conformation of dianemycin, its sodium salt and of lenoremycin-Na$^+$ (Ro 21-6150 or A-130-A). *Bull. Soc. Chim. Belg. 86*:609-631.

Blount, J. F., and Westley, J. W. (1975). Crystal and molecular structure of the free acid form of antibiotic X-206 hydrate. *J. Chem. Soc. Chem. Commun. 1975*:533.

Day, L. E. Chamberlin, J. W., Gordee, E. Z., Chen, S., Gorman, M., Hamill, R. L., Neuss, T., Weeks, R. E., and Stroshane, R. (1973). Biosynthesis of monensin. *Antimicrob. Agents Chemother. 4*:410-414.

Deber, C. M., and Pfeiffer, D. R. (1976). Ionophore A23187. Solution conformation of the calcium complex and free acid deduced from proton and carbon-13 nuclear magnetic resonance studies. *Biochemistry* 15:132-141.

Dorman, D. E., Pascal, J. W., Nakatsukasa, W. M., Huckstep, L. L., and Neuss, N. (1976). The use of ^{13}C-NMR spectroscopy in biosynthetic studies. II. Biosynthesis of narasin, a new polyether ionophore from fermentation of *Streptomyces aureofaciens*. *Helv. Chim. Acta* 59:2625-2634.

Fehr, T., King, H. D., and Kuhn, M. (1977). Mutalomycin, a new polyether antibiotic. *J. Antibiot.* 30:903-907.

Fehr, T., Keller-Juslén, C., Loosli, H. R., Kuhn, M., and von Wartburg, A. (1979). Correction of the stereostructure of mutalomycin, noboritomycin A and noboritomycin B. *J. Antibiot.* 32:535-536.

Gachon, P., Kergomard, A., and Veschambre, H. (1970). Grisorixin, a new polyether antibiotic related to nigericin. *J. Chem. Soc. Chem. Commun.* 1970:1421-1422.

Gachon, P., Farges, C., and Kergomard, A. (1976). Alborixin, a new antibiotic ionophore: Isolation, structure, physical and chemical properties. *J. Antibiot.* 29:603-608.

Grover, S. H., Guthrie, J. P., Stothers, J. B., and Tan, C. T. (1973). The stereochemical dependence of δ-substituted effects in ^{13}C NMR spectra. Deshielding syn-axial interactions. *J. Magn. Reson.* 10:227-230.

Johnson, L. F. (1979). Spin-decoupling methods in ^{13}C nmr studies. In *Topics in Carbon-13 nmr Spectroscopy*, Vol. 3; G. C. Levy (Ed.). John Wiley and Sons, New York, pp. 2-16.

Jones, N. D., Chaney, M. O., Chamberlin, J. W., Hamill, R. L., and Chen, S. (1973). Structure of A204A, a new polyether antibiotic. *J. Am. Chem. Soc.* 95:3399-3400.

Keller-Juslén, C., King, H. D., Kuhn, M., Loosli, H. R., and von Wartburg, A. (1978). Noboritomycins A and B, new polyether antibiotics. *J. Antibiot.* 31:820-828.

Kinashi, H., Ōtake, N., Yonehara, H., Sato, S., and Saito, Y. (1975). Studies on the ionophorous antibiotics. I. The crystal and molecular structure of salinomycin p-iodophenacyl ester. *Acta Crystallogr.* B31:2411-2415.

Lallemand, J. Y., and Michon, V. (1978). [13]C Nuclear magnetic resonance studies on X537A (lasalocid), an ionophore antibiotic: free acid, sodium salt and thallium salt, and behavior in solution. *J. Chem. Res. S* 1978:162-163.

Lallemand, J. Y., Le Cocq, C., Michon, V., Derouet, C., and Rao, R. C. (1979). Etude par résonance magnétique nucléaire du carbone ^{13}C de l'éméricide, un antibiotique ionophore. *C. R. Acad. Sci.* 288C:383-386.

Levy, G. C., and Nelson G. L. (1972). *Carbon-13 Nuclear Magnetic Resonance for Organic Chemists*. Wiley-Interscience, New York.

Lyerla, J. R., Jr., and Levy, G. C. (1974). Carbon-13 nuclear spin relaxation. In *Topics in Carbon-13 nmr Spectroscopy*, Vol. 1, G. C. Levy (Ed.). John Wiley and Sons, New York, pp. 81-148.

Martin, G. E., Matson, J. A., Turley, J. C., and Weinheimer, A. J. (1979). ^{13}C NMR studies of marine natural products. 1. Use of the SESFORD technique in the total ^{13}C nmr assignment of crassin acetate. *J. Am. Chem. Soc. 101*:1888-1890.

Miyazaki, Y., Shibata, A., Tsuda, K., Kinashi, H., and Otake, N. (1978). Isolation, characterization and structure of SY-1 (20-deoxysalinomycin). *Agric. Biol. Chem. 42*:2129-2132.

Mizoue, K., Seto, H., Otake, N., Mizutani, T., Yamagishi, M., Hara, H., and Omura, S. (1978). Studies on the ionophorous antibiotics. 14. Structural studies of minor components of lonomycin. *Abstract 2P-21, Ann. Meet. Agric. Chem. Soc. Jpn.*, Nagoya, Japan, April 1-4.

Mizoue, K., Seto, H., Mizutani, T., Yamagishi, M., Kawashima, A., Omura, S., Ozeki, M., and Otake, N. (1980). Studies on the ionophorous antibiotics. Part XXV. The assignments of the ^{13}C-NMR spectra of dianemycin and lenoremycin. *J. Antibiot. 33*:144-156.

Mizutani, T., Yamagishi, M., Hara, H., Kawashima, A., Omura, S., Ozeki, M., Mizoue, K., Seto, H., and Otake, N. (1980). Studies on the ionophorous antibiotics. Part XXIV. Leuseramycin, a new polyether antibiotic produced by *Streptomyces hygroscopicus*. *J. Antibiot. 33*:137-143.

Nakanishi, K., Crouch, R., Miura, I., Dominguez, X., Zamudio, A., and Villarreal, R. (1974). Structure of a sequiterpene, cuauhtemone, and its derivative. Application of partially relaxed Fourier transform ^{13}C nuclear magnetic resonance. *J. Am. Chem. Soc. 96*:609-611.

Nakayama, H., Otake, N., Miyamae, H., Sato, S., and Saito, Y. (1979). Studies on the ionophorous antibiotics. Part 14. Crystal and molecular structure of the thallium salt of carriomycin. *J. Chem. Soc. Perkin Trans. 2 1979*:293-295.

Occolowitz, J. L., Berg, D. H., Dobono, M., and Hamill, R. L. (1976). The structure of narasin and a related ionophore. *Biomed. Mass Spectrosc. 3*:272-277.

Otake, N., and Koenuma, M. (1977). Studies on the ionophorous antibiotics. XI. The artifacts and degradation products of lysocellin. *J. Antibiot. 30*:819-828.

Otake, N., Koenuma, M., Kinashi, H., Sato, S., and Saito, Y. (1975). The crystal and molecular structure of the silver salt of lysocellin, a new polyether antibiotic. *Chem. Commun. 1975*:92-93.

Otake, N., Koenuma, M., Miyamae, H., Sato, S., and Saito, Y. (1977). Studies on the ionophorous antibitoics. Part IV. Crystal and molecular structure of the thallium salt of lonomycin. *J. Chem. Soc. Perkin Trans. 2 1977*:494-496.

Ōtake, N., Ogita, T., Nakayama, H., Sato, S., and Saito, Y. (1978a).
    X-Ray crystal structure of the thallium salt of antibiotic-6016, a
    new polyether ionophore. *J. Chem. Soc. Chem. Commun.* 1978:875-
    876.

Ōtake, N., Seto, H., and Koenuma, M. (1978b). The assignment of
    the ^{13}C NMR spectrum of lysocellin and its biosynthesis. *Agric.
    Biol. Chem.* 42:1879-1886.

Petcher, T. J., and Weber, H. P. (1974). X-Ray crystal structure
    and absolute configuration of p-bromophenacylseptamycin. *J. Chem.
    Soc. Chem. Commun.* 1974:697-698.

Pinkerton, M., and Steinrauf, L. K. (1970). Molecular structure of
    monovalent metal cation complexes of monensin. *J. Mol. Biol.*
    49:533-546.

Rodios, N. A., and Anteunis, M. J. O. (1977). Solution conformation
    of nigericin free acid and nigericin-sodium salt. *Bull. Soc. Chim.
    Belg.*, 86:917-929.

Rodios, N. A., and Anteunis, M. J. O. (1978a). High-resolution ^{1}H-
    nmr study of carriomycin free-acid and its sodium salt. *Bull. Soc.
    Chim. Belg.* 87:437-446.

Rodios, N. A., and Anteunis, M. J. O. (1978b). Solution conforma-
    tion of lonomycin free acid and lonomycin sodium salt. *Bull. Soc.
    Chim. Belg.* 87:447-457.

Rodios, N. A., and Anteunis, M. J. O. (1978c). Solution conforma-
    tion of septamycin and its sodium salt. *J. Antibiot.* 31:294-301.

Rodios, N. A., and Anteunis, M. J. O. (1979). Lonomycin-Na^{+}. A
    recall of its ^{1}H NMR spectrum. *Bull. Soc. Chim. Belg.* 88:37-41.

Roth, K. (1977). Carbon-13 {^{1}H} off-resonance rauschentkopplung.
    Org. Magn. Reson. 10:56-62.

Seo, S., Tomita, Y., Tori, K., and Yoshimura, Y. (1978). Determina-
    tion of the absolute configuration of a secondary hydroxy group in
    a chiral secondary alcohol using glycosidation shifts in carbon-13
    nuclear magnetic resonance spectroscopy. *J. Am. Chem. Soc.*
    100:3331-3339.

Seto, H., Sato, T., and Yonehara, H. (1973). Utilization of carbon-13-
    carbon-13 coupling in structural and biosynthetic studies. An
    alternative double labeling method. *J. Am. Chem. Soc.* 95:8461-
    8462.

Seto, H., Miyazaki, Y., Fujita, K., and Ōtake, N. (1977a). Studies
    on the ionophorous antibiotics. X. The assignment of ^{13}C-NMR
    spectrum of salinomycin. *Tetrahedron Lett.* 1977:2417-2420.

Seto, H., Yahagi, T., Miyazaki, Y., and Ōtake, N. (1977b). Studies
    on the ionophorous antibiotics. IX. The structure of 4-methyl-
    salinomycin (narasin). *J. Antibiot.* 30:530-532.

Seto, H., Westley, J. W., and Pitcher, R. G. (1978a). The complete
    assignment of the ^{13}C-nmr spectra of lasalocid and the sodium salt-
    complex of the antibiotic. *J. Antibiot.* 31:289-293.

Seto, H., Mizoue, K., and O̅take, N. (1978b). Studies on the ionophorous antibiotics. XVII. The structures of lonomycins B and C.
J. Antibiot. 31:929-932.

Seto, H., Mizoue, K., Nakayama, H., Furihata, K., O̅take, N., and
Yonehara, H. (1979a). Studies on the ionophorous antibiotics.
XX. Some empirical rules for structural elucidation of polyether
antibiotics by ^{13}C-NMR spectroscopy. *J. Antibiot. 32*:239-243.

Seto, H., Mizoue, K., O̅take, N., Gachon, P., Kergomard, A., and
Westley, J. W. (1979b) The revised structure of alborixin.
J. Antibiot. 32:970-971.

Seto, H., Nakayama, H., Ogita, T., Furihata, K., Mizoue, K., and
O̅take, N. (1979c). Studies on the ionophorous antibiotics. XXI.
Structural elucidation of a new polyether antibiotic 6016 by application of the empirical rules in ^{13}C-nmr spectroscopy. *J. Antibiot.
32*:244-246.

Smith, W. B. (1978). Carbon-13 NMR spectroscopy of steroids. In
Annual Reports on NMR Spectroscopy, Vol. 8, G. S. Webb (Ed.).
Academic Press, London, New York, and San Francisco, pp. 199-
226.

Steinrauf, L. K., Pinkerton, M., and Chamberlin, J. W. (1968).
The structure of nigericin. *Biochem. Biophys. Res. Commun.
33*:29-31.

Stothers, J. B. (1972). *Carbon-13 NMR Spectroscopy*. Academic
Press, New York, pp. 55-101, 269-278.

Tanabe, M. (1974). Stable isotopes in biosynthetic studies. In
Biosynthesis, Vol. 2, T. A. Geissman (Ed.). The Chemical Society,
London, pp. 241-299.

Tanabe, M. (1975). Stable isotopes in biosynthetic studies. In
Biosynthesis, Vol. 3, T. A. Geissman (Ed.). The Chemical Society,
London, pp. 247-285.

Tanabe, M. (1976). N. M. R. with stable isotopes in biosynthetic
studies. In *Biosynthesis*, Vol. 4, T. A. Geissman (Ed.). The
Chemical Society, London, pp. 204-265.

Toeplitz, B. K., Cohen, A. I., Funke, P. T., Parker, W. L., and
Gougoutas, J. Z. (1979). Structure of ionomycin—A novel diacidic
polyether antibiotic having high affinity for calcium ions. *J. Am.
Chem. Soc. 101*:3344-3353.

Tone, J., Shibakawa, R., Maeda, H., Inoue, K., Nishiyama, S.,
Ishiguro, M., Cullen, W. P., Routien, J. B., Chappel, L. R.,
Moppet, C. E., Jefferson, M. T., and Celmer, W. D. (1978).
CP-44,161, a new polycyclic ether antibiotic produce by a new
species of *Dactylosporangium*. *Abstract No. 171, 18th ICAAC
Meeting*, Atlanta, Georgia.

Tsuji, N., Nagashima, K., Terui, Y., and Tori, K. (1979). Structure of K-41B, a new diglycoside polyether antibiotic. *J. Antibiot. 32*:169-172.

Tsuji, N., Terui, Y., Nagashima, K., Tori, K., and Johnson, L. F. (1980). New polyether antibiotics, A-130B and A-130C. *J. Antibiot. 33*:94-97.

Wehrli, F. W. (1976). Organic structure assignments using ^{13}C spin-relaxation data. In *Topics in Carbon-13 nmr Spectroscopy*, Vol. 2, G. C. Levy (Ed.). John Wiley and Sons, New York, pp. 53-77.

Westley, J. W., Evans, R. H., Williams, T., and Stempel, A. (1970). Structure of antibiotic X-537A. *Chem. Commun. 1970*:71-72.

Westley, J. W., Evans, R. H., Harvey, G., Pitcher, R. G., Pruess, D. L., Stempel, A., and Berger, J. (1974). Biosynthesis of lasalocid A. Incorporation of ^{13}C and ^{14}C labeled substrates into lasalocid A. *J. Antibiot. 27*:288-297.

Westley, J. W. (1977a). A proposed numbering system for polyether antibiotics. *J. Antibiot. 29*:584-586.

Westley, J. W. (1977b). Polyether antibiotics. Versatile carboxylic acid ionophores produced by *Streptomyces*. *Adv. Appl. Microbiol. 22*:177-223.

Westley, J. W., Seto, H., and Ōtake, N. (1979). Further proposal for polyether antibiotic notation. *J. Antibiot. 32*:959-960.

AUTHOR INDEX

Italic numbers give page on which the complete reference is listed.

SUBJECT INDEX

A

Acanthifolicin, 115-117
Alborixin, 73-76, 88, 117-119,
 201-205, 280, 305-306, 313,
 322, 378-381
Antibiotics (numbered):
 A-130A (lenoremycin), B and C,
 88, 96-100, 205-208, 360-365
 A-204-A, B, 70-73, 88, 100-104,
 224, 231-232, 254, 264, 267,
 300, 306, 310, 312, 322, 366-
 375, 385-392
 A-712, 220, 223
 A-6016, 88, 119-122, 224, 230,
 366-375, 392-394
 A-23187 (calcimycin), 15-20,
 27-30, 49, 88, 103-115, 215-
 219, 255, 263, 268, 281, 309-
 310, 343, 383-384
 A-28695A, B, 224, 232
 BL-580Δ, 224, 228-229
 CP-44161, 353-356
 DE-3936, 228
 K-41A, B, 90, 135-138, 224-
 225, 229-232, 371-375, 391
 X-206, 68-69, 94, 183-186, 201-
 205, 262, 266, 273, 280, 298,
 303-305, 313, 322, 343, 378-
 381
 X-14547A, 50, 94, 185-188,
 215, 219
Aromatic solvent induced shifts
 (ASIS), 307-315
 assignments, 314-315

[Aromatic solvent induced
 shifts (ASIS)]
 distribution of lipophilicity,
 312-314
 fractional lipophilicity, 309-311

C

Carriomycin, 88, 120-124, 224,
 228-229, 256, 268, 300, 306-
 307, 309-312, 314, 322, 366-
 375, 385-392
Chemical synthesis of polyethers,
 1-50
Chemical transformation of polyethers, 50-86
^{13}C NMR of polyether antibiotics,
 335-400
 application of empirical rules,
 392-400
 biosynthetic labeling, 340-341
 chemical shifts, 344-385
 classification of polyethers,
 341-344
 differentiation of signals, 337-
 338
 empirical rules for structure
 elucidation, 385-392
 selective proton decoupling,
 388-340
 techniques used for ^{13}C assignments, 336-341
Coupling constants in proton
 NMR, 284-295

413

Milton Keynes UK
Ingram Content Group UK Ltd.
UKHW021835071024
449327UK00021B/1505